you
are not
alone

The NAMI Guide to Navigating Mental Health

With Advice from Experts and Wisdom
from Real People and Families

you
are not
alone

KEN DUCKWORTH, MD

zando

NEW YORK

Zando
zandoprojects.com

Originally published in hardcover September 2022
First paperback edition: January 2025

Text design by Aubrey Khan, Neuwirth & Associates, Inc.
Cover design by Evan Gaffney
Cover art by June Glasson

The publisher does not have control over and is not responsible for author or other third-party websites (or their content).

Library of Congress Control Number: 2022935062

978-1-63893-097-6 (Paperback)
978-1-63893-001-3 (ebook)

10   9   8   7   6   5   4   3

Manufactured in the United States of America

CONTENTS

PART I

Mental Health and
Mental Health Conditions

PART II

The Recovery Journey:
Evidence from Lived Experience

PART III

Family Matters

PART IV

Best Practices

FOREWORD

As the CEO of the National Alliance on Mental Illness (NAMI), I often describe our organization as "a community that cares." Not only is this our motto, but it is also a goal we aspire to every day. At NAMI, we want to ensure we reach as many people as possible, using as many mediums as possible. With that in mind, we are publishing *You Are Not Alone: The NAMI Guide to Navigating Mental Health*—our first-ever book—which will stand as a long-lasting, physical embodiment of our mission.

While this is a NAMI project, the content is not about our organization. The book offers advice on navigating a challenging and complicated mental health care system, as well as ways of finding a path to recovery, so that everyday people can live *well* with mental illness. The intention of this book is core to NAMI's mission of building better lives for the millions of Americans affected by mental illness—and it is why all proceeds will go back to NAMI in order to support our work.

When Dr. Ken Duckworth came to me with the idea of writing a book that could help people on their road to recovery, I knew it was something we had to do. Those of us who have been impacted by mental illness know what it is like to seek guidance only to receive silence and shame in response. I believe that getting the support and guidance you need should be as easy as entering your local bookstore, asking, "What should I read if my kid is struggling with their mental health, and I don't know where to start?" and being answered with, "This comprehensive guide called *You Are Not Alone*."

This book will help you gain perspective and advice from what we call "lived experience experts." These are people using their real names, sharing their stories, and talking about what they've learned. This is how we break down social barriers—with real people being open and vulnerable. We are also pairing their knowledge with traditional research experts to give the reader the best of all these perspectives.

Our mission is well represented by the stories we share, which focuses on first-person experience from people with mental illness, as well as those of their family members and loved ones. As Dr. Duckworth writes, "At NAMI, family members and peers are joined in the same mission, but not with the same perspective. . . . The belief that listening to alternative viewpoints deepens understanding is at the core of why NAMI has chosen to be inclusive."

Whether you are experiencing mental illness symptoms for the first time, are a caregiver of someone who is struggling, or just a concerned friend or family member, I hope that this resource will help you to determine next steps for yourself or your loved one. There is a whole community of people who care about what you're going through—the NAMI family—and we are here to provide guidance, community, and support on your mental health journey. Indeed, *you are not alone.*

Sincerely,

DANIEL H. GILLISON JR.,

CEO, National Alliance on Mental Illness

INTRODUCTION

I know what it's like to feel alone.

That's why I decided to write a guide on living, and recovering, with mental illness. No such guide existed when I personally needed it, and many other people I have loved—including my father—or who I have come to know as a doctor, colleague, or friend, have been without a guide to turn to as well.

My dad was a fun, charismatic, loving, and generous man who was episodically ill with bipolar disorder. Back when he needed help, our family had no tools to navigate the convoluted mental health "system." When he was hospitalized, we didn't even consider discussing next steps with the professionals who were caring for him, because we didn't know that was something to discuss. We did not have the language to talk with his doctors or with each other. My father's doctors did not offer any counsel about what my dad could do to reduce his symptoms or extend the time between his episodes, and we knew nothing of the science that might help us. There was no book to read that laid out options for treatment. We were ashamed, isolated, and uninformed. When other people were sick, friends, colleagues, and family members sent cards and brought casseroles, but when my father was ill, our family tried to pretend nothing was wrong, and even the people who knew something was wrong did not send or bring anything. No casseroles, no flowers, no cards.

I decided to become a psychiatrist to find answers to my questions about my dad and his illness—to help him, my family, and other families. When I announced that I was applying to medical school, my family was initially thrilled. My older siblings, Sue and Joe, had been the first in our family to attend college; our relatives in prior generations were security guards, seamstresses, salespeople, and ministers. So, my decision to set aside my initial interest in political science and history to study medicine was greeted with praise. A doctor! A (shame-reducing) home run!

However, my choice to go into psychiatry, rather than becoming a successful surgeon or cardiologist, was much less well received. For decades, Dad held out hope that I would choose another specialty, calling me during my psychiatric residency to ask, "How was the operating room?" He loved me deeply, but he didn't want this path for me; it was just too close to his deepest source of shame.

I was also surprised that, at that time, psychiatry was not ready to consider my motivation for entering the profession as legitimate. On my psychiatry residency applications, my essay about my dad's illness and my quest to help him seemed to violate an unwritten rule. It was ignored at programs across the nation, while interviewers engaged with me on topics relating to the practice of medicine, my volunteer work, or even college football. One person at a prestigious hospital told me my reason for entering the field was a "terrible" one but might have been acceptable if my father had been a psychiatrist himself and not just a patient. I was devastated. Only one person who interviewed me, Ned Hallowell, told me that my personal experience could be helpful in my professional life, and so I joined his program at the Massachusetts Mental Health Center in Boston, where I am still on the faculty. Fortunately, sharing one's personal experience of being affected by mental health conditions is becoming more acceptable in applications to the mental health field.

I was a bit lost when neither my dad nor the field of psychiatry wanted me to keep going, but my love for him had set the course: Every professional choice I made was inspired by my desire to learn about the possibility of recovery from mental illness from every possible angle.

Since then, I have worked in almost every kind of role in the mental health field, and in almost every kind of setting and system. If you look at my résumé, you might think I'm either very curious or have trouble keeping a job. I was curious about the two distinct cultures of addiction and mental health, so I worked on a dual diagnosis assertive community treatment team. Because I wanted to improve policies, I became the chief psychiatrist and commissioner at a major state department of mental health. As I began to see how early mental health issues start, I trained as a child and adolescent psychiatrist and had a private practice for adolescents, became a school consultant, and worked to reduce the use of restraints for children in hospital units. After watching the state mental hospitals close in a slow-motion tragedy, I worked in a recovery-oriented human service nonprofit organization helping people with serious mental illness live independently and developed clinical services for unhoused people in Boston. Curious about how we get new medicines, I was part of a research team that studied clozapine's impact on reducing suicide risk. Working at a major health plan taught me how malleable and variable insurance benefits are. After learning there was a better way to serve people early in their course of psychosis, I volunteered for five delightful years at an early psychosis program. Along the way, the National Alliance on Mental Illness (NAMI) found me, and it has been the joy of my professional life to work as NAMI's psychiatrist.

I have, in short, spent my career learning and thinking about life with mental illness, recovery, and what a practical "how-to" guide would need to cover to provide support and guidance to others facing the challenges my family and many others confronted. Now, finally—and with the help of hundreds of thousands of others who have shared expertise, wisdom, and the lessons of lived experience—I have written the book that my dad and family so desperately needed, in the hope that it eases the way for individuals and families everywhere.

This book contains information relevant to people independent of their or their loved one's diagnosis. At the same time, it provides guidance relevant specifically to people with certain illnesses. It also addresses concerns that arise for people of different cultures and identities as they navigate the complex world of mental health treatment. The book will help those affected by anxiety disorders, attention deficit disorders, bipolar disorder, borderline personality disorder, depressive disorders, dissociative disorders, dual diagnosis/substance use disorders, eating disorders, obsessive compulsive disorder, post-traumatic stress disorder, psychosis, schizoaffective disorder, and schizophrenia. Some of the people who share their stories here may have co-occurring autism spectrum disorders or developmental disorders, but I will not be addressing those important conditions in depth, as they deserve a guidebook of their own.

Mental illness and recovery are human experiences, so I consider experience-based evidence an authoritative source for this book. Individuals who have lived with mental health conditions are a source of untapped wisdom on how to build a life and thrive while living with mental health conditions. My goal is to synthesize this anecdotal evidence with traditional research-based evidence; to provide practical, compassionate advice; and to offer the comfort that comes from knowing that, wherever you are in your recovery journey, you are not alone.

For this book, I was fortunate to interview in depth 130 people from Cape Cod to Hawaii, and from Anchorage to San Antonio—all of whom self-identified as having a mental illness or loving someone who does. The age of interviewees ranges from sixteen to one hundred. They are from different races, ethnicities, religions, sexual orientations, socioeconomic and educational backgrounds, gender identities, national origins, abilities, and cultures. Some of the people I interviewed have been unhoused, incarcerated, or lost jobs and relationships. Others work as physicians, carpenters, musicians, schoolteachers, or police officers. Some are on disability, and others are veterans. These people told me about their diagnoses; some have had many diagnoses, and some took a long time to get the one diagnosis that formed a base upon which they could build their recovery. Their journeys were often very trying for them and for their families.

These "lived experience experts," as I think of them, have taken a master class in living with some combination of the extremes of mood, thought, perception, addiction, and behavior while also dealing with the rest of life—things like developing an identity, integrating their experience into their sense of self, building friendships, raising kids, finding love, and establishing careers. Some have used their experience to serve others: volunteering on a crisis hotline, providing mobile crisis peer support, training police officers on de-escalation techniques, or becoming a social worker. The 130 interviewees had on average about twenty years of lived experience of mental health conditions. Together, they have more than two thousand years of experience from which the rest of us can learn. You will hear from them, in their own words, throughout this book.

In the interviews, I asked people who lived with mental health conditions open-ended questions about what they had learned, when they first thought they had a concern, what their experience was of treatment and services, what worked for them and what did not, how their culture or identity impacted their journey, and how they define recovery. I asked family members similar questions. Families are often a key ingredient in recovery, and I was fortunate to learn from many families who have young and adult children living with mental illnesses. I also interviewed siblings and those, like myself, who are the children of people who live with mental illness.

Given the prejudice and discrimination many still face, you might think people would be reluctant to engage in intimate discussions of their experience of illness and their quest for recovery. However, the people I interviewed told me they cared about feeling better, being in less pain, developing coping tools, building a life, and—by being interviewed for this book—sharing their experience to help others. Family members know the trap of isolation and blame, so they also wanted to step forward to share what they have learned. Everyone I interviewed chose to use their real name in this book—to lead with their experience and reduce the shame associated with these issues. Most of the interviewees didn't care much about the imperfect state of neuroscience or the meaning of imperfect terms like "mental illness," "mental health condition," or "brain disorder." When you talk to people, they just want to learn, teach, and connect. They want to stop the cycle of secrecy and isolation. And they want to help you and your family.

In Part I, I review what we know about mental illness, what we don't know, and how our understanding has evolved. I look at mental health conditions through the lenses of development and trauma. Sharing stories from experience, I cover the imperfect science of diagnosis: why diagnosis is a process; how getting an accurate diagnosis can help; and why an accurate diagnosis is not a prerequisite for effective care. And I explain current approaches to treatment and how integrating the best of the traditional "medical model" of care with a newer and evolving "recovery model" offers the best chance for the most favorable outcome.

My perspectives on these topics are intended to frame and introduce Parts II, III, and IV, in which people with lived experience of mental illness and thought leaders in many mental health fields share their expertise. In Part II, individuals describe in their own words what they learned, how their culture or identity influenced their experience, what mistakes they made, and what made a difference during their recovery.

In Part III, we hear from family members of people with mental illness. In this book, "family" refers to people related by biology, caregiving, choice, or community. Families who have learned how to communicate, practice self-care, and advocate for their loved ones serve as beacons of hope for those of us beginning a challenging and unknown journey. Unfortunately, not all journeys end well when it comes to mental illness. Families who have faced the hardest challenges, including the worst possible outcomes, share how they responded.

Finally, in Part IV, we turn to the traditional experts. Mental health researchers do important work every day, but their research is often not well translated to the public. To get this information out to people in plain, nonscientific language, I bring many thought leaders together to answer the questions people most frequently ask me about living with a mental health condition. In this part of the book, renowned researchers, innovators, and activists share wisdom on the "state of the art" of mental health care at the time of this writing.

. . .

Over the years, I have fielded thousands of questions from people seeking insight and guidance into mental illness recovery. And I know that millions more Americans are seeking answers to these same questions every day, whether for themselves or for someone they love. Forty years ago, I was one of those people, desperate for answers I could not find. Even as a young boy, I had understood that something was very wrong with my dad, but I did not know the first thing about what it was. All I knew was that he was taken from our house by a police officer at the front door while he was screaming. After his hospitalization at Byberry State in Philadelphia when I was eight years old, we moved to Michigan. I later learned that Dad had lost his job in Philadelphia after that episode, but that his company, Chef Boyardee, transferred him to another sales job in Detroit. That kind of corporate loyalty is unusual today for people in similar situations. It meant we could count on his job and his income to afford secure housing and food. It meant we didn't have to move from shelter to shelter, so I could go all the way through school in one school district, and there meet my lifelong friend Marty Derda, who has been beating me at Wiffle ball for close to five decades. These fundamental supports—housing, food security, and connection—were part of what we now call the social determinants of mental health, and they were all in my favor. I was also white, which gave me advantages I didn't understand then. Even with all these advantages there was a lot of heartache in my family.

One of my darkest moments was while I was a college student sitting in my car in the parking lot of Northville Regional Psychiatric Hospital near Detroit where my dad, once again, had been admitted as a patient. My loving, playful, generous father struggled all his life with severe bipolar disorder and often required months of state hospital care to bring him back from mania and psychosis. I remember feeling like no one understood my pain, and that there was no one on Earth I could talk to about it. When I later returned to campus, I described the experience to my girlfriend as "not that bad." I didn't say anything to my loving older siblings, who had moved out of the house by then and had formed their own busy young families. Dad's condition was not a secret to us, yet we all felt so much shame that each of us suffered alone, in silence. I was haunted by images of my father full of anger and throwing beer bottles, or drooling while sedated by powerful antipsychotic drugs, but it never occurred to me to see a mental health professional. That night in the parking lot it seemed hopeless for my dad, and for our whole family.

Fortunately, change was coming. At the exact time that I was sitting in that parking lot outside Northville Regional Hospital in 1979, a group of 284 people from around the nation was gathering in Madison, Wisconsin. They were primarily the parents of adult children with severe and persistent mental illnesses, tired of the way they and their children were treated both by mental health professionals and in the world and frustrated by the lack of support services. They were meeting to bring their voices together, and their meeting was the beginning of what became NAMI—an organization that would one day take my life's greatest heartache and, as it has done for millions of others, connect me to a community and a purpose.

Some of the parents at that critical meeting had already formed their own smaller groups at home. The largest such group was in San Mateo, California, where Toni Hoffman, Fran Hoffman, and Eve Oliphant had formed Parents of Adult Schizophrenics (PAS). They had held a conference prior to the Madison convention and were key in creating momentum for a national organization.

The grassroots movement was growing. The late Eleanor Owen, who turned one hundred years old in 2021, had helped to form another early group in her home state of Washington after a tragedy in her local community. "I looked at the headline and I thought, 'I will call that family. I know what they're going through,'" she told me. "Eight strangers did exactly the same thing. Within a week, we met around my dining room table and drafted the outline for the Washington Advocates for the

Mentally Ill, WAMI. That established our local organization." Eleanor, like other early leaders, then connected with people across the country who agreed that a national organization was needed, and they decided to establish the national meeting in Madison.

Laurie Flynn, who would serve as executive director of NAMI from 1984 to 2000, got to know many of the founders, including Bev Young and Harriet Shetler. "They'd had such a terrible time," Laurie recalled. "They'd had so many locked doors. And to be opening some of those doors, just by sharing the truth of their experiences with each other—really felt affirming. They thought they were going to make a difference for the next generation. And indeed, they did." That momentum continues today, and sharing first-person experiences remains critical to NAMI's work and mission.

Every year, millions of people are affected by mental illness. In 2020, in the early stages of the Covid-19 pandemic, that number was higher than ever. In a Centers for Disease Control and Prevention (CDC) study, more than 41 percent of Americans reported clinically significant mental health symptoms that year—double the prevalence in years past. The authors of that study noted an even greater impact of the pandemic on younger people, adult unpaid caregivers, and racial and ethnic minorities. Too many of us—and our families, friends, and caregivers—are confused, afraid, and overwhelmed. We may not know that what we are experiencing is an illness. We may be worried about a loved one who denies that anything is wrong. Some of us know we need help, but we don't know how or where to find it; or we find ourselves scrambling anew when a treatment or medication that used to work no longer seems adequate.

The mental health "system" in the United States is chaotic, underfunded, and often hard to access. Many mental health care professionals and institutions are wonderful, but they're affordable only for the rich. At NAMI, the questions keep coming to me: What does it mean when different doctors give me different diagnoses? When is my adolescent just being a teenager and when is her mood something to worry about? What if my insurance company will not cover my treatment? This treatment/ medicine/community/faith/practice made such a difference for me—how can I share or make a career of my knowledge with others?

NAMI has been helping millions of Americans seeking answers to those and many other questions for more than forty years. Composed of a national umbrella organization and over 650 state and local affiliate organizations serving communities in forty-nine states, it has become the largest grassroots organization in the United States helping people with mental illness and their families navigate recovery. Thousands of members are devoted to raising public awareness and providing advocacy, education, and support so that all individuals and families affected by mental illness can build better lives. At NAMI, we understand that mental illness affects not just the brain but every aspect of human life—social, emotional, vocational, spiritual, even philosophical. We understand that one person's mental health condition also affects the lives of family members, caregivers, and friends.

Why is this book for both people with mental health conditions *and* family members? Because that is who NAMI is now. NAMI was founded as a family group and has, through board elections and intention, become a group for both families and for people living with these conditions. This evolution adds depth, compassion, and, at times, tension to the movement that is NAMI. One of these tensions is how to refer to people who experience mental health challenges themselves, to distinguish them from family members. We now use the term "peers" (though of course if you are a family member you will also have "peer" family members). Many people qualify as both "peers" and "family members."

NAMI embraces the tension that can arise in enacting this radical idea to welcome all into the mental health space. Families and peers may disagree about what is and isn't a symptom of illness, about what treatment is and is not needed, or about the use of leveraged or forced treatment. The belief that listening to alternative viewpoints deepens understanding is at the core of why NAMI has chosen to be inclusive. The collective power of peers and families helps to move legislation and to change attitudes in our society. We also celebrate the richness that flows from these different perspectives. At NAMI, family members and peers are joined in the same mission but not with the same perspective.

I am still at times astonished by the impact of the work NAMI has done to make mental illness something we can talk about openly, so we can recover together. NAMI has developed and offers a set of peer-led support and education programs in a variety of community settings—from houses of worship to schools to NAMI Affiliates—and now online. Much of our programming is offered in Spanish as well as English for both peers and for families. NAMI's national HelpLine, 1-800-950-NAMI, staffed by volunteers aged twenty-one to eighty-plus who have lived experience of mental illness, helps many thousands of people annually find resources, information, and support. NAMI also trains volunteers to become better advocates, and many of the gains in the field are tied to NAMI's advocacy efforts.

We have come a long way. Over the decades, my father fought off every attempt I made to discuss his illness. My choice to go to medical school and then residency was probably more helpful for me than for him. He did take his lithium more often over time, but he never engaged in the kind of conversation about his experience that is common in recovery today. But I think, in the end, he did appreciate in his own way what I had attempted to do. On his death bed, he told me, "I am sorry for all the hard times." It was the only time he ever raised the subject of his illness—a lifelong challenge that had begun for him at age seventeen and lasted for seventy years, until his death at eighty-seven—in conversation. This simple statement was an incredible gift to me. I know how lucky I am to have had that moment.

I am indebted to the people who chose to tell their story in this book and so to serve others, instead of choosing privacy. To be so open and so generous in sharing your experience is a game-changing, shame-reducing way of living. I'm grateful for your courage and leadership.

This book is for my father, Joe Duckworth, and for the millions of people like him and those who love them. I could not have written it without the lifelong support of my often overwhelmed and loving family of origin: my mother, Wanda; and my siblings, Joe, and Sue. I also thank my adopted NAMI family.

There is a NAMI group or organization somewhere near your community, and there is hope. We will welcome you with open arms.

You are not alone.

AUTHOR'S NOTE

Self-Identification

The individuals and families you will meet throughout this book have each provided me with a brief description of who they are and how they would like to be identified. While many included their race, ethnicity, sexual orientation, or other cultural identity in their description, some did not. I intentionally did not offer my opinion on, interfere with, edit, or consider outside opinions on how people chose to identify themselves. The inconsistencies are therefore a reflection of the unique personalities and individual choices of the people who have so generously shared their experiences and perspectives.

Methods

People in the NAMI community and beyond volunteered to be interviewed for this first-person-as-expert book. Before the actual interview, I spoke to each person about the idea of the book and addressed their questions. I used an interview protocol approved by an Institutional Review Board (IRB). After they gave permission, my colleague Jordan Miller and I conducted the interviews in the form of online Zoom conversations (one was done in person). The conversations were recorded and then transcribed. When people elected to share their understanding of their diagnoses, I took them at their word, as no doctor–patient relationship was entered. Given the informality of spontaneous conversational speech, I have taken some liberties in polishing quotes from verbatim transcripts so that they read well and convey meaning clearly as written text. For example, we eliminated some "ums," "likes," and repetitions, and occasionally resequenced sentences to clarify the sequence of events in someone's story. Interviewees were given the opportunity to review the edited quotes to ensure that the text accurately reflected both how they spoke and what they meant to say.

Demographics

In this book, you will meet each person individually as they describe themselves in their own words. Note that not every person answered every demographic question, and there were no pre-written boxes to check.

That said, our community of lived experience experts were from thirty-eight states, of eleven races and ethnicities, and across the spectrums of both gender and sexuality.

Interviewees represented twenty-five different faith orientations, over fifty occupations, and reported ages from sixteen to one hundred, with one person noting that she was "old as dirt."

I am grateful to each of them.

Scope and Substance

Finally, this book addresses the experience of recognizing, getting help and treatment for, and living and recovering with a mental health condition, regardless of the diagnosis. While it does contain some information on treatments, research developments, and best practices for some specific conditions, it is not comprehensive. For example, eating disorders (which can also co-occur with other mental health conditions) and dissociative identity disorder (which can be rooted in trauma) are only touched on in these pages. There are many other helpful and enlightening books and resources available that focus on treatments for and recovery with specific diagnoses and conditions. We guide you to some of the ones NAMI members have found most helpful in the Resources section (page 389).

PART I

Mental Health and Mental Health Conditions

ONE

Do I Need Help?

"I never really believed them to be voices because I knew the people that I was talking to, and they were real people. They were alive. So I thought that it was more of an elevated sense of communication, like we were talking on a different level. Like our brains were strong enough and powerful enough to communicate in a way where we didn't have to use our mouths."

—LLOYD HALE,
South Carolina

"My friends pointed it out to me at first. They would call me hyper, but it wasn't a typical type of hyper for middle school kids. I was frenzied. I felt like I was swept up in a hurricane of sorts, and I kept trying to find a landing, but then I just kept on blowing higher and higher and I couldn't control what was going on. I was twelve."

—DIANA CHAO,
California

"Not only did my son lose interest in all his hobbies, and he'd started isolating and his personality was changing, but he also wasn't taking care of his business anymore. A couple times a week he'd be on the highway somewhere or on the road with his gas tank empty, and we would have to take gas to him. He used to be responsible and could think ahead and plan, and he just wasn't anymore."

—ANGELA BRISBIN,
Missouri, on her son, Michael

• • •

All people experience mental and emotional pain. At times we are sad or anxious, or we feel isolated from others. We may stop finding pleasure in things we used to enjoy, or we find ourselves in jobs, environments, or relationships that don't work for us. We grieve when loved ones die. We have trouble sleeping or getting out of bed in the morning.

For most of us, these difficult experiences pass with time. We work through our struggles, absorb our losses, make changes in our lives for the better. Some of us change our state by exercising, improving our sleeping habits, being with friends, working, or taking a trip—literally getting a change of scenery. Others find their way by talking to family and friends, going to a grief support group, or engaging with their faith community. We find solace in connecting with or giving to others. The fog lifts, the pain recedes; we find ourselves older and wiser, having learned that we can get through something difficult.

But for some of us, sometimes, the mental and emotional pain digs in and grows. We seem unable to make our way through the fog; unable to live life the way other people seem to be able to do. We may feel disconnected from the rest of the world, numb, afraid, desperate, unhappy, or unexpectedly irritable and having paranoid thoughts. Ending the pain may become a recurrent thought. This internal experience may arise not just from our current life circumstances; instead, it can come from something that is happening in our brain, from something that happened long ago, or from some biological or neurochemical process that we have no control over.

Because mental and emotional pain is an inevitable part of the human experience, it can be difficult to recognize the difference between the normal ups and downs of living and a mental health condition—whether in ourselves or in another person. How do you know that you, or someone you love, has a mental health condition? How do you know whether or when to seek help or intervene?

While many physical health issues make themselves known through measurable, physical metrics—blood pressure, high sugar levels—the symptoms of mental health conditions can cloak themselves in emotions, thoughts, perceptions, and behaviors not easily distinguishable from our "usual selves." Mental health conditions may manifest differently from person to person. Sometimes changes are noticeable to others; other times, they're not. It can be easy to miss brain-based symptoms in ourselves and in our family members. It can be difficult to evaluate and critique our own thinking. Someone who is depressed, for example, may think: "My level of unhappiness is keeping me from functioning well and enjoying life as I once did. I better get help." But someone with depression may instead think, "The world is a bleak place; I am a failure and in so much pain. Ending it all may be my only way out."

One of the cruelest symptoms of major depression is hopelessness. People experiencing it may not ask for help because they believe there is no help to be had. When depression is treated effectively, this feeling ebbs over time. But in the moment, we may be convinced that our outlook is a logical response to immutable facts, and that the people trying to tell us otherwise—or, worse, cheer us up—just don't get it. Recognizing "symptoms" in our own thinking is particularly challenging for people experiencing the onset of psychosis, with symptoms such as hallucinations or delusions. One of the people I interviewed, Mike Smith of Wisconsin, reported this exact phenomenon; he was hearing voices for years before he realized this was not everyone else's experience. Mathematician John Nash won the Nobel Prize for developing game theory, which he accomplished while he was ill with schizophrenia. When he was asked why he hadn't seen that his hallucinations were not part of reality, his answer, as Sylvia Nasar reported in her biography of Nash, *A Beautiful Mind*, was that they "came to me the same way that my mathematical ideas did. So, I took them seriously."

In addition to the self-awareness challenge, there is no objective mental health equivalent to blood work or a blood pressure cuff to help us ascertain that someone is ill, or with what illness. We know that mental illnesses are real, and common, but they emerge from a brain with about 100 billion neurons (give or take a few billion) that we do not yet fully understand. We aren't yet able to pinpoint the precise brain elements and processes that contribute to a disordered mood or thought experience. Nor do we fully understand the interplay of genetics and environment in the formation of mental illnesses; we only know that they are both some-how involved and that they interact. Genetic and environmental risk for mental health conditions travels in families, just as it does for diabetes or cancer. But not all members are affected equally. Some are not affected at all; some may have a vulnerability that might be expressed under cer-tain stressful conditions, and some will develop a life-threatening condi-tion. Not only does each of us embody a unique set of genetic influences, we each draw upon or are influenced by a unique combination of strengths, talents, culture, belief systems, and family relationships.

Mental illness isn't always a simple black-and-white, yes-or-no matter. Symptoms and experiences change over time and can improve or worsen as we age. A person living with post-traumatic stress disorder (PTSD) can have a great year and then get retriggered by a specific stress and re-experience symptoms such as flashbacks and nightmares. A person who lives with bipolar disorder will have periods—sometimes years—of high functioning between episodes. People who have a vulnerability to addic-tion or to depression may be prone to a recurrence under stresses, like the loss of a relationship or a humiliation at work. One person told me, "Recovery was perishable—like food in the produce section."

With rare exceptions, we do not know what causes mental health con-ditions, and we do not know exactly how some of the most successful services, treatments, and strategies for helping people recover from these conditions work. We know that traumatic experiences change the body and the brain, but there is much more to learn. Traumatic experiences are the drivers for PTSD, of course, but how exactly do they relate on a biological level to increased risk of other conditions, such as addiction or major depression? We know what the protective factors for mental health and resilience are, such as stability and connection, but we don't know how they contribute to this complex equation or how a person with many protective factors and no trauma can still develop a mental illness.

Truth be told, we don't even have a good term. "Mental illness" is an imperfect label to describe these many-faceted experiences that also often involve the body (e.g., panic, trauma, eating disorders, addiction, depression, and mania). Formal definitions of mental illness have evolved over time but living with a "disorder" or "condition" is an experience that textbook definitions do not adequately describe. For example, is post-traumatic stress really a disorder? The response to traumatic events that we now call PTSD is a series of body and mind experiences rooted in the evolutionary drive to protect ourselves; some argue it may be better classified as an injury response. Nor do these diagnostic definitions incorporate any recognition of a person's strengths and capacities, or of the impact of culture and social norms on our experience of behavior and illness.

It's not just our rudimentary knowledge of the brain that inhibits our understanding of mental illness. What we know, or think we know, has also been limited by an unfortunate historical legacy. For centuries, we have somehow collectively agreed that if the most complex organ in the body has a disturbance and provokes a mood, thought, or perceptual experience that results in behavioral issues, we need to retreat to shame and isolation or to lock the "disturbed" person away in an asylum—or, in more recent times, in a correctional institution. We have had decades of insurance companies failing to cover many basic mental health–related services, thus perpetuating the idea that these all too real concerns are somehow not legitimate. Underfunding, discrimination, isolation, and shame are killers in our society—and these issues all contribute to people being denied help or receiving inadequate services, as well as raising their risk of suicide. In a society that has long sidelined mental health conditions, it can be hard to recognize and accept that you may have one.

Because our society glorifies self-reliance and independence, it can also be difficult to accept the need for help. We must learn to recognize that the common refrains—to "snap out of it," or to "pick ourselves up by the bootstraps"—reflect a lack of understanding about the nature of mental health conditions. The idea that we can get better through sheer force of determination is not entirely wrong; some people do get better over time through self-care, the support of friends and family, or just continuing to live life and put one foot in front of the other. But that model doesn't always work, and thinking about recovery from this perspective in all circumstances is unhelpful. One of the things we do know is that getting help earlier improves outcomes. It is much better to intervene in stage 1 cancer, which is local, than stage 4 cancer, which has spread to other parts of the body. The same early intervention public health principles hold true for mental health and illness.

We have managed to learn a great deal about the brain, particularly in the last half century. For example, developments in imaging that allow us to watch the brain in action and in our understanding of genetics have afforded us new ways of understanding brain function and have increased the potential for identifying biological markers akin to blood pressure. But while these research developments represent a stunning leap forward in our scientific understanding, they are not yet ready for practical application in helping people who live with mental health conditions.

In Part IV, I ask some leading researchers in the brain science field to describe some promising areas of research with potential practical applications. For example, the recognition that circuits are part of the brain's makeup has inspired research into magnetic and deep brain stimulation. There is emerging research on the effectiveness of psychedelics for treating trauma and depression. And researchers are exploring the possibilities for truly personalizing treatment for major depression rather than relying on educated guesswork. All this research is evolving, and the National Institute of Mental Health (NIMH) and NAMI websites are good places to follow new practical developments that flow from this science.

In truth, however, the most helpful things we have learned about mental health conditions are from people with lived experience. They have taught us that mental health conditions are just that, exemplifying that people are not their illnesses. People with mental health conditions also have a lot more expertise than professionals do about the process of recovery—how people survive and thrive not just despite a mental health condition, but in the process of reckoning with it and building a life worth living. As Kimberly Comer of Florida told me, "My meds help me deal with my symptoms, but my skills help me build a life."

People who have "been there" can best articulate what mental illness is in human terms. In reading their stories—shared throughout this book—you may begin to identify with what they felt and recognize yourself or a loved one in their descriptions of their mental illness, their accounts of when and how they knew they needed help, and their journey to discover what worked best for them.

Do I Need Help?

The best way to assess your blood pressure is to take it. It is almost impossible to assess blood pressure without a basic measurement. People used to have to go to the doctor's office to get their blood pressure checked, but now home monitors help make it more accessible, even if they are not 100 percent accurate. Getting a blood pressure reading at home, or at a pharmacy, isn't often precise, but it is informative; it can let you know if you need to get the reading done by a professional and that you may need help to get your physical health in check. Blood pressure can quietly go awry until there is a serious consequence.

Mental health can go awry, too, sometimes quietly and sometimes not so quietly. In either case, you need to get an assessment to figure out what's going on. If you can do an assessment with a professional, that is optimal in terms of quick access to a reliable interpretation and planning next steps, but there are also a lot of screening tools accessible online to help you make an initial directional assessment on your own. These mental health screens help you get a ballpark estimate of what your experience may mean about your mental health, relative to the experience of millions of other people who have taken the same assessment over the years.

Screening tools have been well studied for validity and accuracy, but they are the mental health equivalent of the home blood pressure cuff. When Marty Parrish of Iowa got a very high score of 25 out of 27 on the PHQ-9, the most common tool for depression screening, both he and his psychiatrist saw that he was not responding to the treatments that had been tried and needed an urgent new approach for his very serious depression. He has now had four good years of life and love after treatment with a technique called repetitive transcranial magnetic stimulation (rTMS). The PHQ-9 screening measurement was a turning point in changing his treatment and improving his symptoms, though Marty is clear that his wife, Peggy, is the most important factor in his recovery.

The easiest way to first assess whether you—or a loved one—need a more in-depth mental health evaluation is to use one (or more) of the many validated screening tools now available online. Mental Health America (MHA.org) has collected the best tools for identification of risk for the most common major mental health conditions, including major depression, mania, anxiety, PTSD, psychosis spectrum, eating disorders, and attention deficit hyperactivity disorder (ADHD), among others. These screening tests are often the same ones you'd be given at a clinic or doctor's office. The tests are not "diagnostic," meaning, the test alone is an insufficient basis for determining an official diagnosis. But they may indicate your level of risk for a treatable condition and help motivate you to get a formal assessment.

One way to look at warning signs is to look broadly at the symptoms that can be part of a mental health diagnosis. These can look nonspecific, but a combination of symptoms may indicate a possible mental health diagnosis. There are overlaps with normal behavior in some cases and especially early in the course of an illness process. How long someone has had a particular symptom, or manifested changes in behavior, is also relevant in making a diagnosis; however, not every concern is necessarily part of a mental health condition.

Some symptoms and experiences that could indicate that a mental health assessment is warranted are:

- Feeling very sad or withdrawn for more than a few days
- Change in social drive or interest in connection
- Seeing, hearing, or believing things that aren't real. (Culture is important here. Some people within certain communities and cultures may not interpret hearing voices as unusual.)
- Trying to harm oneself or end one's life, or a preoccupation with this idea
- Excessive use of alcohol or drugs
- Drastic changes in mood or intensely changing moods
- Severe, out-of-control risk-taking behavior that can cause harm to self or others
- Changes in sleeping patterns
- Extreme difficulty concentrating or a change in thinking/ memory
- Sudden, overwhelming fear for no reason, sometimes with a racing heart
- Persistent physical discomfort or pain without a medical cause
- Intense worries or fears
- Significant weight loss or gain

Screening tools are a good way to sort these nonspecific symptoms. If you get a concerning score on an assessment, contact your primary care provider or a licensed mental health practitioner to help answer the questions raised by the screening test.

For Family Members: Does My Loved One Need Help?

Determining if a loved one would benefit from an assessment for a mental health condition is often challenging. It can also be hard to bring up the topic at all. Mental health symptoms can be confusing and nonspecific and are sometimes understandably concealed due to shame or lack of awareness. It can also be easy to overlook slowly developing symptoms. For teens, it can be difficult to discern what is and isn't in the normal range of development. For a while, Karen Yeiser of Ohio thought that her daughter Bethany's increasing withdrawal from family and friends after she went to college was just a sign of emerging adult independence and "her becoming more of who she was," since Bethany had long been intensely focused on excellence in academics and music. Bethany also had good, rational explanations for her withdrawal. It took a long time to get Bethany diagnosed, for her to understand her diagnosis, and to get help that worked. Most people, even some clinicians, would miss these subtle emerging symptoms.

Sometimes the picture is clearer, but the underlying cause is not. A major change in a teen's energy, social drive, and school functioning are indications for concern. This pattern could be explained by a medical condition like mononucleosis, but it could also be symptomatic of a major depression or an indication that the teen is self-medicating or experimenting with mind- and mood-altering substances. Ruling out medical issues can be important, so helping to arrange a meeting with a primary care provider is often a good first step.

Here are some broad principles that may help you recognize that a loved one may be experiencing, or potentially vulnerable to, a mental illness:

Think Young: More than half of all mental health conditions manifest before age fourteen, and three quarters by age twenty-five. Many of the people interviewed in this book could look back and see clearly that they had symptoms (often anxiety, depression, or impulsivity) in their elementary school years. Some noticed nothing until late in high school or in their early twenties. Others used substances to change their underlying feeling state. Some discussed their concerns with their family, though many did not. Chapter 7 focuses on developmental aspects of mental health.

Stressful Experiences Affect Developing Brains Until Age Twenty-Five: Stressors like bullying, divorce, and traumatic events during childhood raise a person's risk for mental health symptoms in childhood and be-yond. The Adverse Childhood Experience Study (ACE), one of the larg-est studies ever conducted on the link between trauma in childhood and later life well-being, highlighted the need to understand these risks and the need to support individuals affected by childhood trauma in devel-oping resilience; this is developed in chapter 6.

Negative Thoughts and Feelings May Be Mistaken for Facts: People who are depressed may feel unlovable or forget that they have many strengths and talents. The cognitive fog of depression makes it difficult to recall these essential and sustaining truths, even if they were well known to them only a few months prior. Negative thinking and hope-lessness are part of the condition of major depression, and it is very hard for someone to critically assess for themselves what is a feeling and what is a fact. This is particularly true when this is someone's first experience with hopelessness and negative thinking, but it can still be the case when symptoms come back after a period of relief. The person may know at one level that their experience marks a recurrence of an illness process that they have seen before, but their dashed hope that symptoms were gone forever may be a more powerful force than intellectual insight.

Take Note of Patterns and Family History: If a person has had a previ-ous episode of depression or mania, that presentation is often going to resemble the next episode. This pattern can be quite specific. A specific sleep change, or the use of particular words or phrases, can be a signal for the recurrence of a manic episode, for example. This signal can help to identify earlier intervention to prevent a more intense episode.

While we cannot pinpoint the exact contribution of genes, we do know that a family history elevates risk. Nikki Rashes of Illinois, who is now a manager of national education programs at NAMI, was finally convinced that she might have bipolar disorder only when her mother, Sally, laid out the extensive family history of mood and related disorders. "My mom is my hero to this day," Nikki told me. "When I was first diagnosed with bipolar disorder, she finally talked to me about my family history. First having that word put to it—bipolar disorder—helped me to see that 'Okay, there's something legit going on.' And then knowing my grandma suffered from extreme depression, my uncle with bipolar disorder . . . This isn't just me being strange and me losing my mind; there's something seriously happening. It all started to make sense."

Nikki's mother also used her knowledge of family history to inform the doctors Nikki was working with—though it took persistence to get them to hear her. "I had explained to that first psychiatrist the family history, that I was sure that it was bipolar because of her ups and downs," Sally said, "and she just didn't believe it. Well, it took four psychiatrists before we found one who did."

Trust Your Gut: You know your child or family member. If you are concerned, don't ignore that. If another family member or someone else you trust is concerned, pay attention. Sometimes we are too close to notice day-to-day changes that someone else may see more clearly.

Listen Closely: People describe emotional distress in many ways—from physical symptoms (often stomachache or recurrent headache) to statements about wishing to be free of pain or fear. Some children and teens are more prone to showing distress rather than discussing it, as every school nurse knows. The safer a family member feels, the more likely they are to share their experience with you. If they do not or cannot discuss it, please remember that these are hard conditions to acknowledge and accept, and this is not a commentary on your parenting or your relationship.

Get to Yes on an Assessment

We are all experts in our own feelings, thoughts, and actions. It is easy for people to feel ashamed of a mental health challenge, and then to act with defensiveness. I encourage you to remember this as you engage a family member on a potential vulnerability; try to focus on an empathic understanding of the distress your family member is showing or telling. Problems with sleep are common, not usually a source of shame in our society, and a key to many mental health conditions, so if the person you're concerned about says they are having sleep trouble, that can be a great place to start a conversation. If you can get to yes on any aspect of what they see that you also see—for example, excessive sleep, insomnia, or fatigue—you may be able to leverage that to get your loved one into the pediatrician's or primary care doctor's office. Some people will openly discuss their persistent sadness, feelings of panic and anxiety or a change in thought patterns; some will not. The key is to keep the conversation going and to remind the person that you love them and are here to help them problem-solve, now or later.

There is a technique called motivational interviewing that can help support a person to move ahead even if they are ambivalent about making a change. In this model, you don't press your loved one into action, but rather engage them in a discussion to help them move ahead in their own way. William Miller, who developed the technique, explains it further in chapter 17.

Knowing how to help someone get an assessment can be challenging and very specific to the individual and the family system. Mental health clinicians have seen the challenge of engaging someone into care before and may be able to offer you specific advice and strategies. NAMI has hundreds of locations around the United States, and people at your local affiliate may be able to provide helpful support, the benefit of their experiences, and knowledge of local services. Chapter 3 addresses in more detail how to go about getting an assessment, as well as longer-term treatment.

Be Gentle on Yourself

There is no perfect way to identify mental health symptoms. You are unlikely to have been given any training in this important area. If you are like many people, you have been taught it is better to keep concerns to yourself or to "power through" in the hopes that, with time, the symptoms will pass on their own. This may work, but often does not. If you are concerned about a family member who is not sharing their experience with you for any number of reasons, it can be hard to have a dialogue. The first presentation of a mental health condition is commonly the most difficult to identify and seek help for. Ideally, that experience can inform discussions, collaboration, and future planning.

Once you recognize that you or a loved one may have a mental illness, the next step is to obtain a diagnosis. A mental health diagnosis—and its ramifications—is a continuous learning process for all members of the family, and the more you can engage in that process together, the better the experience is likely to be. Remember: while diagnosis is often critical to inform decision-making, a person is not their diagnosis. This is the paradox of diagnosis that will be the focus of the next chapter.

TWO

The Paradox of Diagnosis

"You cannot tame it until you name it."

—ANGELINA HUDSON,
Texas

"I finally got to a therapist, finally got a diagnosis of major depressive disorder. It was such a relief to find out that the thing that I had been going through was not just an aspect of my personality, but in fact a treatable condition. Leaving a doctor's office with a diagnosis of 'you've got a chronic mental illness and have had for most of your life,' and just skipping down the sidewalk is sort of an odd thing but knowing that it could get better was really the payoff."

—JOHN MOE,
Minnesota

"When I first received a diagnosis, I was relieved to know that there is a name for this. I decided I was going to break the news to everybody. I said, 'Guys, for quite some time now I've been having some problems. Well, you'll be happy to know, as I was, that I have a mental health diagnosis. I have major depression, along with the substance abuse.' Everybody kind of looked at me and silence fell across the room. Dead silence. Finally, my mom spoke up and she said, 'Honey, don't tell anybody that. They'll think you're crazy.' But I said, 'Mom, I am, in a sense. I have a diagnosis; I have a prescription for some things that are going to help me.'"

—CLARENCE JORDAN,
Tennessee

• • •

I t is not always easy to ask the question, "What kind of illness do I have?" or "What kind of illness does my family member have?" To ask the question is to acknowledge that there may be an illness, and for many people that requires overcoming shame. We have made much progress in the past half century in developing a better and more compassionate understanding of mental illnesses as medical conditions, and as a common human experience. But people still tend to feel shame. The idea that their thinking, mood, and/or behavior might be a problem to work on can be challenging to accept. Family members may feel that they are somehow at fault for their loved one's mood or behavior; they might worry that others will judge them. Shame is a very common burden and a powerful barrier to seeking help. It can take courage to accept that you or someone you love may be affected by mental illness. But once you can accept that possibility, the question "What's the diagnosis?" becomes an important one to ask.

A diagnosis can be a powerful tool in supporting recovery. It provides a preliminary framework, like a rough draft, for understanding what you or your loved one is experiencing. Having a diagnosis also introduces words and concepts that can make the experience feel more manageable and can often help determine next steps. This is true even if—as is often the case—different professionals give you different diagnoses, or you get a diagnosis that does not accurately describe what you are experiencing. Misdiagnosis does happen—the diagnostic system is far from perfect—and ongoing questioning is important, especially if your treatment or services are not helping.

Typically, physicians diagnose illness by looking for the ways in which your bodily processes diverge from "normal." Very high sugar levels mean diabetes; too little thyroid hormone leaves you fatigued. But when it comes to mental health conditions, focusing only on what diverges from normal can feel invalidating and even dehumanizing. Mental illness affects your very thoughts, emotions, and behaviors—things that are highly connected to your sense of self and your self-worth. Your many strengths and talents do not disappear when you have a diagnosis, but it can feel like they do. And this can create a major obstacle in the process of acceptance, and thus in the process of recovery.

This is the paradox of diagnosis: It is helpful to know your diagnosis, even if it is just a rough draft. It can inform your recovery, but you also need to know that your diagnosis does not define you. Your experience is much more than a symptom checklist. You are a person, and your diagnosis is a tool to help you plan to move forward. Mood, thinking, and behavioral symptoms can be powerful and scary, but they do not define you. A diagnostician should not disregard the human dimension of living with a mental health condition during the diagnostic process. If they do, it might be worth considering a different clinician.

Because we do not have blood tests, MRIs, or genetic analysis to help with mental health diagnosis, the lack of hard science compounds the shame often associated with these brain-based symptoms. Broken bones or urinary tract infections do not usually generate shame as they are objectively observable on an X-ray or urinalysis. We do not have a comparable biological test in mental health. Cancer once had a similar "shame and silence" status in our society before we found more scientific understanding and treatments. It's good to remember that we all tend to be afraid of what we do not understand, and we need a better understanding of the brain to help with that challenge.

We still do not know enough about the brain to organize mental health experiences by their neurobiological characteristics and develop a diagnostic framework more informed by neuroscience. The biological response to traumatic events is now well understood, but there is no similar detailed understanding of the mechanism of depression, bipolar disorder, addiction, or schizophrenia. For these conditions, we largely observe that our treatments are often helpful and hypothesize mechanisms from those results. Why is our diagnostic framework still so limited after billions of dollars' worth of research and a series of genetic breakthroughs? Our understanding of the human brain is so much more sophisticated than even a decade ago, yet we cannot currently connect that science to inform individual diagnoses. There is research, such as the Research Domain Criteria funded by NIMH, that is attempting a purely neuroscience-based approach to rethink diagnosis. It is interesting, but in its infancy.

Despite all the obstacles, limitations, and caveats, it is important to get your diagnosis (or diagnoses) as close to right as you can. An imperfect framework can still help a lot of people. So mental health professionals rely on the American Psychiatric Association's diagnostic tool, the *Diagnostic and Statistical Manual of Mental Disorders* (DSM), the five editions of which reflect a constant evolution in how mental illness is recognized and defined, what illnesses are called, and what their symptoms are. The DSM is designed to produce "inter-rater reliability," meaning that a psychologist in Ann Arbor and a nurse practitioner on Cape Cod would add up the same symptoms and both come up with the same or very similar syndrome-based diagnosis. But are the diagnoses valid on a brain-based biological level? We just do not know yet.

A Brief History of How We Got Here

When I was on call as a resident in the early 1990s, I was interested in the history of how we understand diagnoses. I learned that my dad had classic bipolar disorder, now known as bipolar I, with psychosis—experiences such as hallucinations or delusions that others do not perceive as real—intermixed with periods of normal functioning. I also met other patients with symptoms like his. Did this concept of bipolar disorder always exist? I was fortunate to be a resident at the Massachusetts Mental Health Center, which was founded in 1912, so there was plenty of history for me to explore. There was a section of old records in the wood-paneled library. When I was on call, I posted myself in the library, looking—in those pre-privacy-law days—at these records to understand how the doctors thought about diagnoses. I learned that how we think about diagnosis was not at all fixed, but rather it was evolving, based on new science, theory, and social norms.

I found that the medical records of the 1910s and '20s contained exquisite detail on symptoms, such as the speed of speech and the specific kind of delusion or hallucination. There was no speculation, only description, which was closer to the approach used in the rest of the medical field. There were also records of treatment for late-stage syphilis, which can cause hallucinations and depressive symptoms and thus was a very common cause of institutionalization at that time. I noticed a lot of very careful temperature checks filling the records and then saw that the patients were being discharged with minimal symptoms. In the pre-antibiotic era, the German psychiatrist Julius Wagner-Jauregg figured out that if patients who had late-stage syphilis were deliberately infected with malaria, high body temperatures from malarial fever would kill the bacteria that caused syphilitic symptoms like confusion, weakness, hallucinations, and depression, and patients would improve. This malaria breakthrough was used as a successful treatment for the brain-based impact of late-stage syphilis at my mental health center. There were treatments for malaria, so many patients were discharged without symptoms of either syphilis or malaria. Dr. Wagner-Jauregg won the Nobel Prize in Medicine in 1927 and was the first psychiatrist to do so. It must have seemed at the time like scientific cures for other mental health conditions were right around the corner, if only they carefully detailed what they were seeing.

These miracles were sadly not to come. When I looked at later records, that descriptive framework was nowhere to be seen. It was clear the field had taken a hard turn in a different direction. The records from the 1950s, '60s, and '70s were full of observations of the patient's mother. What did she wear? What did she say? What was her tone like? This was the time of the theory of the "schizophrenogenic mother"—the psychoanalytic idea that cold or cruel mothering was the cause of schizophrenia—and multiple leading theorists preached it. This misguided model harmed a lot of people and alienated many families from the mental health field. Laurie Flynn, a former executive director of NAMI and mother of a large multiracial, multicultural family, put it this way: "You had to pay to get blamed."

Today's diagnostic framework is credited to Emil Kraepelin, a German psychiatrist who was among the very first to organize symptoms into patterns to inform diagnosis. Kraepelin's method—categorizing illnesses by describing patterns of symptoms—is still at the root of our current approach to diagnosing psychosis more than a hundred years later.

Psychiatrists made many errors in the latter half of the twentieth century. Incredibly, until 1972, the DSM—the handbook widely used by mental health professionals in the United States—stated that being gay was a mental illness. The framework of psychiatric diagnosis used to posit that children could not become depressed—until some researchers interviewed children and found that they met the diagnostic criteria designed for adults. Given the problem of child and teen suicide, it is troubling that the field held this idea for so long. We now know that these two ideas, just like the one about schizophrenogenic mothers, were simply wrong. It is important to remember that the DSM is a useful but imperfect framework, bound by what diagnosticians can "see" at the time, and can be influenced by societal conventions, culture, and theories of what is and what is not mental illness. These repeated errors speak to the need for a better understanding of the underlying neurobiology of mental illness.

There are still many unanswered questions in the field of diagnosis. Are mood symptoms a manifestation of addiction, or is addiction an attempt to self-medicate an experience of suffering? An illness defined one way in the DSM—for example, major depression—often manifests differently in a child or teen than in an adult. So, is it the same illness appearing differently in different stages of life, or are these, in fact, different illnesses? How many kinds of schizophrenia are there? When does grief become a pathological process requiring treatment? We do not know enough yet to answer some of these important questions, but we need to keep asking them.

Our challenges in brain research and understanding are not unique. Kraepelin used to collaborate with his research assistant, a psychiatrist and neuroanatomist named Alois Alzheimer, who studied dementia senilis, the dementia that can accompany aging. The elusive search for effective treatments for what we now call Alzheimer's disease shares some of the complexity of our quest to design treatments for mental health conditions.

Getting the Right Diagnosis Matters

An accurate diagnosis can help chart a treatment course that supports your recovery. Achieving accuracy can be a process, and an absent or incorrect diagnosis can have serious consequences. On the other hand, I have seen many people improve even while going through the diagnostic process, if they are engaged in therapy, are benefitting from a medication, or have support from family and peers. It is also true that many people will get different or multiple diagnoses over time.

Some psychiatric misdiagnoses are common. For example, borderline personality disorder (BPD) and bipolar disorder are sometimes confused. Cathleen Payne of Virginia is a sixty-one-year-old woman who reports she has lived with BPD for more than fifty years and has been married to her husband for thirty-six of them. Many years ago, Cathleen heard about the then-new diagnosis of BPD and thought it fit her experiences of intense emotional reactivity and self-harming behaviors. She reported this to her psychiatrist but was told that BPD "didn't exist." At that time, psychiatrists were concerned that, because there were no good treatments for BPD, diagnosing it could be devastating to the patient and thus should be avoided. Cathleen was prescribed lithium to treat what that doctor thought was bipolar disorder. Years later, after she found dialectical behavior therapy (DBT)—a structured therapy designed to teach people coping skills to manage emotional dysregulation, now the best studied psychotherapy effective for treating people with BPD—her well-being improved dramatically. By then, however, she told me that the lithium she'd been taking for over eleven years, for no valid clinical reason, had taken a toll on her kidneys. It's only in the past decade that DBT has become a commonly accepted intervention for BPD. Cathleen now volunteers her time for the National Educational Alliance on Borderline Personality Disorder, an advocacy group that connects people with BPD to the evidence-based treatment that helped her, and to other helpful interventions. André Ivanoff describes DBT in more detail in chapter 18.

Similarly, the consequences of missing the diagnosis of obsessive compulsive disorder (OCD) can be severe. Stephen Smith, a twenty-eight-year-old white man who currently lives with his wife, two kids, and two Bernedoodles in San Antonio, Texas, started to experience intense anxiety, recurrent thought patterns, and other associated behaviors at the age of sixteen. The symptoms significantly worsened when he was a college student and quarterback of his school's Division III football team. He did not have a name or diagnosis for this distressing experience, but he could not stop the intrusive, repetitive thoughts, and he knew something was wrong. His symptoms became so overwhelming, he had to drop out of college. He had a supportive girlfriend, now his wife, but she did not know what he was experiencing either. He spent hours each day searching the internet and posting descriptions of his symptoms hoping to get answers, but to no avail. When he went to get clinical help, he was given the wrong diagnosis more than once. One clinician even advised him to move away from his family, as they were deemed the cause of his anxiety and symptoms. (They were not.)

Based on his Google searches, Stephen eventually realized he might be living with obsessive compulsive disorder (OCD). He saved up and waited for many months to see the one expensive specialist in San Antonio who specialized in OCD. Once the doctor confirmed Stephen's suspicions, the diagnosis and treatment made a difference immediately. Stephen told me how much relief he felt: "I thought, 'You're not alone.' I'd had no idea there was a name for this. The fact that it has a name means that it's somewhat normal, right?"

After getting the right diagnosis, the right kind of psychotherapy—exposure response prevention (ERP)—and the right medications, Stephen is now doing very well. He even founded a company called NOCD to give people virtual access to this specific psychotherapy. NOCD trains therapists in ERP, hosts an online support group, and makes resources available to reinforce and support the lessons in treatment. NOCD was inspired by Stephen's experience of misdiagnosis, of getting the wrong kind of care, and feeling alone. He does not want people to lose years like he did and knows from his own experience that there is good care available for people with OCD. NOCD is being added as an in-network service provider to health insurance plans across the country.

Sarah Greulich, a proud wife, dog mom, and aunt who has dedicated her life to working in the nonprofit sector, was born and raised in New Jersey by two parents who both suffered from various mental illnesses. She told me that the misdiagnosis of her mother's mental illness had lifelong consequences—not just for her mother, but also for herself. She recalled that, as a child, when she came home from elementary school, her mother would remain asleep on the couch all afternoon, and that she and her sister were often on their own with their dog. After her father left her mother when Sarah was thirteen years old, her mother's mood symptoms worsened considerably, and Sarah was on the receiving end of her physical and verbal abuse for many years. The abuse continued when later, as an adult, Sarah took on the role of her mother's caretaker. She persisted, though she described the experience as "very difficult to endure." At some point, a physician prescribed her mother opiates, and her mother did not share with the physician or with Sarah that she had struggled with addiction before. Finally, when her mother was in her sixties and in the late stages of cancer care, she had a critical mental health reevaluation. The reevaluation led to her finally receiving an accurate diagnosis of bipolar disorder and a prescription for the appropriate medication. This medicine dramatically reduced her mother's symptoms of irritability and hostility. Her mother also no longer craved the opiates to self-medicate her mood symptoms. Sarah had only two months of peace with her mother before her mother's death, but those months were priceless. She understood that her mother and her illness were not the same thing. "Addressing the illness can bring the real person back to you," she told me.

For Cathleen, Stephen, and Sarah's mother, it took a very long time to get the right diagnosis and effective treatment for that diagnosis. The grace they show about these diagnostic missteps is inspiring, as is their dedication to helping others to avoid these preventable problems.

If your treatment plan is not working, regardless of your age, please reassess both the treatment and the underlying diagnosis. Most clinicians welcome this discussion and will welcome a second opinion if they are not sure themselves or want to support you in your quest for more understanding.

My Blurry Diagnosis

It is also important to remember that the reason diagnoses can be imprecise is because we are human beings. When does a feeling become a mood? When does a mood become a mood disorder? I know from my own experience how blurry the boundaries can be—not just in terms of changing criteria in the DSM, but in terms of the human condition.

When my beloved brother Joe died a few years ago, I was overwhelmed by grief. It was more than I could bear that my older brother and best friend was gone, and that I was now the only living member of our original family, having lost my loving sister Sue to cancer a decade prior. Though my dad had bipolar disorder, and I had always worried I might develop severe mood symptoms, I had never experienced true depressive or manic symptoms before. I was relieved to not have had mood symptoms in my twenties during my cancer treatment when I was given a lot of steroids—so-called "mood looseners." I then figured I was out of the woods on mood disorders. But Joe's death was too much for me. I was having trouble getting out of bed and was unable to sustain attention in conversations and work meetings. It seemed ridiculous that three days is what I was given for bereavement leave; I felt like it would take three years. My experience got worse over the weeks that followed. I was crushed by sadness in a way I never had been before. I lost interest in my favorite activities. This was a classic feature of depression—but even after a career of studying it, I did not have the capacity to notice it in myself.

I had planned to skip my monthly dinner meeting with my friends, but I forced myself to show up. This group of friends from my residency training days are all psychiatrists. They took one look at me and immediately encouraged me to contact my therapist and to get evaluated for antidepressant medication. They were right. Therapy and an antidepressant helped me with this experience. I noticed that, though I knew I was still in tremendous pain, it softened, and I also felt less connected to it after taking the medicine. It felt weird, to feel one step removed from my grief. Joe was still gone, and I felt a little disloyal to him for not feeling quite as much. But it helped me. In the following months, my concentration slowly improved. Given my dad's diagnosis, I knew I needed to keep an eye out for the possibility that the antidepressant might trigger manic symptoms. But they did not. I began to regain some energy. Months later, I noted that I was enjoying walking again. Over many months, the medication, my psychotherapist, my family, and friends, the huge stack of sympathy cards that I read and reread, and talking about my experience with my life partner, Kelly, pulled me to a more functional level. My doctor and I decreased and then stopped the medicine about nine months later and I continued the psychotherapy.

Now, with this difficult period behind me, I note that my diagnosis might have been different, based on the different ways of understanding grief reflected in different editions of the DSM. Was I in a deep state of "normal" grief, or had I crossed a line into major depression? The answer would depend on when I asked. Until the most recent, fifth version of the DSM, grief was not considered to be indicative of major depression for the first two months. This was the so-called bereavement exclusion.

The idea was that grief resembles depression in many ways, but that you could not have both at the same time. Then the thinking changed for the DSM-5 TR. In late 2021, a new diagnosis was added to the DSM called prolonged grief disorder, which again illustrates the evolving way the field has worked to reconcile loss and its role in illness.

The evolution of the diagnostic framework makes it clear that we do not know how to fine-tune our understanding of some of these core human challenges. How do we define and distinguish heartbreak and loss, grief, and depression? And whatever the "right" diagnosis was for me, the tools of time, psychotherapy, medication, community, support, and finding small ways to honor my departed siblings, Joe and Sue, worked to help me move ahead.

The Art of Diagnosis

Given the humbling absence of scientific tools like blood tests or brain-imaging technology to help us make an accurate psychiatric diagnosis, we must use the tools and evidence at hand. Diagnosis remains, in part, an art, informed by experience, culture, and training. Symptoms are symptoms and can be significant, but a good clinician can also look beyond them. Here are some of the factors good clinicians consider in making a diagnosis—and some things for you to consider and do in preparing for a mental health assessment.

Think Below the Neck

We can use those scientific tools to be sure something medical is not responsible for symptoms. When you get an assessment, both you and your practitioner should assess what is happening below the neck. Primary care doctors and pediatricians are skilled in this, and so are psychiatrists and nurse practitioners. You may have taken medications or have a medical issue that mimics mental health symptoms. Amphetamines (as well as LSD and, for some, use of marijuana) can cause paranoia; a steroid treatment can cause mania or intense sadness. Symptoms of thyroid disease can look just like major depression. Autoimmune disorders, substance use, and infectious diseases are all examples of health concerns that need to be assessed in a person who is presenting with mental health symptoms. Bear in mind there is a body-mind connection that can add complexity to the diagnostic picture.

Think Movie, Not Snapshot

People can look different in different "snapshots" of their life. The same is true in a psychiatric interview. That is one reason so many people note that their diagnosis has changed over time. It is also a reason that clinicians try to sort out when symptoms first appeared and how they developed. The "movie" can be much more helpful than a "snapshot." There are many different possible underlying conditions that could explain why a person has paranoia and hears voices—from substance use to severe mood disorders, to schizophrenia, to a medical cause. It often takes time to rule out some of the alternative hypotheses, and to see developing patterns, before a clinician can make the correct diagnosis.

The course of your symptoms over time can also lead to a change in diagnosis, like a plot twist in a movie. For example, many people who seek help for a depressed mood do so because they have experienced an episode of major depression. From there, the course varies from person to person. Some people will have only one episode of major depression, and some will struggle with a recurrent vulnerability to major depressive episodes. A smaller group of people will later experience a manic episode, which changes their diagnosis from major depression to bipolar disorder. That is why a diagnosis of bipolar disorder can surprise both a clinician and the person diagnosed. Knowing your family history can help you to better understand your risk of this kind of change in the diagnostic picture. A diagnosis of bipolar disorder has clear implications for your medical treatment plan, since the most effective medications differ from those that target major depression.

Family History

It is helpful to know your family's mental health history, as history can provide useful clues in informing your diagnostic process. But family history does not definitively determine what condition you have, how you experience it over time, or your outcome. Genetics are not destiny. People ask if mental health conditions are genetic, and the answer is more complex than a simple yes or no. Based on what we now know, risk exists in the interplay of nature (genetics) and nurture (stresses, trauma, infections, and more). The study of this interplay of genes and environmental stressors—from flu in pregnancy to bullying in grade school to a legacy of alcoholism—is called epigenetics.

Mental health conditions can run in families, the way diabetes and heart disease can also run in families. Information about the past is useful. Knowing that a parent or grandparent experienced manic episodes is helpful in treatment planning. If your diagnosis is major depression, for example, you will be more alert for manic symptoms and your doctor may want to prescribe a mood stabilizer in addition to or instead of an antidepressant. Because of my family history of psychosis, I encouraged my children to be careful about early use of marijuana since early use and family history of psychosis increases risk.

But there are no straight lines in the genetics of mental health. Of all mental health conditions, ADHD is among the most likely to run in families, but that does not mean that it is 100 percent transmitted genetically. The identical twin of a person who has developed schizophrenia has about a 50 percent chance of developing the same illness. The complexity of the human genome and how genes interact is beyond our current knowledge.

I encourage people to have conversations about their family history of mental health and substance use. It can be helpful to know family members' diagnoses, as well as medications and treatment interventions they tried and whether they were effective.

People from prior generations and from certain cultures may be reluctant to discuss mental health histories in the family, but if the shame and secrecy can be surmounted, history can be illuminating. Trish Lockard is a sixty-six-year-old woman who works as a freelance nonfiction book editor, with an adult son and daughter. Trish told me she has depression on her mother's side, including her maternal grandmother, her mother, herself, and her son. She described to me her own journey to understand the impact of mental illness in her mother and grandmother, and how noticing patterns across generations eventually helped her and her son to seek care:

> Every time my mother was upset at me about something, this tells you her mental state, she used the threat of taking her own life while I was at school. It wasn't until I went away to college that I realized that my mother was not a well mother.
>
> I began to recognize that I had genuine mental illness in my family because I had not understood that depression was a mental illness. I didn't think of myself as having mental illness. I didn't really think of my mother as having mental illness. So, it was an interesting revelation to realize I was one of those people with a mental health disorder. My son, who is thirty, has been diagnosed with depression and social anxiety. I too have been diagnosed with depression. I don't know if it's a genetic component, a cultural component, or both. Probably both.

It is sometimes helpful to do this sleuthing in the context of other aspects of family health history that are easier to talk about, like heart attacks or cancer. Whatever you can learn, remember that there may be errors in what people think they know, and there are also likely to be unknowns—for example, what the diagnosis was for an ancestor who spent time in a long-term psychiatric hospital.

Take Notes and Keep Records

By working proactively and keeping records of family history, you can help to reduce the chaos and errors that often complicate mental health care. The care "system" is fragmented and disorganized. One facility may do one thing well, but rarely connects or communicates to the next fa-cility or outpatient practitioner involved in your care. Each clinical site can feel like an island. When I was an outpatient doctor, I had patients admitted to and discharged from a local hospital without my knowledge. The hospital even started one of my patients on a medicine he and I knew did not work. My patient did not recall this or advise hospital staff when he was ill, and they did not contact me. Precious time was wasted.

Here is a proactive way to organize your (or your family member's) information so that the diagnostic snapshot has more context and history—whether in an old school binder or on a digital document:

- Gather records. When you stop care with a clinic or clinician, ask for a summary of your work together. They may be surprised, as few people ever ask for such a thing. But remember, they are working for you.

- Gather discharge summaries. When you are discharged from a hospital or detox, ask for the discharge summary, which will list their diagnosis of you and your treatments. This summary is a very helpful document in your course of care. Even if their diagnosis was incorrect, the record of treatment may offer valuable information.

- Prior neuropsychological testing. This kind of testing evaluates aspects of how your brain works—such as working memory and executive function (the ability to organize)—in doing cognitive tasks like reading or absorbing visual information. It is often done to help understand why a child may be having difficulties in school and can help families to understand challenges like distractibility and the best approaches to learning.

- Meds that worked—and did not. For each medication, note what dosage(s) were tried, and for what duration, to target what specific symptoms. Your current medications and prescriber are also important.

- Psychotherapies that worked—and did not work. Was it the clinician, or the kind of therapy, or both that helped—or that had no impact?

After Diagnosis and Beyond Shame

Getting a diagnosis, a name for something that may have seemed intangible and indescribable, may feel like a relief. It may also feel troubling or dispiriting. And the truth is, it can be a mixed blessing. An illness can be treated; but no one volunteers to have it. And while you may have found the courage to accept the reality of mental illness, the rest of the world is not yet a prejudice-free space.

It is tempting to imagine such a world. Once I even glimpsed it with my own eyes. In the 1980s and '90s, I was a consultant to a private boarding elementary school, supporting the administration and parents when concerns arose about a child's mental health. At one treatment planning meeting I attended, I was among a group of educators there to support and encourage the parents of a nine-year-old boy who had developed OCD. The boy had been washing his hands incessantly, to the point where his hands were bright red, and he was in a lot of distress. This was a completely new condition; he had no prior history of compulsive behavior. The educators at the meeting were warm and kind, open to anything they could do to support the boy and the family. The family was forthcoming and engaged with the educators without defensiveness. It was a beautiful moment. All agreed that, after the boy's long absence due to getting medical treatment, he and his family would be welcomed back to school and supported. The meeting felt different from others I'd attended.

It took a while before I figured out the difference. The boy's OCD, unlike almost all other mental health conditions, had a clear medical cause. The boy had PANDAS, a rare condition that occurs after a streptococcal infection (strep throat), where children develop antibodies that attack parts of the brain and cause OCD. And because the boy's OCD had this rare medical cause, everyone in the room, including the parents, were absolved of any concerns, or any unconscious beliefs, about whether the family environment or some genetic legacy had contributed to the symptoms. PANDAS was a no-fault diagnosis—it was like he had bronchitis!

This rare moment gave me more insight into the added problems we face with mental health diagnoses. This dynamic could have happened at any school and is in no way unique to the one I happened to consult. Based on my experiences at other treatment planning meetings, if the boy just had OCD, not PANDAS, the family would have been more guarded; the school's support of him and his family more muted. As more people tell their stories and choose not to hide from shame, and as science helps us understand more, there will come a day that mental health conditions will be treated equitably to medical concerns. But we are not there yet.

Working to get a diagnosis can help you, but it is only a beginning. Your journey will likely require courage. But as you will learn in the pages ahead, from some of the millions of people who have traveled this path before you, this is a journey with many rewards. You can feel better. You can feel connected to a community. And there is much to learn, meaning to find, and maybe even unexpected joy to experience on your road to recovery.

THREE

How Do I Find Help?
Minding the Many Gaps

"There was one licensed therapist in my area who was specialty-trained in exposure and response prevention (ERP), the gold-standard therapy for OCD, and she was cash-pay. She charged about $350 a session, and she had a waitlist about seven months long. So, the only chance to get better was to basically wait for months and find resources to pay for the therapy, which my family didn't have. It was a total nightmare."

—STEPHEN SMITH,
Texas

"Not one doctor—and I'm talking about seven doctors, maybe four clinicians—nobody ever had a pamphlet or said, 'Have you looked into NAMI? They have some classes and support groups.' Nobody."

—SHIRLEY HOLLOWAY,
Alaska

• • •

Let's begin by acknowledging reality: The mental health "system" throughout the United States is chaotic and full of gaps. It has long been broken and fragmented, and if you try to wait for the system to be less confusing and frustrating, you will be waiting a very long time. So, I encourage you to start seeking care as soon as you are ready, to give yourself as much time as possible to find the help you need. It is easier said than done, of course, but there is good care available, and strong evidence that getting help earlier leads to better results for all mental health conditions.

There are very good, experienced, compassionate people out there who want to help: physicians, nurses, clinicians, case managers, social workers, counselors, and others. But finding them, and paying for them, can be very challenging. Health care is rife with inequities, and care for mental health and addiction is no exception. Try to hold on to the fact that the chaos, inaccessibility, and disparities that characterize the mental health system are real, and no reflection on you. If you can't find quality care that you can afford, it's not that you haven't tried hard enough or that you don't need or deserve that care. It's that what you need is hard to find.

Why does this chaos persist? I learned some of the reasons during my stint as acting commissioner of the Department of Mental Health (DMH) for the Commonwealth of Massachusetts. Even before my first day on the job, I had a sense of foreboding. It was 2003; the state was facing an enormous budget shortfall, and newly elected governor Mitt Romney had vowed to cut spending. Considering the dire financial situation, no one else wanted the job I'd just taken. Even I had accepted it against my better judgment. But I cared a lot about mental health services, and I'd been a political science major in college, and so I was curious. How did policy decisions get made?

In the first meeting I attended, on my first day on the job, I found out. After brief introductions, the administration official running the meeting passed around a proposed organizational chart that eliminated the Massachusetts Department of Mental Health. No one said anything about it or asked my opinion. I had lost an essential mental health department on day one, before I'd finished my first cup of coffee. The next piece of paper I got listed the many DMH programs I was being directed to cut to help close the enormous budget gap. I felt sick. I knew these were programs that people desperately needed.

The idea to close the Department of Mental Health was not the outcome of a thoughtful planning process involving the community; nor did it reflect input from the many thousands of mental health professionals working in the field. It was a panicked retreat to meet a budget shortfall in the wake of an economic recession. No one enjoyed the process. None of the programs were cut with malice. And while the decision to close DMH was ultimately reversed months later, there were some programs I could not save despite multiple efforts at advocating for them. The Commonwealth of Massachusetts was broke.

This misadventure gave me insight into both the extreme fragility of public mental health services, and why there are so many gaps and so much variability in what the system offers. DMH was just one of the pieces of the mental health system, and it was just for one state. The same recession that walloped Massachusetts was having a similar impact in nearly all fifty states. Those states were undergoing a similar service reduction process to close their own budget gaps, each of them likely cutting different services. When states are short of money, and must balance their budgets, allocations for mental health and addiction services are often the first to be cut. In the Great Recession of 2008 to 2011, the United States lost more than three thousand long-term state hospital beds, which never returned. Recessions and budget shortfalls are to mental health services what hurricanes are to sand dunes on a beach. The dunes erode and don't get rebuilt when the weather clears.

There is no singular authority or coordinating body overseeing maintenance of a quality mental health care system that provides equitable access. The gaps in services move around as decision makers make changes that work for their small piece of the puzzle. For example, let's say your employer changes health plan coverage to save money, but your therapist does not join the lower-paying network, making your costs to see that therapist too high and unaffordable. Or your local Medicaid director develops an innovative program for pregnant mothers with addiction, then leaves for a better job and her successor defunds the program. Or your local court institutes a progressive jail diversion system, which could keep you out of a correctional setting, but if you are arrested in a different county, you may not benefit from the same compassionate response.

People and families already overwhelmed by a mental health crisis are thus faced with the hardest obstacle course in American health care. We know that more than half of all people who have mental health conditions get no help at all. What we don't know is how much of that has to do with internal barriers, like distrust or lack of awareness, versus how much is related to the cost of care or the confusing "system" of care. Leaders often tout aspirational models where there are "no wrong doors" to enter care. But given the absence of coordination from state to state, system to system, institution to institution, and profession to profession, there are still plenty of doors that lead to long waitlists, ineffective or unaffordable care, jail, or homelessness—and some doors that do not open at all. People who do not speak English or who are not citizens face even higher barriers to access care.

Due to the patchwork history of mental health funding, your options for care will be informed by many variables. These variables include your age, financial situation, insurance coverage, zip code, local leadership, underlying conditions, economic recessions, state law, employer (if you have a job), the severity of your condition, and, of course, luck.

Having the ability to pay privately makes some aspects of getting help easier, but it does not solve everything in terms of access to care or the quality of care available. American health care is expensive and does not have a stellar or equitable record of outcomes. The private pay market in mental health care is another reflection of this inequity and misallocation of resources. Even private pay may not make a difference: A fancy rehab in California or Florida may or may not be able to help you achieve long-term recovery from a substance use disorder.

So, where do you start? How *do* you go about finding and accessing appropriate and affordable help? That depends on your situation:

1. Do you need help handling a crisis or emergency?

2. Are you seeking to make first contact with a mental health professional for an evaluation or diagnosis?
3. Are you looking for effective longer-term care?

Finding Help in an Emergency: Acute Crisis

A mental health crisis is usually defined as exhibiting behaviors that may lead to endangering yourself or another person. The danger could be self-harm, suicidal planning, or high-risk behavior, like wandering in traffic when hallucinating, or unsafe use of potentially fatal drugs or other mind-and-mood-altering substances. If you're not sure whether thoughts about suicide qualify as urgent, ask yourself or your loved one if you have thought about what method you would use. If you've thought about where, how, or when you would end your life, that means you've begun developing a plan. That's a crisis.

If you or a loved one is having a mental health crisis, safety is the most important outcome. If, for example, you have developed a plan to take your own life, you should go to a hospital emergency room or call 988, a new three-digit resource line. When you call 988, you will be connected to a trained person who knows of and can point you to local resources. If a loved one has a plan, and they will not agree to go to a hospital emergency room, call 988 for help determining appropriate next steps. Hospital emergency rooms can assess you medically; this is an essential first step in many cases. Some medical problems can create mental health crises, and a medical setting is the best place to evaluate whether there is an underlying medical issue. Overdoses and cutting can also be acutely managed in the emergency department. Again, safety is the important outcome in an acute crisis.

If you are already in treatment and face an urgent crisis, your mental health professionals are trained to help you navigate it and should have a process in place. If you reach out and they do not answer the phone, their voice message or service should advise you of next steps.

Life-Threatening Emergency Telephone and Text Resources

The new centralized system for handling mental health crisis and suicide prevention responses in the United States can be accessed by dialing 988. Calls to 988 will be routed to the caller's local crisis center and connect them to a crisis counselor for immediate assistance.

Calling 988 should be your first choice if you or your loved one is at imminent risk of suicide, or if you or someone else is experiencing a mental health crisis. The 988 service is operational twenty-four hours a day, seven days a week. As crises are so individual, and services variable by locality, a call to 988 will get you to a crisis counselor who will assess your level of need, help you sort out the options available, and initiate actions that will provide help. Local crisis resources and services might include some combination of mobile crisis response team, walk-in emergency psychiatric services, crisis stabilization center, hospital emergency room, community-based peer respite house, or peer-run emotional support warmlines, where trained volunteers can offer empathy and support. For people more comfortable with texting, Crisis Text Line connects individuals in crisis with crisis counselors when they text NAMI to 741741.

If you are a parent, and your child or teen states that they are suicidal, it may help to call 988 with your child present. Their staff are trained to help in these challenging situations. A safe outcome in a crisis is critical, and then the planning for a longer-term strategy can begin.

There are also suicide prevention and crisis intervention support services that focus on offering a peer response to individuals within specific communities. The Trevor Project provides crisis and suicide prevention support to LGBTQ+ people by phone, web chat, or text messaging. At Trevor, volunteers understand the unique needs of help seekers because they share many of the same life experiences. Veterans Crisis Line specially serves the crisis and suicide prevention needs of veterans by phone, at 800-273-8255, by text, to 838255, or via online chat at veteranscrisisline .net, and many of the responders are veterans themselves.

If you're hesitant to go to an ER, ask a friend or family member to stay with you while you may be at risk. Call 988 as soon as possible. The 988 responders will know if there is mobile crisis service in your area, which can come to your home or wherever the crisis is occurring. This option, part of a growing initiative to offer a less institutional and more welcoming model of assessment and care, is available only in some places.

Care After Crisis

The period after an acute crisis is critical. It is a time to make decisions on next steps in treatment, to attend to your self-care, and to plan proactively as you develop more stability.

Clinical Decisions and Finding the Right Level of Care

Whatever the origin of the acute crisis, you will need a plan to address both immediate and longer-term needs. For example, identifying the underlying stressors and triggers of the crisis is important. Many possible pathways can follow, and they will be driven by many factors, including your preferences, clinical situation, available services, and insurance coverage. For example, if you are admitted to a hospital, options for next steps may include step-down to a residential facility, an intensive outpatient day program, or returning home with outpatient follow-up. At this point, it is important to engage your support network. Some hospitals handle discharge planning better than others. Sometimes discharge plans fall apart right after—or even before—discharge. Other times, discharge planning can be "lost in translation" between programs. Be vigilant and proactive in communicating with your support network and with the professionals on duty. There should be a plan for your next steps and follow-up care, and you should know what it is. Ideally, you should have a voice in planning for yourself or your loved one. You should be able to ask questions and understand the reasoning behind professional recommendations and decisions.

Take Care of Yourself

If you are the person experiencing a mental health crisis, think about what has helped you feel better—or, if you've had mental health struggles before, what helped to stabilize you—in the past, and create a "toolbox" of coping mechanisms. Would it help to talk to a friend? To meditate or take a nap? To exercise or go for a walk? Take action to help yourself, even if you doubt it will work. Doubt and feelings of helplessness may be symptoms of a mental health condition. Do something that might make you feel better and observe how you feel afterward. In difficult times, many people benefit from reaching out to friends, family, and support groups for encouragement.

The NAMI HelpLine—800-950-NAMI or info@nami.org—can offer you empathy and support and provide you with information about resources in your community. The HelpLine is not a suicide prevention resource, but it is staffed by trained volunteers, many of whom have their own lived experience. It is because of this lived experience that they can empathize and effectively help. They know what works and what hurts. The NAMI HelpLine also maintains a comprehensive directory of nearly eight hundred trusted, peer-informed resources that are known to be helpful to the mental health community, and volunteers can guide you to the ones likely to be most useful to you.

It can also be helpful to call a warmline—a phone number where trained peer volunteers offer empathy and support. To find a warmline in your area, and information on local social services, dial 211, or go to www.211.org. These support lines are usually staffed by peers living with a mental health condition who are likely not trained crisis counselors. They are great resources, especially for people who are isolated and want to talk through options with someone who "gets it." Please note that warmlines are not for an acute crisis, such as suicidality. As warmline operator Ky Quickbane, a twenty-eight-year-old queer trans man residing in Pittsburgh, Pennsylvania, told me:

> On the warmline, I have folks who just want to talk about what they had
> for dinner and their pets. An invaluable question that I think needs to be
> added or recognized in the mental health system is, What do you need

right now? Do you need to talk about it? Do you need space? Do you need to try a coping skill?

Remember that you are not alone, and help is available. If you've had experience with this mental health condition before, you may already have a long-term treatment plan in place and may already have experienced how it has helped lessen your symptoms. Try to remind yourself that what worked before can work again; and that the way you feel now is not the way you'll feel forever.

Proactive Planning

If you or your loved one live with a mental health condition, it's important to plan for a potential crisis. Developing a crisis response plan can help you and your family make decisions when no one's thinking is at their best. Talk with your treatment team so you can think about where to go for intensive treatment and how to get there; how to take time off work or explain your absence to others; and what methods you can use to calm yourself in an emergency. You and those closest to you should know how to reach your mental health professionals in case of an emergency. The Wellness Recovery Action Plan (WRAP), developed by Mary Ellen Copeland, is a great tool that helps people identify triggers, stress, and coping strategies in the process of developing a plan. Copeland talks about the evolution of WRAP in chapter 4, and explains how to create your own plan in more detail in chapter 17. Also in that chapter, Jackie Feldman offers additional guidance on creating a crisis plan.

Another tool some people find helpful is a psychiatric advance directive (PAD) that outlines what steps you want to take during an emergency or if you are incapacitated due to a mental health condition. Note, however, that it is enforceable only in some states. It is best to create a PAD when there isn't a crisis, when you can think things through. An example of a directive you might include in your plan is "I was mistreated at Hospital A, and even if I don't or can't say so clearly while in crisis, I do not want to go there." This helps you retain more control of your outcomes in the event of a future crisis.

Planning can also involve learning and training. For example, if opiates are part of the clinical picture, it can be lifesaving for families to learn how to recognize the symptoms of an overdose and how to administer naloxone, a medicine that can treat narcotic overdose. Naloxone is available from pharmacies in most states without a prescription, and often for free or at low cost. It comes in several forms, but the easiest to administer is a nasal spray. You can ask a pharmacist to demonstrate how to use it when you pick it up. The American Red Cross offers a First Aid for Opiate Overdoses online course that covers the use of several different naloxone products.

Important But Not Urgent Situations: Getting an Evaluation and Finding Care

There are important situations that are not acute emergencies—when you need help, but there is not a threat of harm to yourself or others. One common example is the worsening of mood symptoms and sleep changes with a decline in functioning. These are situations in which a mental health issue has compromised your or your loved one's ability to successfully manage daily life, is causing profound emotional pain or feelings of hopelessness, or has manifested in thinking or behavior that is irrational, unusually isolating, or secretive. It may feel like the need for help is urgent, though you may not know exactly what kind of help is needed, or even what exactly is wrong.

If you know you need help, but emergency measures for safety aren't necessary—or if you or your loved one is troubled by a mood state, thought pattern, feelings, or symptoms that you don't understand or know what to do about—then your first step is to connect with a clinician who can do a mental health evaluation. If you have been treated for a mental health condition before, or are currently in treatment, call your treatment team and let them know what's happening. If your health condition has grown worse recently, it could mean that you need a new evaluation, or need them to help make changes to your treatment plan. Don't be afraid to speak openly and honestly about what is and isn't working for you. It may be the case that you need a new treatment, service, or strategy to help you avoid a crisis.

If what you are experiencing is new to you, then you need to get an initial evaluation; this will then point the way to what kind of care you need. In the United States, where there is no single organized system for mental health care, there is also no one place to obtain an evaluation, and the path to obtaining good mental health care is often unclear. Options will differ depending on what is available in your community, what your health insurance plan covers, whether you are enrolled in Medicare or Medicaid, what you can afford, and where and with whom you feel most comfortable. If you have been hospitalized, or even been seen in an emergency room, then you should have a first draft assessment to help inform your future planning. Be sure to ask hospital staff for a copy of that assessment and recommendations for follow-up care postdischarge.

Below are some ideas for where to begin when you need a mental health evaluation. I'll discuss other resources for getting evaluations for kids in chapter 7.

Consult a Primary Care Physician, General Practitioner, Pediatrician, Nurse, or Physician's Assistant

If you have a relationship with a general practitioner, primary care physician, clinical nurse specialist, or physician's assistant, you can start there. Primary care providers (PCPs) are an underappreciated backbone of the American mental health patchwork. These doctors and nurse practitioners are often well informed about resources in your community and may be connected to a network of practitioners in mental health fields or know someone who is. PCPs and general practitioners can also check whether there are medical causes for your psychiatric symptoms (such as hypothyroidism masquerading as depression) and assess the impact that any medications you are taking could be having on your mood and thinking.

Many health insurance plans require you to select a PCP, and some will ask you to consult with that person before you can obtain a referral to an in-network specialist. If you haven't already established a relationship with a PCP or general practitioner, and your insurance plan hasn't assigned one to you, you may be able to find one who is a covered provider at a community clinic, medical offices connected to hospital systems, or in free-standing practices.

A significant percentage of primary care services are directly related to mental health. As a result, more adult and pediatric PCP offices have added a social worker to their staff or offer other resources as part of an integrated or collaborative care model. It can feel like a lot to ask of some of the busiest people in health care to be the front door to the confusing mental health system, but it is a door that nonetheless might lead to help. Many cases of anxiety, depression, and substance use can often be addressed directly, if not always exclusively, through the PCP's office.

Kelly Pavelich, a twenty-six-year-old white woman living in Arlington, Virginia, had a good introduction to mental health care through her PCP. Kelly said she would not initially have considered going to a therapist because she felt too ashamed to talk about her eating issues or acknowledge her depression. Fortunately, she trusted her PCP, who noted that Kelly's weight loss and liver trouble could be a consequence of an eating disorder and her low mood and prescribed her an antidepressant. Kelly reports that in just a few days, her mother noticed an improvement in her mood, and though Kelly herself didn't notice feeling any better, she did regain just enough energy and perspective to reconsider her reluctance to seek help. The PCP's awareness that Kelly was struggling, and the prescribed medication, were key factors in Kelly's ultimate decision to find a therapist to help her understand her experience and address her mental health condition. Her trusted PCP was the right door for her. Kelly shared the story with me in more detail:

A doctor weighed me, and I started crying. Six months later, my PCP said, "I think you just have an imbalance in your brain. It's not that bad.

Just try this medicine and see if it helps." I think she prescribed it because she knew I wouldn't go to a psychiatrist. This was my doctor at home; I've known her for a long time. When I first moved [to the East Coast], I was having a rough time because I didn't know anyone. I called my primary care doctor in Seattle and the nurse that picked up the phone was so nice. And she followed up with me a week later, "Just want to check in to see how you're doing."

My first time getting on mental health medication, my mom said she noticed it right away, me improving. But for me, honestly, it's hard to explain. I never felt like I fell back into that low point, but I also wasn't like, "I'm so uplifted." I was level, which is good. I feel like I needed that to put me in a place where I could think about mental health, like therapy and just daily taking care of myself. Before that I was so deep into depression and anxiety that I couldn't even see clearly all these other options available to me.

University-affiliated graduate departments of psychiatry, psychology, and social work have expertise in mental health, and often offer evaluation services. For example, if you live in Atlanta, one option might be the Emory University Department of Psychiatry and Behavioral Science. Academic institutions found across the country often have long waitlists and may require you to be connected to their system (usually via your PCP) to get access. It may make sense to get in line there while you are sorting other options. Some offer sliding scales for services and accept lower fees, and some offer free care with trainees. These trainees are typically young and enthusiastic and are supervised by more experienced clinicians. You should get more precise details about how the supervision process works before you accept help from a trainee, so that you know you're getting the best care.

The Elusive "Covered Provider"
Unfortunately, there are multiple funding streams in American mental health—and this only adds to the confusion when it comes to finding

help. Private insurance covers about half of Americans' health care services. All insurance companies are not equal, however, in how they approach mental health coverage. Under current law, as an insurance holder, you are paying for the right to get a mental health evaluation and, if needed, ongoing care. But obtaining the services can be more difficult than advertised. The health plans offer online directories of providers in their network. However, these lists do not usually distinguish which provider is expert in what treatment, or what facility serves what population. The directories can also be out of date and inaccurate. These so-called ghost networks frustrate people looking for help; they have attracted the attention of regulators and been the subject of lawsuits and settlements.

You may have to research each provider to determine whether they provide what you need. Then you may have to spend time calling places only to find out that they only serve veterans, youth, or people referred by city agencies. You might also find that if you call individual practitioners, almost no one in the directory returns your calls. That is because the mental health clinicians who work in private practices, but sign on as preferred providers for insurance plans, often work for themselves without support staff, in small, individual practices and are often overrun with demand. These clinicians focus on helping one person at a time, which is great if you are the one person getting care. But, of course, this is not a wide-scale formula for broader public health access.

If your calls aren't returned, you can call the health plan's customer service line and ask for their help. Be sure to get the name of a particular person at the health plan who can help you with your search. After your call, send them a follow-up email. If that does not work quickly, establish a paper trail—this is a record of the date and time you placed or received a call, the names of anyone you spoke to, and brief notes on every interaction, including any voicemail message you leave that goes unanswered. Health plans are highly regulated, and a record is helpful in getting results either in finding a practitioner, appealing a denial of care, or appealing an absence of care.

If you can't find an appropriate practitioner to do an evaluation in your insurer's network, you can request that the insurer direct you to one or provide coverage for a provider who is not in their network by filing a formal appeal. A good appeal letter can get you connected to an appropriate provider; I have seen firsthand that this can be an effective way to get a health plan to pay for care. The best letters I have read lay out your or your family member's needs, detail your efforts to find someone on your own, and state clearly what you are asking for. Do not accept the first or even the second no. Follow the entire appeal process in writing, as frustrating as that may be. In the interim, work with your primary care provider (if you have one). Then seek peer support: your local NAMI, Mental Health America, or Depression and Bipolar Support Alliance affiliate may offer support or be able to send you in the right direction. Peers can be a great resource on how to gain momentum in your process of getting an evaluation, and they may have firsthand insight into the quality and compassion of specific practitioners or programs that they can share with you.

While regulations are different in each state, there is usually some sort of process for an independently approved reviewer to make a binding decision on whether a private insurer should pay for an out-of-network clinician (and other services). In some cases, challenging insurance companies legally may be necessary to get results. Unfortunately, this aspect of access often requires relentless and time-consuming self-advocacy or connection to a group who is willing to help, like your state or local NAMI.

Historically, private health plans failed to pay for most mental health care. In the early 2000s, my private insurance outpatients were provided only $500 per year of outpatient care and up to two hospitalizations or detoxes for mental health diagnoses. That was the limit of their "coverage." The same patients had no such limits on health care coverage for treating their diabetes or cancer. As a health care provider, and as a patient, I saw this disparity up close. As mentioned earlier in the book, I had cancer during my residency. My dad and I both had life-threatening conditions, and we were given the same antipsychotic—his for psychosis, and mine for nausea associated with chemotherapy. The similarities ended there. My problem was medical, so I was treated in a beautiful, well-lit facility full of well-trained staff, the walls festooned with banners from famous athletes telling me I was a hero. His was mental health, so he was treated in an overcrowded, understaffed, and dark hospital. There were no cheerleading athletes, no hopeful banners, and the unspoken societal message was "Pretend you were never here."

Many advocates and legislative leaders noticed the same discrepancy. The Mental Health Parity and Addiction Equity Act of 2008 was the first major step to address this structural discrimination. *Parity* means equality, and the law is designed to mandate insurers to treat mental health and physical health equally. However, it does not yet constitute a definitive solution. There are many exceptions built into the law; and payment sufficient to cover the actual costs of care in the private pay market is not currently considered a central part of what is meant by parity. Addressing true parity is yet another advocacy challenge in the field.

Even if you have top-tier, employer-provided private insurance, you may still struggle to find a covered, in-network licensed practitioner to do an assessment. Underpayment by insurers is the lead reason half of the licensed psychiatrists in the United States report they take no insurance at all. Depending on the city or state, many other mental health practitioners may not participate in health insurance networks, either. Fundamentally, the problem is that they are undercompensated by health plans relative to the investment they have made in education and training, the value of their years of experience, and their operating costs. Private pay cash rates are frequently higher than what most insurers are willing to cover. It is the health insurance companies' problem—not yours—that they do not have the right kind of provider in the network for you or your family member.

Some insurance plans that have out-of-network benefits will reimburse some percentage of fees you pay directly to providers, if you are wealthy enough to pay for care out of pocket and diligent enough to deal with all the paperwork. Out-of-network deductibles also can present challenges to access. During open enrollment, make sure you understand how the health plan approaches mental health.

From Assessment to Treatment

While licensure rules differ from state to state (including what supervision non-licensed professionals require), and private insurance companies may also have different requirements on licensure for their networks, broadly speaking, most independently licensed clinicians—meaning practitioners with a wide range of academic training, clinical training, and forms of licensure—can help you with a first assessment, evaluation, or question. I think of the initial evaluation as a rough draft assessment of your challenges, helping to inform what kind of services would help you. The recommendations for treatment suggested in any evaluation may or may not constitute your final or only treatment plan.

The clinician who first evaluates you is not necessarily the right provider for longer-term treatment. Someone with excellent qualifications for doing an assessment may still not have the qualities you want or need in a therapist. For example, the psychiatrist who is an expert in prescribing medications may not be a skilled practitioner of cognitive behavior therapy (CBT). Similarly, a practitioner of eye movement desensitization and reprocessing therapy (EMDR) for PTSD is often not licensed to assess the need for, or prescribe, the medication you might need. Or the clinician who evaluates you may not speak your language or understand your culture. To establish trust, an effective working relationship, and the right therapeutic environment to support your recovery, you must find providers who are not just knowledgeable and experienced in treating people with your particular mental health condition but are also a "good fit" for you. Not every clinician with the right credentials is someone you might feel comfortable talking to about your most intimate personal struggles.

If you have worked with a mental health practitioner in the past, it is often best to start there. Most practitioners can treat anxiety or depressive disorders, but not all will be able to manage an early onset psychosis, bipolar disorder, or opiate addiction. To find someone who can, you may have to engage with local resources, such as your community health center, state mental health authority, or local NAMI.

How to Assess Your Clinician

It is important to find someone you connect with, who listens to you. Studies show that having a trusting relationship with a therapist is a crucial factor in successful treatment. When it comes to the right "match" with your clinicians, trust your experience and instincts.

You may place a priority on finding a clinician of a specific race, ethnicity, gender identity, sexual orientation, or cultural background, or one who at least has experience working with someone "like you," whatever way you define that. Finding that person may be challenging, however, given long-standing structural barriers that have discouraged people of color from becoming mental health professionals. Another challenge is the traditional belief within the field of psychotherapy that therapists should remain "blank slates," that revealing too much about themselves could interfere with the therapeutic process.

But the field has been changing. The rise of relational psychology— the theory that healing happens interpersonally, through the development of a trusting and mutually respectful relationship between therapist and patient—has encouraged therapists to be more transparent about their own identity when appropriate. Therapists are now trained to be more culturally humble, working to cultivate sensitivity to people from cultures or belief systems different from their own. However, in part because there is no easy way to assess what training the clinician has received, and in part because human beings all have blind spots, a good therapist is one who considers their understanding of cultures other than their own to be a perpetual work in progress. If you can't find a good match in terms of a therapist's own background or identity, you should certainly raise the question in an initial interview and assess their openness to, interest in, and experience with treating people "like you." (We will explore this idea further in chapter 10.) *Psychology Today* and *Zen Care* are two online forums where practitioners pay to promote themselves. Their profile pages often include a photo, a description of their identity, clinical interests, training, and information about fees or what insurance they accept. This can be a good way to find specific Latinx, Indigenous, Asian, Black, and queer clinicians and get a better sense of their background, experience, and approach.

One other consideration is whether the therapist has experience working with people who have your mental health condition, and if they have been trained to provide any of the specific treatments shown to be effective for that condition. Sometimes these specific treatments— particularly those that focus on very particular "targets" or that are time-limited by nature—may be a complement to "regular" talk therapy, but sometimes you can get empathy and well-studied treatment from the same person or system. Altha Stewart and Jen Leggett discuss therapy choices and culture in chapter 17.

When you first meet with a provider, here are some basic questions to ask:

- What is your training and philosophy of care?
- How many people have you treated with my diagnosis?
- Do you have any experience working with people from my culture or identity?
- How do we arrive at a treatment approach and plan together?
- What is your after-hour coverage?

Remember, you can decide that a clinician is not a good match for you for any reason, and you can always begin the process again. This is true whether you are in a clinic, a hospital setting, or are seeing someone in private practice. When I was the medical director of a community mental health center, I regularly worked with people who had no insurance or Medicaid to find new therapists in the same mental health center who were better matches for them. The clinicians usually did not take it too personally; we know we cannot all be a good match for everyone.

Start at the Program Level

Another approach to finding quality treatment is to look for the programs you think you need and sort out payment and availability later. What follows are a few ways to begin to implement this approach.

Substance Use Treatment Locators

If substance use is a factor in your or your loved one's mental health condition, the Substance Abuse and Mental Health Services Administration (SAMHSA) treatment services locator provides a geographic map of care sites specializing in substance use disorder and mental health treatment. It does not, however, specify which facility offers what treatment approaches. It also does not categorize them by quality, insurance, philosophy, or bed availability. The SAMHSA treatment locator does list MDs who are licensed to prescribe Suboxone, a well-studied and effective medication for opiate use disorder. Cross-matching your insurance plan network with the SAMHSA treatment locator will give you a list of possible providers for you.

Knowing a program exists near you is a good start, but it's not the same as knowing if it has what you want. A creative advocacy group, Shatterproof, is working to make substance use disorder treatment programs more transparent by establishing quality metrics and providing transparent feedback from patients. These are not definitive ways to assess a program, as not all reviews are objective or reflective of the quality of care. Yet they are data points that are currently hard to find in an opaque culture. Shatterproof's addiction treatment locator, assessment, and standards platform, called ATLAS, is currently available in California, Connecticut, Delaware, Florida, Indiana, Louisiana, Massachusetts, New Jersey, New York, North Carolina, Oklahoma, Pennsylvania, West Virginia, and Wisconsin, with plans for continued expansion to additional states. (See chapter 17 for info on Shatterproof's mission by its founder, Gary Mendell.)

Community Health or Mental Health Centers

The 1963 Community Mental Health Act was meant to build community mental health centers so that people could be treated at home instead of in institutions. This endeavor is now viewed as a failure. It did not anticipate the many needs of formerly hospitalized patients and has resulted in homelessness and criminalization for many. There is, however, a frayed network of Community Mental Health Centers (CMHCs) that resulted from that legislation that provides team-based outpatient care. There is also a network of Community Health Centers (CHCs) that focus primarily on physical health, but also offer some resources for mental health care. The Indian Health Service (IHS), for example, offers free care to populations on reservations. CMHCs, CHCs, and the IHS are often well connected in local communities and offer language- and culture-specific resources. They are, by and large, mission-driven organizations often staffed by altruistic people, although turnover among clinicians can be high given the heavy workload and modest pay. In addition to private insurance, they accept Medicaid, providing free care for those who qualify.

Public Mental Health "Systems"

Each state has its own way of attempting to serve people who live with serious mental health conditions. There is usually an eligibility process, and waitlists for services and housing. Around the United States, many state hospitals have been closed. Indeed, it is a national shame that prison beds outnumber mental health hospital beds in most counties.

The public system is, again, a frayed patchwork. A local resource will know what is available and how to navigate local and regional resources to obtain care. You can always try your local NAMI office; they are likely to have a good handle on what can be found in your state, and how to best connect to it. If you are eligible, then the case manager's job is to help you sort through the options available.

A Public Health Approach to Early Psychosis Care

For people, primarily young people, who are having their first experience with psychosis, coordinated specialty care (CSC) is an excellent example of a well-researched and compassionate service model that marks a big improvement over "treatment as usual" for dealing with a complex set of symptoms at a critical time in life. This model provides strength-based care, helping young people learn how to manage their experiences and to focus on leveraging strengths and to develop positive roles for themselves in school or work, and supports the thoughtful use of medication only as needed. CSC also engages families early on, working collaboratively in attending to the young person's experience of psychosis. These programs are generally open to all regardless of insurance or resources.

I volunteered at one such program in Boston for five years and had a wonderful experience focusing on young people's strengths and helping them pursue their goals. It was strength-focused, not disability-focused. Families were welcome, and the young people involved valued being part of a community with shared experience. Early Psychosis Care is also discussed in chapter 7, and in chapter 18, Matcheri Keshavan explains more about the CSC model.

The VA system

The US Department of Veteran Affairs is the nation's largest integrated medical system and cares for many who have served our country—about 8 million veterans every year. The VA has a particularly strong interest in helping traumatized veterans. There are eligibility rules for obtaining services from the VA that have expanded in recent years. The VA's National Center for PTSD provides educational materials and consultation to providers inside and outside the VA, based on the most current and compelling research findings. PTSD specialty services are available throughout the VA health care system at both outpatient and residential levels of care that emphasize the provision of studied treatments.

Help Not Handcuffs: Police Training and Jail Diversion

There is a national movement to train police officers in de-escalation and to improve the quality of response to people with mental health and addiction issues. This is an important issue, and NAMI is working with other organizations to help police departments get their officers involved in Crisis Intervention Team (CIT) programs.

In addition to the mobile crisis and CIT approaches, diverting people living with mental illnesses from jail can be accomplished at the court level. This is explored in chapter 13.

Alternative Approaches to Care

Workplace Resources

If your employer's benefits offer you access to an Employee Assistance Plan (EAP), this is one resource for opening a conversation about accessing a mental health evaluation and effective care. EAPs can offer support and may have referral information to professional clinicians if needed. EAPs are underutilized, perhaps because employees have privacy concerns. You can ask your EAP or employer how scrupulous they are about confidentiality.

In the wake of the mental health challenges of the Covid-19 pandemic, business leaders are recognizing the need to offer more mental health resources to their employees and are adding additional services options to help expand access. For example, some companies now offer cognitive behavioral coaching models—typically, an online resource connecting employees to a coach who is not a clinician. Though convenient, these online resources are not the same as therapy; they are usually best for mild symptoms, and, in some cases, while you are still searching for or waiting on accessing clinical care.

Faith and Counseling

Faith is powerful for many people, and it sustains many through hardship. Many faith leaders provide support, and your church, synagogue, temple, mosque, or other setting may be a safe and helpful place to start your process of seeking help. Your faith leader may also be able to help connect you to a licensed professional for an evaluation. In addition, there are clinicians who employ a specific faith-based model in their approach to therapy.

Be aware, though, that not all spiritual advisors are knowledgeable about mental health conditions or treatment options. We will hear more about the interplay of faith and care in various sections of this book.

Mental Health Apps and Other Tech Approaches

There are more than twenty thousand mental health apps on the market—and that number is only growing. This is a relatively new and largely unregulated space. Some apps and websites offer peer support and connection, whereas others offer treatment services. Few are FDA-reviewed, so it's important to note that how they handle data and protect privacy are not standardized. Many people also report that it is easier to download an app or browse a website than to engage with these resources over time. For others, though, it offers convenient access and connectivity to someone else so they can feel heard.

There are also new models of support with video- and text-oriented services like Talk Space and Better Help. These novel approaches are challenging traditional ideas of what constitutes therapy and are opening new pathways to access support. We have a lot to learn about these models in terms of safety and effectiveness. However, ongoing innovation will be needed given the supply versus demand mismatch, and technology like these apps may be one way to help address that gap. John Torous provides information on evaluating new mental health technology in chapter 17. Remember that a licensed clinician is an important aspect of any professional care you may get regardless of how it is delivered.

Peer Support

One resource that is usually available and can be effective as you navigate the treatment maze is the power of peers.

Whatever mental health condition you are dealing with, either for yourself or as a family member, remember that isolation can work against recovery. Feeling heard is very important, especially when it comes to intimate and emotionally charged matters. "Pain shared is pain halved" is an old expression that predates psychotherapy by hundreds of years, and one that reflects the common experience that a person in pain often feels lighter when they feel heard.

Peer support may be more accessible than professional help and offers something unique and vital. For many, feeling heard by someone who has "been there" can make all the difference. The addiction recovery community has long recognized the power of peer support. Bill Wilson and "Dr. Bob" Smith cofounded Alcoholics Anonymous, the model for all 12-step fellowships, after recognizing that talking to each other helped them both stay sober. Fortunately, the peer movement in mental health recovery has grown considerably in the past decades. Certified peer specialists and peer navigators—the specific terms and certification process differs from state to state—represent a growing and important resource in mental health care and substance use recovery, and I discuss this peer role in addiction and co-occurring mental health more in-depth in chapter 5, and more generally in chapter 9.

Support organizations and initiatives for mental health recovery are now proliferating across the country. There are support groups offered by your local NAMI affiliate (for both families and peers), Mental Health America, the Depression and Bipolar Support Alliance (including Balanced Mind Parent Network for parents of children under age eighteen), Obsessive Compulsive Disorder International, the Anxiety and Depression Association, and other organizations. Some people find community in meetings of Emotions Anonymous, "an international fellowship of men and women who have emotional difficulties and want to live more manageable lives." The National Educational Alliance on Borderline Personality Disorder and Emotions Matter focus on education for individuals and families with borderline personality disorder. Ivory Garden provides forums, chat rooms, and support to people living with the effects of childhood trauma. Hearing Voices Network supports individuals who hear voices, see visions, or have other atypical experiences, and runs in-person groups in many states nationwide as well as online. Peer support for people recovering with both mental health and substance use conditions is covered in chapter 5.

Keep Going

This is a lot to navigate—but there is often quality help available. You may struggle to find it, at least initially, but it is out there. The key is to keep looking. I know this is not easy to do when you are having mental health symptoms or you're in crisis. But as UK prime minister Winston Churchill said during World War II, "When you are going through hell, keep going." Your frustration is justifiable. The mental health care "system," unfortunately, is fractured and hard to navigate. But navigating it as best you can is ultimately worthwhile.

We as mental health care providers know this sad fact, too. One of my teachers, Matcheri Keshavan, noted, "I have trained and practiced psychiatry in three continents: first in India, then in Europe—UK and Vienna—and finally in the US for the past three decades. In my experience, mental health care in the US is the most fragmented of all the countries where I have seen the practice of this profession. However, I may be biased. There are also pockets of excellence in this country."

Finding the pockets of excellence won't be easy. There is no clear path and many gaps. But whether it involves connecting with a local support group, asking a primary care provider, connecting with your local NAMI affiliate, engaging with your insurance carrier, or making fifty phone calls, you *can* make your way toward recovery. Keep asking questions and engaging in the process. Over time, you will learn every option available in your locality and state for you or your family member. Start anywhere—but, most important, keep going until you find what you or your loved one needs.

FOUR

Pathways to Recovery: First Steps

"Knowledge without treatment is like knowing the brand of refrigerator you're locked inside. 'Oh, that's interesting.' It's not going to get me out of the fridge."
—JOHN MOE,
Minnesota

"When I say better, I mean I'm able to manage . . . because everybody's not well every day. So, I have wellness tools that I use. The huge one is mindfulness and meditation. It changed my life. But it doesn't work by itself. I have to take medication."
—BRENDA ADAMS,
Kansas

"The first couple years of my diagnosis, I saw it as a burden. I saw it as a failure. I saw it as a flaw. But over the years it has transformed into something that has made me do things I could only have imagined."
—POOJA MEHTA,
North Carolina

• • •

There is good reason to have hope. People very often get better—no matter what mental health condition they have. The tools and proven strategies to help people thrive while living with a mental health condition range far and wide: Some are very specific to one condition, and others are general; some are rooted in medical and professional interventions, and others draw on human strengths—be they artistic, athletic, spiritual, or vocational. Only you can discover which tools and strategies will work best for you. Every person's pathway is unique. However, communicating with and connecting to peers is a powerful tool for recovery for everyone. People who have taken the journey before you can offer a lot of ideas about where to begin, what you might try, and what has worked most effectively for them.

It's often best to take the long view, and if putting any of these ideas into action isn't something you feel you can do now, that's okay. You are not doing anything wrong. Many people find that having the energy and motivation to engage more proactively in recovery comes with time. The people I talked to for this book shared stories of very difficult experiences along their recovery pathways, including overdoses, job loss, homelessness, incarceration, and more. Each of them also talked about how they eventually found recovery on their own terms. This chapter focuses on the more positive elements and most useful tools they discovered to help them navigate these challenges over time.

This chapter can share only a limited number of stories, just to give you an idea of the diversity of successful approaches to living and recovering with a mental health condition. But some common elements and themes emerge that may be helpful to keep in mind as you begin your own journey. A central theme is that no one medication, therapy, lifestyle change, or relationship is likely to be a magic wand. For many people, recovery involves assembling a tool kit, and learning which tools they need to use, how to use them, and when; and then using these tools to sustain recovery, which is an ongoing effort.

Corinne Foxx, a twenty-eight-year-old biracial woman residing in California who works in the entertainment industry and as a NAMI ambassador, provides a great example of how to build and personalize your tool kit; it can be as simple as opening a note on your phone. She explained:

I'm so about building out a toolkit that works for you. I have my toolkit on my phone. It says: Corinne's Guide to Wellness, How I Beat Mental Illness Every Day. Over the years as I was going through the trial-and-error process of figuring out what actually worked for me, I would write down the things that did:

Working out, I have four to five times a week. Meditation, every day. Therapy, weekly. Journaling, writing affirmations, workbooks. Socializing with my friends two times a week. Expressive art: I must dance or write or act. I even have sleeping on this list. Giving back. Connecting with God. And I have it written down so specifically for me, because when you're going through a really tough time or an anxious period, it's hard to remember any of the tools you have.

And I can ask, if I'm not feeling well, what haven't I done in a while? I know that these tools are tried and true.

Often, tools come from two different worlds: the medical model and the recovery model. I explained in chapter 2 how the system of *diagnosing* mental health conditions is rooted in a medical model, focused on identifying symptoms or "deficits" from "regular" functioning. The professional approach to *treating* mental health conditions is rooted in this model as well. In the medical model, the deficits and symptoms of mental health conditions are managed with medical tools. Medications are a classic "medical model" tool, and they can often help with symptoms when used thoughtfully. Neurostimulation and some kinds of psychotherapy are other examples of important medical model tools. In chapter 18, leading experts summarize recent thinking on some of the most effective and well-researched tools in this category.

Mental health conditions are multidimensional human challenges, however, and "whole person" recovery, meaning recovery that goes beyond symptom relief, is often a long-term endeavor. A mental illness may be chronic or cyclical; it can remit for long periods and then reappear in response to the inevitable stresses and changes of life. Medications and treatments that reduce symptoms can make the journey easier, but they are not cures. And while reducing symptoms is vitally important, it's often not sufficient.

Just as important to recovery are the pathways people have found to achieve the good things in life—such as peer support, relationships, vocation, spirituality, purpose, and fun. These creative approaches are strength-based and peer-driven, rather than symptom-based and professionally driven. They focus not on targeting isolated symptoms or deficits but on building and living a good life. I'll refer to these as "recovery model" tools. Experts also develop these ideas in more detail in Part IV.

In my experience, the most effective path to recovery often involves combining the best tools for treatment of your mental health condition that the medical model has to offer, with recovery tools that focus on building and living the best possible life. This powerful "both/and," rather than "either/or," approach has been transformative for many of the people I interviewed for this book, and for so many others I know.

Recovery Tools: The Both/And Approach

In this chapter you will hear in more detail how people define, describe, and conceptualize their own recovery. Broadly, recovery involves building a life, discovering one's strengths, finding a purpose, and being connected to a supportive community that can sustain you despite the symptoms you experience. When people are directly involved in designing their own plan—including defining recovery and wellness goals, choosing services that support them, and evaluating treatment decisions and progress—both the experience of care and outcomes are significantly improved.

The "recovery model" concept in mental health was led by the late William Anthony, founding director of the Boston University Center for Psychiatric Rehabilitation. I was fortunate to work in Boston and to learn from Dr. Anthony and his mentees. He focused on people's strengths, not their deficits, and on providing them with the supports they needed to create the life they wanted—as a whole person. Time has proven him right. After all, most people want to live a fulfilling life, not just experience symptom relief. Focusing too narrowly on alleviating symptoms—essentially, on achieving an absence of a deficit—rather than on creating a life, is the primary risk of a medical-model-only framework. Fortunately, many mental health care professionals are now combining medical model tools and recovery model tools creatively and intentionally in developing approaches to treatment.

Medical Model Tools

There are a vast number of professionally driven approaches to addressing some of the symptoms and experiences of mental health conditions, largely rooted in research. Broadly, they fall into one of two categories: medications and neurostimulation. Talk therapy is a kind of bridge between medical model and recovery model tools in that it can be focused on symptom reduction, on self-understanding, or on both. Here I have framed talk therapy as a medical model tool because it is delivered by professionals. These professional model tools also often work better in combination than they do individually to effectively treat mental health conditions.

Medications: These are tools that may help with specific symptoms and are prescribed by specific types of providers: primary care physicians, nurse practitioners, psychiatrists, and, in a few states, psychologists. Before taking medications, I encourage people to have a good understanding of the potential benefits and risks. One way to do that outside of the prescriber's office is at NAMI.org, where you'll find information on medication created by an independent group called the College of Psychiatric and Neurologic Pharmacists (CNPP). Information pages can be printed so that you can have them in hand when you meet with your prescriber. They offer easy-to-follow information about what uses the Food and Drug Administration (FDA) has approved a particular medication for, what its intended effects are, and what side effects you might encounter.

The more you know, the better prepared you will be to make informed choices about medications in a shared decision-making process with your prescriber.

The FDA has a formal approval process for each medication, and they approve medications to treat specific conditions, according to specific criteria. The FDA also mandates that the company producing the medicine indicate the side effects and risks of taking it. The most concerning are summarized in what are called "black box warnings" included in packaging for any medicine that requires them—a kind of stop sign for people to see before they proceed. It is legal for prescribers to prescribe medicines "off label"—meaning, to treat conditions that the FDA has not approved them for—but you should be sure to discuss with your prescriber why a medication is being recommended for you off label, and what is and is not known about it. Most medicines are studied short term, but they are taken over longer periods of time, so this creates a gap in knowledge. All medicines have side effects, and some of these effects—for example, the risks of weight gain and diabetes that can accompany the use of many antipsychotics—may require a proactive approach and is discussed by Gail Daumit in chapter 18. How to balance the effectiveness of certain medicines against their potential for side effects is another key issue to consider when assessing and developing your medical toolbox.

Neurostimulation: This tool includes repetitive transcranial magnetic stimulation (rTMS), electroconvulsive therapy (ECT), and other approaches, and works off the theory that there are brain circuits that can be activated to reduce symptoms. Sarah Hollingsworth Lisanby of NIMH discusses this in chapter 18.

Talk therapy: Also called psychotherapy, this tool can be focused on helping you reduce symptoms (medical model focus) or on helping you establish goals and deepen your understanding of yourself (recovery model focus). Talk therapy can take many forms. Some talk therapies were developed to treat specific conditions; for example, exposure response prevention (ERP) for obsessive compulsive disorder. When that is the case, getting the right form of therapy from a formally trained professional matters.

For many people, though, their relationship with the therapist is just as important as the type of therapy. There are different kinds of therapists with different kinds of training, and many of them take a unique approach, drawing on training, continuing education, practice, and experience. Research also shows that you will likely benefit from therapy, regardless of what type it is, if you trust and feel understood by your therapist.

Recovery Model Tools

Recovery tools are activities and endeavors outside of professional treatment that help people with mental health conditions to care for themselves and build better lives. Some have been researched rigorously, and are proven to be effective, including self-determined **peer-led support models** like the Wellness Recovery Action Plan (WRAP). **Employment** is another powerful recovery tool for many, and we now have an evidence-based, cost-effective approach called individual placement and support (IPS supported employment) that helps people with disabilities to become successfully employed. **Cognitive training** is also a powerful and well-researched tool that promotes success in employment. These recovery tools are also covered in more detail by experts in Part IV.

Other recovery tools are more custom-designed and utilized by individuals in light of their own unique circumstances, interests, abilities, passions, and preferences. There is no easy way to summarize the long and beautiful list of recovery tools people have found, or created, to help themselves deal with mental health challenges while remaining fully engaged with other aspects of their lives. These tools don't easily lend themselves to research study, but almost all the people I interviewed for this book discussed at least one that they have found helpful. Their stories convey the diversity and importance of these tools and how they work, alongside the right tools from the medical model, to provide relief and facilitate healing.

Among them are **regular exercise**, which has been shown to be effective for alleviating anxiety and depression states, and **healthy sleep patterns**, which support regulation and overall health. Though historically underfunded, **music and art** interventions helped many of the interviewees. In future chapters, I'll also introduce people who have found healing through **service and advocacy**, by being part of something bigger than themselves and giving to others with purpose. **Faith and spirituality** have a special place for many, and some of the interviewees draw directly upon faith to help them make meaning of their experiences and their lives. **Meditation**, **crafts**, **hobbies**, and **peer support groups** are examples of recovery tools discussed in the coming chapters.

The Wellness Recovery Action Plan (WRAP)

One of the true pioneers in identifying recovery tools and creating a recovery tool kit is Mary Ellen Copeland, now semi-retired and living in Vermont. She describes herself as a psychiatric survivor and a family member who has spent almost forty years learning how people recover from mental health issues and sharing that information with others. Copeland started to develop what would become her signature contribution to that tool kit—the Wellness Recovery Action Plan (WRAP)— when, relying solely on medical model ideas, she hit a dead end in her own recovery journey. "It really started in the late 1980s when I was looking for answers for myself," Mary Ellen told me:

> I was having really extreme moods; a lot of deep, deep depression. . . . I needed to find out how other people were dealing and coping and getting on with their lives with these kinds of things going on, these kinds of moods. After I was discharged from the hospital, I asked my doctor, "How do people cope?"

The doctor admitted he really didn't know. Copeland continued:

I thought a lot about it. And I thought that the way to get this information was asking people like my mother, who was hospitalized for years,
and others who have gone through this and figured out how to cope and
gotten their lives back.

She designed a study, recruited more than a hundred volunteers, and
began compiling data about what they thought had helped them. "And
I saw a structure to it," she said, "that there were five key recovery concepts everyone talked about: hope, personal responsibility, education,
self-advocacy, and support."

What evolved from this research was WRAP, which has become the
best-known proactive peer-support model in existence, shown to be effective in research studies and used by millions of people around the
globe. WRAP provides a format for identifying risks and symptom patterns; considering and assembling recovery tools; keeping track of what
has or hasn't worked in the past; identifying supportive people, networks,
and environments; clarifying priorities and preferences to loved ones in
event of crisis; and helping to frame thinking about goals. It can be used
and revised to best serve the person who designs it.

The essential insight Copeland embodied in WRAP is that there *are*
strategies that help people cope; that someone with a mental health condition is the foremost expert on what works best for them; and that taking
agency over one's own recovery is one of the most powerful recovery tools
there is. Copeland discusses WRAP in more detail in chapter 17.

Don't Believe a Negative Prognosis

One of the core tenets of the recovery model is that recovery is possible.
With the right care or tools, someone with a mental health condition
can find their way to mental health and well-being. This premise is not

just theoretical. Even people who have been told their odds of doing so are low can recover and build fulfilling lives. One of the first important steps on your or your loved one's recovery journey is allowing yourself to think positive and long term. Definitive negative prognoses are a dark thread in the history of the mental health field, and unfortunately, even today some care providers have not yet adopted a recovery-oriented mindset.

Some of the people who share their experiences in this book faced debilitating prognoses—and chose to fight for their own recovery anyway. Chrissy Barnard, a white forty-four-year-old living in Superior, Wisconsin, was one of them. Chrissy now works as a certified peer specialist and as the grant project coordinator for Douglas County Behavioral Health Crisis Response. She has a meaningful purpose, a strong community, a partner, and a dog. She told me she'd lost all these things earlier in her mental health journey. Her recovery began in defiance of years of pessimistic pronouncements by the mental health care professionals who treated her. "When I was committed to the state hospital, no one said recovery was possible," Chrissy told me. She went on to say:

> They acted like, "You're never going to get out, actually." That was their attitude. They were like, "You're always going to live with this." And I was like, "What do you mean?"
>
> Even when I was in my thirties, at the state hospital, I got a piece of advice I never forgot. My doctor told me, "You'll never get in a relationship because you have your problems, his problems, our problems, and sometimes kids' problems." And that really deterred me from relationships for a long time.

Then Chrissy found the NAMI support group in Wisconsin, where people told her she could start her road to recovery, and that they could help. She recalled thinking:

"Recovery? What do you mean? Is it possible?" I was just floored. I couldn't believe that somebody would say that, because I was told it wasn't possible. I was totally shocked. And then I was like, "Wow. Okay. Now what do I need to do next? If this is possible, give me the action steps I need to take to get there." NAMI Wisconsin introduced me to the recovery concept, defined it as best they could, and encouraged me to grow. A few years later, I was on the steering committee to help start the NAMI Douglas County Wisconsin affiliate, and I was just elected president this January.

Chrissy has become a "both/and" thinker and teacher to others in her rural community. She described tools that made a difference for her, including dialectical behavioral therapy (DBT):

I think it's a combination of medication and DBT, because DBT helps me manage my stresses better so when I feel low or something bothers me, I can manage the stress. Doing mindfulness for me each night is important. And then medications really help me with my manias and long-term depressive episodes. And every night, I do my prayers and I come up with five things I'm grateful for. I feel like that changed my whole outlook on things. Once I started thinking more positive, it got easier, and more and more good things just started happening.

Charita Cole Brown, a sixty-two-year-old widow who is Black and the mother of two exceptional daughters, told me she has lived in bipolar I disorder recovery for more than twenty-five years and now serves on the NAMI Maryland board of directors. She was told during and after some difficult years at Wesleyan College in the 1980s that she should not expect to ever get better:

I was committed to state facilities three different times. I never felt as if anyone in authority was trying to empower me with positive coping strategies during those stays. At the end of each commitment, the doctors' prognosis for me was always, "She's okay right now, but don't expect her to be okay in the long run." In 1982, a therapist told my parents, in my presence, that given the severity and frequency of my manic and depressive episodes, I would likely need a custodian at some point. That was the psychological death knell over my life.

Instead of accepting these negative prognoses, Charita took agency over her life, sought treatment, and with her pastoral counselor's assistance created a personal wellness plan. Instead of needing a custodian, she eventually managed care for her elderly parents:

> My recovery has exceeded my expectations. I have two daughters who have not been negatively affected by their mother's illness, as my own mother was by my grandmother's bipolar illness. I am amazed by and grateful for my extended period of recovery and am enjoying my life.

Charita published her award-winning memoir, *Defying the Verdict: My Bipolar Life*, in 2018.

How "Both/And" Can Work

Once you can believe that you can feel better and move ahead, it is wise to explore a combination of approaches, supports, and treatments that pull from the best of what both the medical and recovery models have to offer. Many of the people I interviewed did just that over the course of their recovery journey; you will hear more throughout the book. Here, just to give you an idea of what is possible, people with different diagnoses and backgrounds, from different parts of the country, share stories about how they assembled their own multipart, "both/and" tool kits to move forward in life. The tools they found represent a small fraction of the tools available but may give you some ideas for what you might try on your own journey.

Sierra Grandy, a bisexual law student from Minnesota in her mid-twenties, serves as a presenter for NAMI's In Our Own Voice program. She speaks to groups of people at workplaces and in organizations about her own mental health journey, teaching others and starting conversations about mental health issues. As both an avid student of positive psychology and spirituality and a leader in the expanding peer movement, she educates others about mental health and how recovery support enhances and deepens the impact of medical model tools. Sierra believes that those medical model tools have affected her both positively and negatively.

Treatment with ECT, sometimes called shock treatment, "saved my life," Sierra told me, but also caused unsettling memory lapses. She worked to find another treatment tool to help with her depressive symptoms and learned via a newspaper clipping her mother sent her about promising research on the effectiveness of a powerful anesthetic called ketamine. Ketamine's potential is still being researched, and so far it has only been approved by the FDA in the form of a ketamine derivative called esketamine, administered as a nasal spray, to be used as an adjunct to other antidepressants to treat people with treatment-resistant depression. Sierra found that a combination of talk therapy and as-needed ketamine treatments was the right course of medical model treatment for her:

Ketamine helps the depression. How I've explained it in the past is, ketamine has helped me see neutral, and then pull myself up from the pit into a neutral or even a positive space, if that makes sense. It didn't get me to neutral; *I* had to get me to neutral. But it gave me the rope to pull myself up. Ketamine did not do that for my anxiety . . . *that*, I still have.

I verbally process things. So just talk therapy in general is really helpful. Group therapy is also helpful. I'm a big fan of "take what you can, leave the rest." Really, one of my biggest coping skills is reading positive psychology, religious, or spiritual books. On my bookshelf, you'll see everything from Ayurvedic to Buddhists to Christian.

When my suicidal thoughts come back, though, I know to go in for ketamine treatment. If I'm starting to feel overwhelmed, or I'm drowning . . . I know my self-care plan.

Many people report that a combination of medication and therapy helped them manage symptoms and move forward, but that using other recovery tools made an important difference. John Henley, a thirty-four-year-old musician and facilities crew member from Connecticut who reports he lives with schizophrenia, has put tools from several different categories—traditional medicine, new science, creativity, and family support—into his recovery toolbox. They include clozapine, the only FDA-approved medicine for treatment-resistant schizophrenia; talk therapy that helps him critically assess his experiences; and family support. Yet what John loves is music, which has also played a significant role in his recovery and helps regulate his thinking. As he told me:

> Clozapine's cool. You take the medications at nighttime, which makes you drowsy, leading to a great night's sleep. You wake up the next day, you feel really refreshed. Like a computer—you turn it off and then turn it back on again the next day, almost like the slate was clean from the day before. It resets you.
>
> Before I took clozapine, I experienced a lot of paranoia and people talking about me, hearing things on the radio, the television talking to me. Now, it's almost like the clozapine gives you an ability to control your thoughts. Voices come up once in a while, but I'm able to control them. Another practice that I have is called rational thinking: "Does this make sense?" "Does this have any foundation in reality?" I stopped creating something that isn't real.
>
> I also feel like some of the cognitive training I did at the research center I went to for treatment helped my brain. My time there was very valuable. I am a musician now, so I try to practice every day—acoustic guitar in the morning, bass guitar at night—and I think that's cognitive training as well. This is what I enjoy; this is what is going to make me feel

good for the day, and just exercising my brain helps it have more control in the real world and not let my thoughts get the best of me.

Haley Amering of New York, a graduate student in her twenties, has also put together multiple tools for recovery. Unfortunately, she spent two years without effective medical tools because she was misdiagnosed and, as a result, was taking the wrong medication. Nevertheless, she found recovery tools of her own. One tool was drumming, a creative outlet that she used both to express her emotions and to regulate them:

Drumming was a huge way that I coped with mental health. It definitely worked for me, for the mood dysregulation I found, especially when I was feeling negative, feeling angry. I was able to just go and drum for however long I wanted, to some of my favorite albums. Playing the drums made me feel very connected just to the music itself. It was very cathartic for me.

I never got lessons; I was self-taught; but then I went to college for drum set performance. I was having more and more mental health issues and I realized, "Hey, this isn't what I want to be going to school for anymore, but now what am I going to do?" That part of my identity was just shattered for a little bit.

Although drumming had been a good tool for mood regulation, Haley still felt she wasn't getting the full treatment she needed:

It had been probably two years at this point that I had been on a bunch of antipsychotics and medication, and I was just lying in bed one night just thinking, "This is not working for me." There's something else. I don't know what it is, but this diagnosis, this treatment is not working for me.

Getting a diagnosis of borderline personality disorder (BPD) marked a turning point for Haley, enabling her to find new, more effective tools—and a new sense of identity and purpose:

Oh my God, everything just clicked for me, which I'm so grateful for, because it's not like that for everyone. I immediately wanted to research everything about it—to become a master in all things BPD. It was very relieving for me.

The most reassuring aspect was feeling as though I could trust my therapist, and that it was possible for these symptoms to go into remission. It was just knowing that it was possible; that there was going to be a plan and that it was going to make more and more sense, especially if I dedicated myself to understanding it.

I had gone to group therapy, which was DBT-based (though I didn't realize it), about six months before my diagnosis. I realized, wow, this is working and is helpful. It's not what I expected it to be. Then we started practicing more and more DBT things.

Haley has worked with an advocacy and support group called Emotions Matter to raise awareness and support for others living with BPD, and also as an intern for NAMI in New York State. She told me she values talking about her experience "as a means to let someone know that they aren't alone and that they're not the only one going through it."

Trevor McCauley of Michigan discovered his difficulties when he was in college, using a medication that wasn't right for him. He also ended up discovering a new path to building a life he loves:

By the end of September, I started on Prozac to treat what they believed was depression. Then, in the beginning of November, strange stuff started happening where I could not sleep or eat normally and was talking a lot. That's when the manic stuff started creeping in. I didn't know that's what it was; I'm just living my life. I didn't sleep for three or four nights, and then I knew something was wrong. I called my dad and I said, "Come pick me up. I need to go somewhere."

Trevor was admitted to a hospital and was diagnosed with bipolar disorder. He left college and found himself back in his family home. He had lost all his momentum and wanted to get going somewhere. In addition to a medication regimen that was helpful, his recovery began with water and movement:

> I would bike or walk to the YMCA. Swimming became my baptism, my healing. Swimming in that pool, it was just water, it was movement. I felt like I was going somewhere. And so, after all these small little pieces started going into place, then it's like, "Okay. Well, maybe I can handle going to work." I didn't even have my driver's license yet. So, I can walk to work. And then it gets to be about going to the library, and finally reading books again.

One book made a pivotal impact:

> I found an old copy of *The Power of Positive Thinking*. I absorbed it. I believed in it to the point that I would take quotes from the book or quotes from the Bible that are in the book, and I would write them down on cards and stuff them in my back pocket, and I would walk a half mile to Kroger [a supermarket] where I found my job. And the only thing that would motivate me to keep going to that store, even though I felt terrible still, was to take those flash cards out and read and recite them. I would just absorb it and believe it. And it would be the gasoline to my tank. That's how I got to work and figured out that I could actually work again, and I could make some money.

Trevor went on to reflect about the incremental changes he made:

> So, I just incrementally built up this life where, eventually, I could do all those things that I was doing before my manic episode. I could actually be functional. And I eventually did go into a classroom setting again. I eventually built a life, but it was all about starting quietly and finding that creative self and then finding a way to relate to my world creatively and finding that traction in the pool, finding exercise as a healing mechanism. That's how it really began for me.

Trevor used professional and medical tools, and he also found other creative recovery tools to help advance his momentum toward a life he wanted. He is now married with children, employed, and loves the outdoors.

Josh Santana, a twenty-five-year-old youth community educator and real estate agent in Massachusetts who was born in Puerto Rico, told me he has been able to integrate his Latino heritage while growing up in the United States as well as thrive as a gay member of the LGBTQ+ community. Josh used traditional medical tools like psychotherapy and medication in his recovery, but he also found an active, adorable, four-legged recovery tool: a dog he named Koda. "A coda is like an additional part of music at the end to signal it's rounding out," Josh explains. "She rounds me out. You get it?" People who live with bipolar disorder benefit from keeping a regular daily schedule. But for many people—including Josh, who is a musician and graduate student—establishing that regularity isn't easy. He found that having a dog helps:

> I invested all my focus on Koda. As someone with ADHD, it was one of the things that I could hyper-focus on. I don't regret it because I get comments day-in and day-out about how well she's trained, how impressive some of the tricks are that I've taught her, and all the other stuff I've been able to focus on with her. She helps me a lot, from managing my sleep, to eating regularly, to exercising and getting fresh air. These things help me maintain my bipolar episodes, too. One of the things that I knew about bipolar before being diagnosed is that routines and regularity are very important and here I am, experiencing that firsthand.

Josh told me that Koda had three previous owners, but they couldn't handle her energy. But this didn't deter him. He recalled:

> I worked on her diligently and in return she helped me form new habits and routines, like falling asleep at a reasonable hour, that gave back to me more than she can ever know. Even beyond this, there was a time I had an

anxiety attack, and was crying and panting on the floor of my room for like five minutes straight. Koda's reaction was very interesting. She seemed really confused and was pacing back and forth, while nervously whimpering. In order to comfort her, I brought her over and said, "It's okay, it's okay." And once I started comforting her, then I sort of started coming out of it too.

For Josh, daily regulation is important. Suzanne Vogel-Scibilia, a sixty-three-year-old married psychiatrist and mother of five who reports living with bipolar disorder, learned to manage the seasonality of her symptoms as she was going through college and medical school:

I'd learned that if I just gutted it out until about April, I got better spontaneously, and the world was right again—until the next winter. Every winter I would get seriously, psychotically depressed, and by April I was okay again. I realized when I went to college that I was going to make sure that I took classes in the spring that were heavily loaded with final papers and final exams.

Janet Berkowitz is a sixty-three-year-old heterosexual white woman with bipolar disorder. She lives in central New Jersey and was born into a Jewish family. Having struggled with recurrent suicidal thoughts, she is now a peer specialist, designing and facilitating creative arts workshops for people dealing with mental health conditions. Janet has relied heavily on medical model tools, including medication and both CBT and EMDR (eye movement desensitization and reprocessing) therapy, but she found that integrating theater and art into her recovery was essential:

Three days after I was home from the hospital, I was determined to take my life because I knew my husband Phil would be out of the house. That morning, before I opened my eyes, I heard the words, "Suicide denied," in my head. I opened my eyes, and I knew God was talking to me, and I said, "All right, I'll take my life tomorrow." And for several days in a row, that kept happening when I awoke. Then, soon after that, I had a lucid dream of me leading a workshop on suicide prevention with teens. I woke up and I said, "Phil, we have to do something about this. I have a feeling that our relationship will only work if we work together on suicide awareness."

Together, they designed a workshop on suicide prevention called Suicide Denied: Taking Suicide Out of the Closet, using creative arts, games, interactive exercises, art, and writing:

I went to the self-help center where I worked and had attended as a client, and asked, "Can I do this workshop here?" It was such a success that it popped me right out of the suicidal thoughts. Afterward, someone came up to me and said, "You saved a life today. You saved my life." So, I noticed that if a long period of time went by during which we didn't do any of this work, I would start getting suicidal again. I'd say, "Phil, we've got to do another workshop," and it would pull me right out of it when we did.

We started teaching and asking if we could teach at different self-help centers; we traveled with our workshop and presented at conferences. Everywhere we went, people were blown away by what we were doing. Since then, I've created many other workshops involving this topic and mental health in general.

Sascha Biesi, the proud mom of one daughter and lots of animals who lives in the Texas Hill Country, underwent ECT to help her with severe depression, and then had cognitive problems related to it. But her need to improve her thought process would ultimately lead to her discovery that baking was a wonderful recovery tool for her:

After I had electric shock therapy, I weighed less than one hundred pounds, and I couldn't remember my daughter's name. I had this recipe box, and since I'm trying to remember things, I started baking. I'm going through my grandmother's recipe box. The handwriting is familiar. My grandmother is familiar. Nothing else is familiar to me. I couldn't even find my way to the store, but I knew I needed to gain weight, get healthy again, and start working on my memory.

I really used baking as a way to not only heal myself physically, but it was also this mental thing too, where I'm trying to relearn how to hold more than one thing in my brain. There are so many treasures in this box, things that I remember my grandmother making for us, I always remember my grandmother had distinctive handwriting, and so I found that super comforting during that time when nothing made sense to me. My father had just passed away. My cousin had just killed himself. I had just split from my husband. I had just had electric shock therapy. Nothing made sense. But this handwriting on this card, and my partner at the time telling me, "Just keep going. Just keep baking. Just keep cooking. Just keep doing it." I found my way out of the dark.

Sascha's bakery, Skull & Cakebones, which she co-owns with her partner of twelve years, has an electric bolt on the logo to remind her that it was her capacity to find a way to overcome side effects of ECT that helped her to become a baker. She is eloquent about what recovery means to her:

For me, it's the difference between trying to avoid living with something and embracing living with something. In terms of recovery, what that looks like to me is: I'm taking my meds; not screaming at anyone. I'm living with my mental illness; it's not dragging me around by my tail. It looks like getting up every day and deciding to breathe and do my tool bag of whatever I need that day because every day is a different day. It's like getting on a surfboard and riding the waves.

Lloyd Hale, who now runs a peer support organization in South Carolina, told me he took clozapine for many years, then was able to slowly taper off that medication. He also used peer support extensively. Lloyd started fasting to connect to his father, who is Muslim, and found unexpected recovery benefits:

> Through fasting, I found a clear mind. It strips me of all of the garbage that I carry around all the time. And it helps me narrow in on what's truly important. Meaning, the Swiss rolls that I love so much, that I go to get from the store all the time, are not important. The time that I spend watching this television program, the same time every day, every night, in the grand scheme of things, it's just not important for my well-being. It really narrows things down, and it strips me of all of that stuff that I carry around as though it's important.

· · ·

These stories show us that people find a way. Today there are more tools available than ever before to help people manage symptoms, grow in self-awareness, find support, and create fulfilling lives while living with a mental health condition. Again, the stories in this chapter represent only a very small number of the endless variety of pathways to recovery. They also reveal that, for each person, it took time and patience to figure out the best route for them. There are no one-size-fits-all solutions, and finding the tools most useful for you is neither simple nor quick. Being open to learning, being willing to try something different, and being persistent may be the most valuable recovery tools of all.

FIVE

Added Complexity: Co-Occurring Substance Use Conditions

"When my family member went to mental health providers, they would say, 'Get your addictions treated.' And the addictions team would say, 'You have a mental health problem.' It was many, many years before she was able to get really targeted treatment that combined interventions for mental health conditions, substance use conditions, and trauma."
—DANNA MAUCH,
Massachusetts

"The cultures collided. When AA people found out I had a mental health condition, they wanted nothing to do with me. Early on in my recovery, they didn't actually tell me not to take my medication. But the message, when I was hearing people talk, was 'don't take meds.' So, I was resistant in early treatment to take meds; I refused. It's hard to get help when you're trying to get well as quick as you can because you want to look okay."
—NADINE LEWIS,
Oklahoma

. . .

F or anyone with a mental health condition, it is a process to find the right combination of medical and recovery tools to manage symptoms and forge a creative path in life. When a person has a substance use condition that co-occurs with a mental health condition, that process can be riskier and more complex. It can be hard to know which issue came first in many instances, and it can be difficult to find a path or program that can help you deal with both conditions. We now know about the concept of "self-medication," but it can be hard to draw the line between a comforting or social habit, and an unhealthy coping mechanism. Substance use conditions also often overlap with psychological trauma, which presents its own challenges, and will be addressed in the next chapter.

Dealing with co-occurring conditions—also referred to as dual diagnosis—involves navigating within and between two distinct and, at times, conflicting cultures. The philosophies that shape approaches to addiction treatment don't always fit easily with approaches to mental health care, and the professionals involved in them don't always talk to each other or work collaboratively. If you or a loved one are straddling these two worlds, and experience that culture clash, you are not alone.

While most professionals would agree that these two cultures are moving toward each other, the pace is too slow for many. About 8 million American adults have both a mental health condition and a substance use condition, so the challenges involved in treatment and recovery are common. Unfortunately, many don't get the integrated care they need. Some practitioners and programs are very forward-thinking in their approach, but some have not been trained in integrated care. If you or your family member have a dual diagnosis and are seeking help, it is best to keep shopping for the right people and programs.

Given that it may be up to you to navigate the system as it is and to find or create integrated care for yourself, you can learn from the experiences of other people who have contended with these additional obstacles to find recovery. I share a few of their stories below.

What Is the Co-Occurring Culture Clash?

When I was a doctor on an intensive community treatment team for people with co-occurring mental health and substance use conditions, I was impressed by the influence the different cultures of addiction and mental health had on my work, and how they influence what people experience when they have both conditions.

Addiction recovery culture, and the majority of addiction treatment facilities in the United States, have been shaped significantly by the 12-step philosophy of Alcoholics Anonymous (AA), an approach to remaining abstinent from an addictive substance and building a meaningful life. AA and its offshoots are distinctly nonmedical and nonprofessional in nature; they do not offer medical treatment but are rather fellowships of people who share a common problem and band together to support each other in "working" a 12-step recovery program that is spiritual in nature. In 12-step fellowships, a person is thought to be the "agent" of their own recovery. While having a substance use condition is not the person's fault, and there may even be a genetic component, it is critical to acknowledge one's own addiction and become accountable for it. The person with the addiction needs to make the decision to get better and act themselves. Consistent with this model, families in the AA community are taught that they cannot cure their loved one or force them into recovery; feeling responsible to do so, or continually attempting to do so, may in turn complicate the problem. As a result, letting your loved one "hit bottom" is risky, but it's sometimes considered necessary. Accountability and agency are a core feature of traditional 12-step addiction recovery. This model works for many people and has saved many lives.

The culture of mental health care is historically very different. Broadly, the assumption is that you are living with a brain-based vulnerability that can be diagnosed, in medical terms. As a result, treatments and services are prescribed, which may include medications, psychotherapy, and supports, such as housing, employment services, and/or visits with an outreach worker. The idea of accountability, while important, isn't as central to mental health treatment culture as it is to substance use recovery culture. Behavior and choices matter, but not in the same way as in the addiction community.

While working on my treatment team, I noticed that when a patient had co-occurring conditions—for example, both a serious alcohol use disorder and bipolar disorder—my own reactions could be mixed: How much was that person able to "own" and be accountable for their addiction, and how much should I simply offer support and resources? I felt confused. My colleagues, the families of the individuals we treated, and the individuals themselves also experienced this culture clash as they weighed these issues.

Addiction was long considered a moral failing, not a treatable brain disorder. This view ultimately inspired the evolution of substance use treatment as a field at odds with the medical model of psychiatry. For example, the abstinence-based "Minnesota Model" of substance use treatment, adapted from 12-step recovery, is still sometimes at odds with the medical model tool of medications for opiate-use disorder (MOUD), also known as medication-assisted treatment (MAT), which employs medicines along with other supports to help people with addiction. The use of MOUD like methadone and buprenorphine (medications that work on opiate receptors in the brain and often diminish withdrawal symptoms from, and cravings for, more potent opioids like heroin or fentanyl) to treat people with opiate addiction is in some circles a fraught subject.

The conflict over MOUD among advocates of abstinence-based recovery is not new. There has been controversy in the past over the use of other psychiatric medications, including even SSRI antidepressants or lithium. While many 12-step groups and most treatment facilities have evolved in their thinking on this subject, there are still people who believe that reliance on any medication at all reflects denial of one's addiction, or failure to "work the program." This can lead to unfortunate circumstances in which 12-step fellowship members may advise people with dual diagnosis to stop taking helpful psychiatric medication in order to be considered truly sober. On the other hand, it can also be hard to find support for faith, religion, or belief in God or a higher power as a viable path to recovery in mental health programs.

Thanks to some leadership on both sides, there are signs of reconciliation between these two cultures and acknowledgment of what the other has to offer for people with dual diagnoses. For example, the addiction culture has increasingly come to understand the potential benefits of MOUD. Self-Management and Recovery Treatment (SMART) Recovery, for example, encourages people taking MOUD to participate in their recovery program. Psychiatric professionals no longer routinely tell people to get sober and come back for their depression treatment, as I was once was taught to do. Modern best practice is to help people deal with both conditions at the same time. The medical framework of addiction has slowly evolved from seeing addiction as a moral failure or a personal weakness to thinking of it as more of a biological and neurological process. For example, to reduce the association of morality and addiction, the DSM-5 in 2013 changed the diagnostic names from "substance dependence" and "substance abuse" to a more neutral "substance use disorder." In this chapter, I prefer to use the term "substance use condition," parallel to mental health condition.

Substance use conditions are now increasingly being understood as a public health problem and not a criminal problem. But this recognition is not yet reliably reflected in codes of law or in the practices and procedures of our criminal justice system, and it comes too late for many individuals and families—especially people of color, who are disproportionately targeted by police for drug-related crimes. Criminalizing people living with addiction and mental health conditions is ineffective—and it doesn't ensure people get the help they need. Drug courts, which focus on helping people with substance use conditions get into or stay in treatment rather than prisons and jails, now exist in all fifty states. But these programs are not universal (not all municipalities, court systems, etc., have them); moreover, abstinence-only treatment protocols can turn a relapse—or even drinking one beer—into a serious parole violation or rationale for imprisonment. Unfortunately, it is still common for prison or jail to be part of the journey for people with co-occurring conditions.

In the stories below, people who have dealt with obstacles due to the clash between addiction and mental health treatment describe what happened and what they did about it. These stories do not cover all potential obstacles nor all potential paths to surmounting them, but I hope they provide examples that may be helpful if you are confronting a similar challenge.

Co-Occurring Substance Use Treatment

One of the first challenges people with dual diagnosis may face is finding a substance use treatment program that is capable of effectively treating someone with both conditions. And the more complex the mental health condition, the more difficult it can be to find appropriate care. Many substance use condition treatment facilities claim to treat people with co-occurring conditions, without specifying which diagnoses they mean or what expertise they have in addressing specific co-occurring conditions. Anyone seeking help will soon find that a fundamental and frustrating lack of transparency is an endemic problem in the treatment industry.

For example, knowing how to select the right residential substance use condition program is challenging even for people for whom the substance use condition is the primary treatment concern and who do not (yet) have a mental health diagnosis. In many states, substance use treatment is a competitive industry, and has become a lucrative business. Significant sums are invested in marketing and advertising—not just to recruit private-pay patients, but any patient with access to insurance benefits, including Medicaid. Many of the programs you see or hear advertised may well be excellent, but who they are expert at treating, and through what means, is not necessarily clear. Many programs know to employ the terms that appeal to consumers—such as individualized, personalized, evidence-based, state-of-the-art, continuum of care, medication-assisted treatment—and they claim to treat co-occurring conditions. But what these terms mean may be fuzzy in practice. Licensing and staffing requirements differ from state to state, so some of these terms mean different things in different states, too.

Different treatment programs have different philosophies. Some are rooted exclusively in the 12-step framework and may or may not offer MOUD. Those that do provide MOUD may do so only as part of a detoxification process. Other facilities may view MOUD maintenance as the goal of care. Other questions are also hard to assess from the outside: Do these programs employ peer recovery coaches? Do they meaningfully engage family members? Do they also treat comorbid mental health conditions, and, if so, which ones and in what way? Do they offer step-down care in an intensive outpatient program? Do they direct program graduates to after-care housing or employment support?

You may get answers to some of these questions by talking to program staff, but can you trust the answers? The lack of an organized database about available programs that provides clear and reliable information beyond the programs' own marketing copy is an additional burden on top of the perennial issues of cost and insurance coverage.

Some innovators are working to address this problem. When Gary Mendell lost his son Brian to addiction, he set about working to solve these common problems that he and his family had encountered when looking for help for Brian. The goal of his nonprofit organization, Shatterproof, is to help people learn what evidence-based treatments can be found in different programs—to improve transparency in order to inform choices. The Shatterproof ATLAS (Addiction Treatment, Locator, Assessment, and Standards Platform) tool can help people see in advance what various programs have to offer, but only in some states. Mendell is working to scale ATLAS nationwide, but in the meantime, see his piece in chapter 17 for more detail, as well as some guidance in how you might apply the ATLAS approach in your own search for care.

Insurance Coverage Gaps

Mental health parity legislation forbids many health insurance plans from benefit discrimination. This means they aren't supposed to charge higher copays, offer skimpier coverage, or require you to jump through more hoops for mental health and addiction care than they do for other medical or surgical services. I recall a pre-parity world in which my patients' insurance covered only $500 worth of outpatient visits per year and two hospitalizations or detoxes, whereas visits and hospitalizations for physical care were unlimited. Health insurance coverage for addiction care has moved forward since parity legislation, to be sure. But it still does not apply to all types of health insurance, and it doesn't fund some models of care or programs that help people recover.

Benefits may also be limited to care at "in-network" facilities—which may or may not include the best facility for you or your family member. Even if your insurance plan offers out-of-network benefits, the costs it covers may only be a small fraction of program costs. Even then, insurers will sometimes authorize treatment for only days at a time. People often experience a parity violation, but don't know that it is happening or where to go for help. The work to ensure everyone receives parity in their mental health/substance use care is far from finished, and legal cases to establish clearer guidelines are ongoing.

Though detoxification programs and residential substance use disorder treatment are usually covered, the extent of that coverage varies from insurance plan to insurance plan, and access to beds can be impacted by both narrow networks of covered treatment providers and facilities and shortages of staffing. High deductible plans create financial barriers to care that often discourage people from seeking help. It can be hard to get what you need, and having to advocate for care during a crisis inevitably makes the crisis even more stressful than it would be on its own. Be prepared to advocate with your insurance company for better coverage if you run into this problem. This may require appealing decisions with your insurer. To learn more about how to improve your odds with insurers, see the list of resources for chapters 3 and 5 in Resources (p. 389).

Danny Anastasi is a husband, father, and skilled construction worker in Massachusetts who, at a critical moment, found an excellent sober house where he could live long term to stabilize his recovery. Danny had been homeless and spending his days at the corner of Mass and Cass Avenues, an area in Boston known for drug trafficking. While living at the sober house, he was able to get a job. He believes the sober house saved his life. "I wouldn't be here today if I didn't go there," he told me. "The place was awesome for me. It was perfect."

Danny's insurance had paid for detox and for residential treatment, but it covered none of the costs of living in a sober house, and it would be hard to find any insurance plan that would. He needed family financial support to help pay for this critical aspect of his recovery.

At the sober house, he was also introduced to a person who told him he needed faith in his life. "There again, God was putting things in my life," Danny told me. "A volunteer at the sober house was like, 'Well here's your problem. You don't have God.'" He found that the 12 steps, a belief in God, and his faith community were his keys to sustained recovery with a substance use condition. Ultimately, he managed to find his footing and build the life he wanted:

The steps are important to my recovery, too, because I got to let all this stuff out. After the fifth step, when you share everything about your past and what you feel bad about with someone else, it was just like, "Don't you know I just did my fifth step? Like how much better I feel right now?" You think you're glowing. It was really strange. The steps helped me a lot.

I have a great life today. Through doing all these things, I was able to get married. We wanted to buy a house; my credit score was a 530. I told myself, I'm going to start working on this. So, I started paying off all the stuff that I had bought on credit. I could save my money by this point. I got my credit better, now we're in a house that we own. We have a baby.

I could finance stuff right now if I want. I rebuilt my family, started speaking with my father and my brother again.

Recovery for Danny is not a completed task. "Actually, the funny thing, you could say recovery is almost like a perishable item, believe it or not," he says. Meetings, church, and engagement with his faith community remain regular parts of his schedule. While insurance coverage did help Danny with the basics, he had to find his pathway with help from his family, paid employment, and the community he began to build while in sober living.

Racism and Addiction

The current public and medical health approach to opiate addiction is beginning to follow the movement away from moral blame and toward biological framework. In the so-called War on Drugs—first launched by President Nixon in the early 1970s at a moment of conservative, and racist, panic about the use of marijuana and LSD—the United States spent hundreds of billions of dollars attempting to eradicate the trafficking and use of illegal drugs, in part by declaring war on growers and traffickers abroad and amping up penalties for possession and use at home. They doubled down on this approach during the crack cocaine epidemic in the late 1980s and '90s, unjustly imprisoning a staggering number of people. People of color in poor, urban communities were targets of the War on Drugs, and racism was a significant factor in the classification of marijuana as a Schedule 1 drug in the 1970 Controlled Substances Act. Penalties for possession and use of crack cocaine— often used with higher frequency in Black communities—were vastly higher than penalties for possession and use of powder cocaine, which was more frequently used, and even considered chic, among the white population.

Substance use conditions do not discriminate—people are vulnerable to addiction regardless of race, class, religion, or nationality. But many believe the move to treat the ongoing opiate epidemic as a public health issue rather than a criminal justice issue could occur only because it was primarily white people using the drug.* So rather than being criminalized, as people of color were during the crack epidemic, the white communities impacted by the opiate crisis were treated more gently, with concern, and with the goal of reducing the number of overdoses.

We know today that a public health approach to drug use not only reduces criminalization of people for a mental health condition, but it is also more effective in stemming drug use. But the impact of the failed War on Drugs is still being felt, racism persists, and growing consensus about the need for both court reform and more treatment capacity have not yet completely transformed laws and policies.

Cathy Guild describes herself as a fifty-six-year-old statuesque Black woman who is the mother of three and mother figure to many others. She works in health care in Massachusetts and has experienced the addiction treatment double standard firsthand, through family and as someone recovering from addiction and PTSD. "There's been an opioid epidemic for years," she told me, "but now because these young white women were getting pregnant and ODing, *now* it's an epidemic. No one said that when my aunt got entangled in heroin and ODed. It was just another Black woman that died, another heroin addict. That's all."

Cathy now sees the trend in reducing jail time for people with substance use conditions, but when she was sentenced, the trend was criminalization. She has developed compassion for the women she visits in jail:

I mean, look at the modern focus in the jails. I remember being on the streets. I remember getting high on those streets, and then I remember my recovery, and then going back and mentoring those women in jail. And I remember seeing some of those women that I used with in that jail who

---

* In 2014 and 2015, 82% of all opiate overdose deaths in the US were of non-Hispanic white people (by 2019, that percentage had fallen slightly to 72%).

could not look at me because they were still using. They couldn't understand how I stopped. Then they thought that I looked down at them. I was like, "How can I look down at you when I used to be you?"

The key tool for Cathy in sustaining recovery was psychotherapy. She got help from many therapists, learning to understand herself and the roots of both her PTSD and her substance use condition. In learning to problem-solve and maintain sobriety, she also gained stability. "Everything starts with a goal, and changing your goals will change your life," she said. "Having a therapist to help you and draw out and say, 'What can we do with that? And there's a reason behind this,' is amazing."

The Pharma/Medical Contribution to the Opiate Epidemic

Many people addicted to opiates have co-occurring mental health conditions. When looking at the recent history of rising opiate overdose deaths in the United States, it is impossible to not discuss the tragedy of the false marketing of OxyContin as an opiate without addictive potential. This lie—and the profits to be made not only by the company that created it but by prescribers and pharmacies—drove the US opiate addiction crisis for two decades. Most people who are addicted to heroin today started with prescription opiates. The United States has about 5 percent of the world's population and consumes over 80 percent of the world's opiates, and the Covid-19 pandemic has added to the crisis. Opiate overdose deaths totaled over 100,000 in 2020 in the United States, which is a substantial increase from prior years. Multiple and unrelenting pandemic stressors, and the addition of fentanyl—a synthetic opiate many times stronger and more lethal than heroin—into the illicit opiate supply have been the likely culprits behind this increase. Yet it is also true that medical prescriptions inspired by false marketing fed the flames of this crisis as well.

Haley Comerford is a straight white woman in her midthirties who grew up in a small town outside Boston. She is single, has no kids, and works for a health insurance company. Haley wanted to share her journey to provide hope for others living with opiate use disorder. She had a stable, happy family but remembers that she developed what she would later learn was called social anxiety around age eleven or twelve. She told me that she started using alcohol after discovering that it helped to alleviate her anxiety; it also gave her a peer group. Later she became addicted to prescribed opiates. In our conversation she referred to Oxy-Contin as "OC":

> Opiates came into my life at the age of sixteen, when I had wisdom teeth removed. They had prescribed Vicodin, and that was kind of the start of the euphoric feeling of opiates. I fell victim to the whole OC thing that happened. I remember the euphoric feeling, and not wanting to come off them. They became a significant problem when I turned seventeen, eighteen years old. From sixteen to twenty-four, when I got clean, the entire time, I searched for that feeling I'd had when I was sixteen years old.
>
> I was born in '86; I graduated high school in 2004. Pharma really started pushing OC in the late '90s, early 2000s. Everyone was prescribed OCs. I got them from my friends, my friends' parents. We would raid their medicine cabinets. It was very easy to come by. All I had to do was just make one phone call and someone's parents were prescribed it for minimal things like stubbing a toe. It was marketed as the one thing that's not going to get addictive. It was outrageous. OCs are what took me to my knees faster than anything else did.

Haley reports she has lost over 150 people she has known to opiate overdose deaths, many during the Covid-19 pandemic. She now carries naloxone with her everywhere she goes, so that if she encounters someone who has overdosed, she can help save their life. Haley found her way to sobriety with the help of Narcotics Anonymous, her family, friends, and her cat. She believes that being employed is important to sustaining her recovery. She even found a way to use probation as a tool, in that it forced her to reconsider her drug use. Her anxiety, which initially led her down her path of substance use, is something she has learned how to manage:

> I think what happened over a period of time was that I started to live myself into a new way of thinking. I started noticing personally that once I had put the drugs down, I no longer needed to steal. I was no longer getting arrested; I was keeping $40 in my pocket longer than twenty minutes; I was building a relationship back up with my mother and father, slowly but surely. I had friends again who would ask me if I wanted to go out to eat, as opposed to if I wanted to go use or find the means to use. I was starting to live a little bit of a better life.

Transcending Shame

Shame is a challenge for many people who have both mental health and substance use issues. Having both challenges can intensify reluctance to seek help or to get support. And delaying treatment and care leads to many adverse outcomes.

Margaret Curley is a nineteen-year-old student studying public health at American University in Washington, DC. Margaret teaches in a creative program in greater Boston called Drug Story Theater (DST). DST is an educational program for middle school students that is akin to NAMI's Ending the Silence program. Many of the teens and recent high school graduates who teach in DST have had both mental health and substance use conditions, and work to integrate their experiences onstage to model recovery for others. DST was started by Joe Shrand, a friend of mine who is an addictionologist and child psychiatrist. DST's tagline is: "The treatment of one becomes the prevention of many."

In pre-pandemic times, I went to a DST presentation in a middle-class suburban community not far from Boston. After the play, in which the presenters act out what they experienced, they then engage with the audience for Q&A. After one middle schooler asked a question about how to deal with an overdose in his family, a presenter asked the other students to raise their hand if they knew someone who had overdosed. Almost half the hands went up. That was a wake-up call. But the real message was the healing power of openness. This middle schooler, and every student who raised their hand, learned that they were not alone. Their willingness to identify themselves and share their experience signifies a hopeful culture shift for those of us who have lived with shame and silence around addiction and mental health.

Margaret talked to me about how her father's death from alcoholism, and the complexities of her experience of shame, influenced her decision to volunteer for DST. She wanted to teach middle schoolers that it's okay to talk about the experience of loving someone who has mental health and addiction issues, or of being someone who has mental health and addiction issues—and that they can get support. She weighed the problem of silence versus the challenges of having difficult conversations, and chose sharing:

It's inherently embarrassing for me to talk about my dad being an addict. It's something that I've been trained and conditioned to be embarrassed about. We didn't even write it in his eulogy.

Something that's difficult with Drug Story Theater is coming to terms with sharing those experiences. When I'm at Drug Story Theater, and I'm standing up in front of an audience and I feel ashamed about this, I also know if I don't say it, then I'm passing that shame down onto the next person in this audience who experiences this. Maybe that kid could have gone to a school counselor and gotten help before their parent passed away from alcoholism. Maybe they could have been connected with resources earlier.

In Drug Story Theater, there is some serious courage, especially from the individuals who have firsthand experience who are able to go onto a stage and say, "I used heroin, and I'm here. I'm alive, and I'm now going to college. I'm trying to become a teacher." It's really powerful. That's what drew me to getting involved. Just bringing light to those experiences and making our programming more accessible for people who are seriously affected by the stigma of addiction.

Signs of Integration

There are signs of hope and integration between the worlds of mental health care and substance use disorder treatment.

Nick Emeigh is a thirtysomething, white, gay man from Bucks County, Pennsylvania, who works as NAMI Bucks County's director of outreach and development. He is also a stigma-crushing mental health superhero, NAMI Man. Nick told me he has lived with co-occurring mental health and substance use conditions for many years. He has experienced psychiatric hospitalizations and had several near-fatal overdoses after the deaths of family members. The program he was in was addressing his substance use disorder, he told me, but finding NAMI marked a moment of integration that made a key difference in his life:

> You think of a recovery house, and you think, it's a house of addicts and everything, but all of them have mental health issues. All of us had things that happened to us in our lives that we were just trying to manage with the drugs and alcohol.
>
> Everybody thinks it's so great and wonderful that I do all this stuff for NAMI, but I do it for me, as well. Nothing has kept me sober, and nothing has kept me treatment-compliant, like knowing that I could use all the stuff that I was the most ashamed of to help people.

· · ·

The long list of hurdles faced just by the people who shared their stories in this chapter include conflicting cultures, shame, loss, racism, inadequate insurance coverage, fraudulent marketing, homelessness, and a punitive criminal justice response to health problems. Despite these hurdles, each person found ways to move ahead and to learn. The Resources section includes a model for doing this systems-level integration developed by Ken Minkoff, a leader on this issue.

This integration is happening in different ways and at different speeds in places across the nation, but there is much more to be done. After you have made some headway in your own recovery journey of navigating these two worlds, sharing your lived experience will be invaluable to others. Your expertise can also be helpful in the bigger effort to integrate the best of both worlds and to move systems forward. When you are ready, we want to hear from you.

SIX

The Impact of Trauma

Note: This chapter includes content that may be distressing to some people. If you begin to experience discomfort or anxiety as you read, please just set this chapter aside for now. You may find the content more helpful to you at another point in time.

"I think I spent quite a bit of my childhood in a ball in the closet because of the violence in my house. My mother was very physically abusive. I think I was like, 'I'm trapped.' And I still, at sixty-six years old, had to explain to my newish boyfriend that when you put pots away and they clank together, that I could actually throw up. I'm shell-shocked. My PTSD is really bad. Loud noises, door slamming—everything activates me."

—SUSIE SELIGSON,
Massachusetts

"I was around the age of twelve or thirteen, and I got molested by a couple of the boys in our neighborhood, older boys. And immediately, as it was happening, and after it happened, I viewed it as a third party. It was happening to somebody else. It wasn't me. That didn't happen to me. I remember distinctly thinking I was watching through the kitchen window. And so, that was a secret that I kept hidden way, way down."

—SNAKE SABO,
New Jersey

. . .

Traumatic experiences affect people's mental health in complex ways. It can be challenging to recognize the impact of trauma, to discern its role in or relationship to other mental health conditions, and to find effective ways to treat or manage its symptoms. An important first step is to consider whether responses to trauma may be part of your or your loved one's story. For some people, that's a question with a clear answer. Others may not yet see, or want to acknowledge, how trauma has affected them.

Human beings are biologically "wired" for survival. In the face of a real or perceived threat to our lives, natural defense mechanisms kick in that focus body and brain acutely and exclusively on dealing with that threat. For example, to prepare for assault, the body moves blood to muscles to help with running, and readies blood clotting materials in case we bleed if attacked. Our sympathetic nervous system goes full throttle, our "options" are limited to "flight, fight, or freeze," and everything else our bodies and brains can do switches off.

This response can save our lives, but it has other consequences that endure long after the immediate threat is gone. While our brain is fully occupied directing so many resources to our survival, it doesn't do other things that it usually does, including processing our experiences into memories in the usual way. As a result, our experience of being threatened—the traumatic event—remains "undigested." This results in symptoms of post-traumatic stress like flashbacks and nightmares. We may feel psychologically removed from the trauma—as if it happened in a movie, or that we were outside observers of ourselves—and cut off from our own emotions. Our supercharged nervous system, so protective in the moment, can remain on high alert for the next threat for a long time, which leaves people with an intense "startle response."

While we have learned a lot about some of the impact of traumatic events, we still have more to learn. The classic model of trauma response described above is an acute model. In the acute model, a person with no prior history of trauma faces a life-threatening experience and, for reasons we don't fully understand, may develop symptoms. People's lives are of course more complex than that, and they can have more and different symptoms than acute trauma responses.

Developmental Trauma/Complex PTSD

Some trauma experts have advocated for a distinct diagnosis for recurrent childhood trauma, sometimes called developmental trauma or complex PTSD. Children who are repeatedly abused or neglected often have different responses to trauma than the acute model just described. They will often have difficulties self-regulating their emotions and impulses or maintaining stable and mutually fulfilling relationships. They may have learning challenges. They may have trouble recognizing their own positive qualities or feeling good about who they uniquely are. While a child's brain is developing, it stands to reason that recurrent trauma often has a different and more fundamental impact.

In Vincent Felitti's groundbreaking Adverse Childhood Experience (ACE) Study, adults insured in a large health plan were asked to report on their childhood experiences. A strong correlation was noted between the amount of childhood adversity and their use of medical and mental health services as adults, and between exposure to childhood adversity and common adult causes of death. The findings provided significant support for the idea that developmental trauma impacts people in many ways throughout their lives.

While complex PTSD is not yet recognized as a distinct diagnosis in DSM-5, it is a diagnosis in the International Classification of Diseases 11, a diagnostic tool developed by the World Health Organization that is used internationally in countries other than the United States. Among those I interviewed for this chapter are people who experienced a single trauma as an adult, people who had repeated childhood trauma, and someone who had both experiences.

Fortunately, finding new and creative approaches to treating trauma is now an active area of inquiry in the mental health field. Traumatic events impact mind and body, so it isn't surprising that many of the successful approaches to trauma work on both. If trauma has a role in your mental health condition and you are seeking help for PTSD, you might find it helpful to hear from other people who have also experienced trauma and found strategies that worked for them. The list is long for what helps people, including multiple integrative psychotherapy approaches, body-based or somatic approaches, meditation, medications, service animals, and community. We will hear from some people who used these techniques in this chapter, but their experiences reflect only some of the tools available. For example, new research on the effectiveness of guided psychedelic psychotherapy for treatment for trauma is being fast-tracked by the FDA after some promising early studies (I haven't had a chance to interview anyone who tried that). A summary of research on this promising idea of guided psychedelic use in psychotherapy and other treatments is found in chapter 18.

. . .

Why did it take so long for professionals to recognize trauma as a major factor in mental health? Unlike the cultural divide that too long separated the fields of mental health and addiction, integrating what we were learning in the field of trauma into treatment of mental illness presented a different set of problems. We lacked language and tools to understand and help manage trauma, both in our patients and in ourselves. When I first spoke about trauma at NAMI, I forgot that there was a long history of people like me—psychiatrists—blaming parents for their children's schizophrenia. No wonder the audience folded their arms across their chests when I mentioned childhood trauma.

We learned together. When NAMI adopted PTSD and borderline personality disorder (BPD) as core concerns in 2007, it opened the conversation in the NAMI community. Trauma was then something to learn about rather than hide from and associate with blame.

The psychiatric field was also slow to integrate the impact of traumatic experiences into its framework. I got a window into this firsthand in 1988, during my psychiatric residency. One of my professors was Bessel van der Kolk, who taught us about both the body's and the mind's responses to psychological trauma. He was focused on understanding the impact of trauma and what to do about it, which led him to write what became his bestselling book, *The Body Keeps the Score*. After his lecture, I traveled up four floors to the inpatient unit in that same building to check on patients who had been placed in restraints. They hated it, and some told me it reminded them of being hurt before. It didn't take a genius to see that they were being retraumatized.

We had in that same residency training program a genius in the lecture hall waking us up to the impact of trauma, meanwhile patients were subject to the routine use of force and restraint on the inpatient unit upstairs. The inpatient unit was run by smart and compassionate people, so that wasn't the problem. The problem was that we were not integrated in concept and action, and we lacked tools. This problem wasn't unique to my hospital. It pervaded the entire field.

While I knew something was wrong with all this, I couldn't put my finger on what to do about it. It was just accepted practice, part of daily life, to use such techniques to limit "out of control" behavior by patients of all ages. The work was overwhelming in terms of volume and severity, so I remain sympathetic to all the people who also couldn't figure out a better solution. To be sure, restraints do stop out-of-control behavior, but they also weren't teaching patients anything about managing their own behavior; instead, they were reactivating trauma responses. I had come to a dead end in my career in inpatient psychiatry. It just wasn't for me.

Fortunately, other people were able to conceptualize a preventive framework and create strategies and tools to help practitioners. After an exposé by the *Hartford Courant* on the overuse and dangers of restraints, the National Medical Directors of State Departments of Mental Health released a groundbreaking paper on prevention of restraint use in psychiatric hospitals. They stated clearly that the use of restraints was a treatment failure. They offered instead a public health framework designed to reduce this practice with prevention, teaching patients what worked to help them calm themselves and training staff to de-escalate difficult situations. By helping people recognize what helps them and what upsets them, you are giving them tools they can use after they leave the hospital—not just to stop one incidence of out-of-control behavior. Most important, the staff are not retraumatizing them.

By this time, I had become the chief psychiatrist for the Massachusetts Department of Mental Health. Finally, I had a framework and tools, and the authority to apply them. My team at the Massachusetts Department of Mental Health set out to help child and adolescent hospitals reduce the use of restraint and seclusion for kids and youth. We used our licensing authority to get their attention, then we worked collaboratively. Next, we engaged occupational therapists, who helped us see the idea of a sensory diet—a personalized activity plan that provides the sensory stimulation some kids need to best regulate themselves—and other techniques to help the kids calm themselves, like weighted blankets, music, and exercise. We also wanted the kids to know what calmed them and what upset them, so they could learn to handle distress.

Together we were able to reduce use of restraints across all child and adolescent hospitals in Massachusetts. Staff from the hospitals that made the change first began to teach the others; it became a peer teaching experience. The initiative didn't cost much and involved teaching kids how to manage feelings and behavior. It wasn't perfect, and it still requires ongoing focus, but child and adolescent hospitals eventually realized that there were ways other than restraints to help kids who behaved impulsively or aggressively.

At about the same time, NAMI had begun to advocate to reduce restraints in hospitals everywhere, and to provide more humane alternatives. They focused on sharing first-person experiences of how restraints had impacted people. The field was moving slowly and unevenly toward understanding how this practice contributed to traumatizing people and doing something about it.

The hard truth was that the field did not have the tools to make a difference. We had a lot to learn about trauma. The federal mental health organization, SAMHSA, later came out with a model of trauma-informed care; this was an important first step in raising awareness of how to think about reducing re-traumatization in many care settings. The next step—learning how to promote resilience and strengths in people who had been traumatized—came later.

The same challenges are still before us in many other places where restraints are still used, like corrections facilities, residential care settings, and in police work. An overburdened workforce has more tools than I did to prevent overuse of restraints, but it takes adequate staffing and training to make this effort work. These can be in short supply, so the risk remains.

Tools That Helped People

As I talked to people, one person at a time, for this chapter, I wanted to learn from them: "What helps people in the aftermath of traumatic experiences?" Their answers reveal many tools that could potentially help you. Some are specific types of psychotherapy; others are more creative, non-professional approaches. In attending to traumatic experiences, there is every reason to adopt once again a "both/and" perspective: Find the most effective tools for you, from both the medical model, and the recovery model. Your own treatment plan should work for you. It is my hope that hearing other people's strategies for how they have addressed trauma will inspire some promising new ideas about how you might move forward on your own path to recovery. Remember that trauma interventions may work at one time but not another, depending on where you are in life and in your recovery. Persistence can pay off in the quest to find treatments.

To learn more about the different kinds of trauma responses and approaches that might be tailored to different types, I recommend reading *The Body Keeps the Score* by Bessel van der Kolk.

Consider the Possibility That Trauma Has Impacted You

Acknowledging the possibility that you are struggling with traumatic stress responses isn't always easy. Robert Cubby is a seventy-two-year-old retired police captain and father of two sons who lives in New Jersey. He was diagnosed with PTSD after a significant acute traumatic event he experienced in the line of duty, while supervising police officers who suffered severe injury after a standoff became a shooting scene.

The biggest initial challenge was considering the idea that he, a police leader, could have PTSD; it was feedback from his wife that accelerated the process toward recovery. In our interview, he reflected on what he now knows were PTSD symptoms:

> I thought: "All of this will pass. I just need a good night's sleep, to stay home for a couple of days." The chief said, "Don't hurry back. Stay home, just decompress, and call if you need to talk to someone," and so on. I didn't pull out. I'm ranting and raving at home now. I'm screaming at my wife, I'm screaming at my kids, I'm crying uncontrollably, I can't sleep. The nightmares are too horrific, I can't eat. This went on for three days.

Finally, his wife said, "If you don't take care of this, if you don't go to see someone, you might as well pack your bags and leave. Because I will not live in a house with you acting this way."

"Well," Robert said, "that snapped me out of it." After that, he called a therapist, a dear friend of the family, and said, "I need to see you right away."

Thankfully, this therapist had some background in PTSD. Robert recalled:

> And about five or ten minutes into the interview, she said, "I've got good news and I've got bad news." And I said, "Okay, hit me." She said, "You have PTSD." And I knew it. But it's one of those things that, like, "It's not me, it's them. It can never be me. Me? No, I'm Superman, it can't be me."

And then that hit me. And I said, "Okay, what do we need to do?" She said, "I know what to do, that's my job. You just need to listen, and we'll get through this." And we did. We got through the turbulence, the real ups and downs that I was able to calm down.

Exposure Therapy

Robert was fortunate to find a psychotherapy based in the model of exposure therapy, which is a well-studied approach to cope with traumatic symptoms. In a nutshell, the basic idea of exposure therapy is that by mentally returning to the trauma in a safe space with a therapist, your body and mind can slowly begin to process the traumatic event.

Exposure therapy underlies many of the therapies that have been developed for PTSD. It helped Robert that the therapist was also a member of his Catholic church; he felt safe with her. He described his experience:

> It was talk therapy. She wanted me to recount the incident in first person, and don't edit or try to explain anything, just as it is unraveling in your mind right now, as you're reliving it, as you're picturing it, every single detail, I want to hear. I want to hear about the blood on the wall, every single detail. And that felt relieving. That felt like I was purged, that the demon was no longer on my back. To be able to do that was taking a burden off, and [so I was] not carrying that anymore.

Cognitive Behavior Therapy/ Cognitive Processing Therapy

Another kind of talk therapy for PTSD with good research evidence of effectiveness is a variation on exposure therapy. It helps a person revisit trauma and focuses on changing the person's perspective on the trauma. This is called reframing. How might it work for a real person?

Nadine Lewis is a sixty-year-old, single, multicultural woman who lives in Oklahoma, and is retired from the Coast Guard after twenty-six years of service. She reports she grew up in a dysfunctional family where undiagnosed mental illness and alcoholism were prevalent. Nadine experienced repeated trauma in her childhood, and reports she began drinking alcohol at age seven to deal with the abuse. In addition to her childhood trauma, she told me she later developed PTSD following military sexual trauma in the Coast Guard. Nadine described how alcohol stopped working as self-medication, so she sought help for her PTSD and substance use:

> When I got to the Vet Center, they started doing cognitive behavioral therapy with me. That helped to start me talking about reframing. They figured that it was the best treatment for me because of my long-term abuse, because I would have to take it in pieces. And it was like an onion. We started peeling it back little by little by little.

Nadine found CBT, medications, and sobriety support all essential tools to recovery. Today, she finds purpose in sharing her recovery journey with others.

Neurofeedback and EMDR

Neurofeedback is a kind of brain retraining that has a growing research literature. Eye movement desensitization and reprocessing—better known by its acronym EMDR—is a specialized psychotherapy technique that uses a focus on an external stimulus (for instance, eye movement) to help with the process of discussing trauma; it is a kind of exposure treatment with a body dimension.

Susan Smiley is the mother of one daughter and is also a neurofeedback practitioner in her midfifties living in California. She told her story of growing up with, and taking care of, a single mother who suffered from schizophrenia in the groundbreaking and acclaimed film *Out of the Shadow*. She told me about growing up in a traumatizing home environment:

My earliest memories are of my parents yelling at each other and having terrible fights. They could get violent, things being thrown, and me hiding behind the sofa, terrified and crying. All throughout my elementary school years, it was mostly just my mother around because my parents divorced when I was four. And that's when her illness really was exacerbated. She was a young mom with two small children and very alone; she lacked support. All the neighbors turned a blind eye. There was a lot of screaming. My mother was completely psychotic and dysregulated. The slightest irritant would set her off. And so, I learned to be as "not irritating" as possible, and therefore to disappear. I can't blame my mother. She was very ill, and it was during a time when the public mental health system was in shambles. She had a good heart and needed proper help that didn't exist at the time, no matter how hard we tried.

Susan described how she put the puzzle pieces of her recovery together over time. She also emphasized that timing is important, in terms of whether a given tool or technique is effective. Something that didn't work early on in recovery might be worth another try later:

Over the years, there's been no one thing that's solved everything. That's one thing I learned suffering from early life trauma due to a mother with untreated schizophrenia. I think my lifelong depression and anxiety were most debilitating. I was in psychotherapy for twenty years before I started looking at other modalities. "Here I am in my late thirties. I've been doing all the things I'm supposed to do. Why is nothing working?" It was clearly my nervous system, and my ability to regulate was really out of whack, and no amount of psychotherapy taught me that.

Susan went on to share:

I see now in my own healing journey of forty years of trying various therapy modalities that they vary in terms of their efficacy, based on a person's ability to take it on at that time in their life or the quality of the practitioner. It's about the right fit of the right type of therapy at the right time in your recovery, whether it be psychotherapy or neurofeedback, EMDR, or yoga therapy. There's no one answer for everyone, and that element I think is important as someone in recovery.

Timing is important. In Susan's case, EMDR didn't work the first time, fifteen years ago:

I thought, "This is silly." It simply did nothing for me at the time. I wasn't able to find my safe space for it to be effective. Now I understand it's because I was too frightened, too hypervigilant. It took doing neurofeedback to help my whole self, brain and body, to calm down to a steady state where I could move through the world with an ease and a sense of safety that I had never felt before. I was way further along in terms of building resilience in my brain and nervous system, and then was able to handle the work EMDR could do. If something doesn't work at a certain stage in your life, maybe it will down the line. I think when someone suffers from serious developmental trauma, it's like piecing together pieces of the puzzle, the recovery puzzle. Certain pieces don't fit until other pieces are put together first.

Skills and Community

Susie Seligson is a sixty-seven-year-old journalist, author, and longtime Samaritans volunteer who lives on the tip of Cape Cod, Massachusetts. She describes a childhood marked by recurrent physical abuse. Susie has created multiple ways to work with her traumatic past. These include dialectical behavior therapy (DBT), telling her story, and creating a strong community. She told me:

Looking back on it, I think I do feel grief about why it had to be so damn hard. *Why*, you know? I think there is a sense of loss. Who would I have been otherwise? I think when I talk about this, I experience a little bit of that. But here I am doing this advocacy work, by sharing my story for this book, because it is hard for so *many* people. And they don't recognize it or they don't ask for help. I think if you have that awareness, you should be doing this, telling your story. It's something you need to share because people are so confused.

I do think that all the meds in the world, in my case for depression and PTSD, would not be enough if I didn't have an incredible, huge circle of loving friends, a dog, a range of passions, and children in my life. And I really need community. That's definitely part of it. And then it's also learning. And it's funny with the DBT because it doesn't come instantly, but I realized how it's kind of woven into my life that I think, "Watch this thought float by." The DBT has really helped me.

Internal Family Systems Therapy

Internal family systems therapy (IFS) is a well-studied model for helping people who have survived traumatic experiences and can also be helpful for treating other conditions. IFS focuses on the idea that we can have a family of experiences within us—parts of us. One excellent use of IFS is to help people with dissociative identity disorder, which often has roots in childhood trauma.

Nancy-Lee Mauger is a fifty-eight-year-old musician and artist. She has two children and lives in Massachusetts. She was diagnosed with dissociative identity disorder in 2010. She described how IFS helps her make sense of her experiences:

Why this affects me in my life now is because, as a little girl these things happened to me. Now I'm out in the world, and I smell something, and it reminds a part of me that's still inside me, of an experience I had. If I'm not prepared for that, that part of me comes out and takes over and then I'm dissociated. That's how it works. It's not this crazy monster thing. I just want to normalize it. We all have the capability to dissociate, we all can be overtaken by parts of us.

When you're angry, really pissed off, and you're spewing things, and you don't even know what you're saying, that's not *you*, that's a part of you. That's normal; everybody does it. I remember being in a doctor's office and she's like, "Well, you had a lot of childhood trauma, so you were once a whole and then you split into all these parts to take care of the trauma. This is how it is and you're going to integrate these parts." And I'm like, "Hell no. You're not going to get me to integrate anything. I'm going to live with all my parts and make them all happy." Integration was just a concept. I didn't really understand at the time the idea that I had to be put back together into a "whole" person—you can't.

Nancy-Lee went on to share:

I didn't like the hospital telling me that I was once whole. But when I walked into IFS, and my therapist said, "Well, okay, here's the deal. This is what IFS believes that we *all* are built in parts." What? Wait. From the day I walked in, he spoke in parts. He would say "A part of me feels this way."

Don't let anybody tell you you're broken. Nothing that has happened to you has broken you. I mean, honestly, that was the worst thing I ever heard about myself. We all go through horrible things. If we don't have the adults to help us through it, it's still there, and we must just go deal with it. I don't have a disorder. I just have to put my parts in order and help them."

Nancy-Lee credits the framework and support of IFS and her talented therapist with making the biggest difference for her of all the approaches she has tried.

Creative Practices

Many nonprofessional approaches also support people as they work to live with the symptoms of traumatic experience.

Breathing Exercises

When something happens that retriggers a trauma response, it also reactivates symptoms. When retired police captain Robert Cubby experienced a reactivation of his symptoms, he found real-time help for himself. His preferred tool is breathing:

> Two years ago, I watched another incident involving police officers on TV as it was unfolding. I was triggered. Badly. It was a flashback, a huge flashback. I started shaking, I felt the symptoms coming on. I'm thinking like, "I've got to find something to do." I started washing dishes, I figured the water hitting my hands, splashing my face might bring me out of it. Nothing.
>
> And so, I got down on my knees, and I'm praying to God. I said, "Please pull me out of this. I don't know what to do." And then I hear a voice on my shoulder, my little guardian angel, and he says, "Breathe, stupid." And I said, "Okay!" And I took a deep breath, and I went through the deep breathing, and it just reset. I pulled out of it, and I said, "Damn, this stuff works!" These are simple things, that's the simplest things that we do.

Our nervous system is divided into two main parts: the sympathetic, which amps us up and gets our bodies ready for action (fight or flight), and the parasympathetic, which slows us down and helps us return to a state of calm (rest and digest). When people experience trauma, the sympathetic nervous system can become turbocharged and overshadow the parasympathetic nervous system, resulting in common post-traumatic symptoms like agitation, irritability, and hypervigilance. Through deep breathing, we can activate the parasympathetic nervous system, and help to slow our bodies down. Meditation, a practice dating back thousands of years, is a great way to practice deep breathing; yoga and other timed breathing exercises are also great ways of engaging the parasympathetic nervous system.

Moving Meditation

Bessel van der Kolk taught me that "the body keeps the score." But how do you use your body to help with trauma? Robert Cubby, who started a support group through NAMI for veterans and first responders, told me in our interview about how mindfulness and movement worked together as an effective technique to help them open up about their experiences:

> A lot of people can't sit still, especially when they're going through PTSD and the monkey mind's jumping all over the place. Like, you expect me to sit still and go over my thoughts when my thoughts are plaguing me to begin with? So, we found that with veterans particularly, they like to move around. Rather than sit still, we do walking meditations. I teach them mindfulness exercises. What can I do mindfully? Mindfully wash the dishes. Mindfully brush your teeth. Just think about every little step that you're doing and keep your mind on that single activity. We found that, by teaching veterans and first responders activities where they can do that, where it's singly focused, it was extremely therapeutic for them.
>
> A woman I know does cooking with veterans. And she said, "I could sit them in a group, and they would say nothing. They'd just sit there and stare, and I would try to evoke things from them, and they wouldn't co-operate: 'I'm fine, everything's good, everything's cool.'" And that's it, that's all they'd do. She put them in the kitchen, they're peeling potatoes, and they're chopping carrots, and they're talking about everything that's bothering them.

A Service Animal

Nadine Lewis, the Coast Guard veteran in Oklahoma with a traumatic history of people mistreating her, has found great support from her service dog, Nara. Nara helps Nadine feel protected and loved:

> Nara helps me with my PTSD by blocking and calming me down when I get anxious or agitated. One of the things she does is, when I interact with other people, she'll sit right in front of me or next to me. If she feels

a person is not a threat, she'll sit next to me and just observe them. If she feels me getting anxious or agitated, she'll move in front of me and create a barricade between me and the individual. Now, if they start getting really aggressive, she'll glare at them. And she'll take a couple steps forward to make the distance between us bigger. If my back is exposed to everybody, she'll sit behind me. And if somebody starts approaching, she'll lean into me, to let me know that somebody is coming too close, and I need to turn around.

Nadine went on to explain Nara's importance in her life:

Nara is very critical for me to function in my daily life. At first when people were getting service dogs, I was like, "No, I don't need one." I didn't realize the difference a well-trained service dog can make for somebody with PTSD and the trauma that I've suffered. Because when you don't trust people, and the only thing you do trust are animals, and to have one like this, that is so gentle, so caring, it's life changing.

Creativity in the Arts

Snake Sabo is a guitarist and founder of the hard rock band Skid Row. Married and the father of twins, he lives on Long Island, New York. Snake reported he has been dealing with bipolar disorder since adolescence. He told me he has guitars throughout his house in case he wants to play one on his way to get something in the kitchen. His love of music comes through in our conversation.

Music also was healing for him. Snake was molested when he was about eleven years old. He didn't tell anyone for a long time, and he believes this event was central to his life experience. I asked him how he coped. He told me, "I figured out ways to mask all of that by being funny." He went on to explain:

Anytime I'm feeling a certain way, I'm going to use humor as a defense mechanism and to deflect any attention to what I was going through internally. No one would ever know. When I started playing guitar, it was the only way I figured out how to voice and release my emotions, because I couldn't verbalize anything. I was slowly releasing stuff that was bottled up inside me, through music. It was my language. Because I would pour out my pain into writing.

Decades later, he spoke to his band:

I finally had a talk with my band and explained to them what had been going on, about the molestation and the other stuff. And that this is who I am for real; that I need therapy and medication. Coming clean about that, all of it, makes it so real. And that was the real beginning of acceptance. And then, with that acceptance, came me being a little bit more vocal about it, telling my story a little bit more.

Snake is still a touring musician, and now a proud NAMI ambassador.

Chess

Jeremiah Rainville is a thirty-six-year-old from Rhode Island who has worked as a certified peer recovery specialist, a certified community health worker, and a peer program manager at NAMI Rhode Island. He now serves as chair of NAMI's Peer Leadership Council. Jeremiah spoke with me about experiencing trauma during his youth in the child welfare system and finding an outlet in the game of chess:

During my first hospitalization, my adopted father taught me chess. Chess was very important because I couldn't play contact sports because of my PTSD. I couldn't be near people. I couldn't have them touch my shoulder.

Playing chess was a lifesaver because I got to compete with something that wouldn't interfere with the PTSD. I had something I could do. I got into it, and I did competitions with it. The other thing that was neat was, when I was growing up in a residential treatment facility, my psychiatrist would play chess with me. That's how we would talk, while playing chess.

He believed that the voices and seeing things was the result of my trauma. I've heard different things about that, but that's what he thought, and I kind of accept that.

In our interview, Jeremiah reflected on how his traumatic past and his present fit together. "I transcended from a life of trauma and sickness to actually doing well," he told me, adding that he is now "helping others and supporting others to move forward the best I can because of my experience."

Mastering Trauma by Teaching

As people engage in therapy, find support, or use recovery tools, promoting change through teaching can also be a healing tool. Teaching about lived experience often becomes an empowering way to help cope with challenges.

Kimberly Comer, a fifty-seven-year-old woman who lives in Florida, now leverages her first-person experience of coping with both a trauma history and bipolar disorder in helping to train correctional officers. Her own experience in corrections was as an inmate, incarcerated in a maximum-security prison after she attempted to embezzle money from her employer during a manic phase of her bipolar disorder. Kimberly was sentenced to three years and served seven months. She also faced time in solitary confinement, which she found traumatic:

> I'm already not properly medicated; I'm already traumatized. They stick me in solitary, and the voices get worse, and the delusions get worse, and the psychosis gets worse. So, while you think you're going to get to speak to somebody that has calmed down, my symptoms just got worse in solitary confinement.

Kimberly met her fiancé on her first night in a homeless shelter after her release from prison. He was a volunteer there, serving her first meal and playing cards with her. Their relationship began seventeen years ago. But that same day, on her journey from prison to the shelter, something else significant happened:

> I served my sentence and was released from prison. The corrections officer who transported me from the prison to the train, as he was helping me down out of the van, said, "You know, it was really nice to meet you. I'll look forward to seeing you again real soon."

In that moment, Kimberly thought to herself, "Whoa." But, as she was happy to tell me, she did see him again eight years later—just not in the capacity he thought. Now, she's involved with NAMI and with Crisis Intervention Training. During a training, she looked over at her co-presenter and said:

> Do you know who that is sitting over in the right corner? She said no. I said, "That's the corrections officer who transported me from a maximum-security prison to the train station. He told me he was looking forward to seeing me again real soon." I said, "So I think I'm going to help him with that," and I did. I went up and introduced myself. Yes, you are going to see me again.

She reflected that: "It was pretty sweet, not going to lie." Kimberly is now an award-winning national certified peer specialist who has worked for NAMI in both Indiana and Florida, and currently serves as the peer mentor program manager for NAMI Palm Beach County. She continues to teach as well as to advocate and work to reduce the impact of trauma for others in the correctional system.

Traumatic experiences and their aftermath can be significant factors in your mental health journey. This is a complex topic, and there are many more treatment approaches and non-treatment strategies available than those described in this chapter. The Resources section at the end of the book suggests other books and organizations where you can learn more.

SEVEN

Helping Your Child, Teen, or Young Adult

"Listen to that gut feeling that you have. You're going to be in denial for a little bit but try not to languish there for long; try to get help as soon as you can. Like any other illness, you want to catch it at a stage one versus a stage four. Ask your pediatrician, 'Where can I go? I'm starting to see some things in my child that are a little unusual.' Acknowledge issues as soon as you can, get through that denial phase and be ready to move on and try to find some help and hope." —**BETSEY O'BRIEN,**
mother, South Carolina

"I was eight years old. At the public-school library, I forgot to check out a book. When I got home that night and I read it, and I looked in the back, there was still a card in the back. I was beside myself. I was up all night. I couldn't tell anyone; like it was a crime. That is my first memory of really being consumed by anxiety." —**PAM GOLDMAN,**
Massachusetts

"In the fifth grade, I experienced what I presumed to be an anxiety attack, a panic attack. I ran away from school; ran I think three miles down to the reservoir where I knew there was this huge rock and I laid there. I built myself a little fort and I hid in there, and I swear to God, I said to myself, 'This life is going to be hard.'" —**MICHAEL HAUCK,**
Connecticut

. . .

It can be hard to reconcile the idea that childhood, ideally a time of wonder, learning, and growth, is also commonly the time when emotional and behavioral concerns first manifest themselves. This chapter provides a general overview of the "lay of the land" of youth mental health concerns, some key strategies, and how to begin getting help. There are many books that address various developmental, behavioral, and mental health challenges in youth. NAMI plans to develop a guide for parents in the years to come that will include developmental issues such as autism spectrum disorder, but I will not be addressing them here, as they deserve a guidebook of their own.

For ethical and consent reasons, I didn't interview children about their experiences. Yet many adults I spoke to describe the onset of behavioral and emotional symptoms when they were young, and parents added important perspectives on what they have learned in supporting and advocating for their kids.

One key takeaway from my interviews—and my career—is that people experience the onset of symptoms earlier than you might think. Half of mental health conditions start by age fourteen, and three quarters by age twenty-five. My father, in an astonishing moment of vulnerability, told me that he was first hospitalized at age seventeen. After his death, I found an honorable discharge paper from the Army, the consequence of an episode he had at age twenty-two. It read "Health: Poor. Character: Excellent." I am not sure I have seen a better expression of the distinction between the person and the illness.

No matter your child's age or developmental stage, the realization that they are struggling is unsettling for parents. It's natural to be concerned when your child is hurting, and to worry when you can't instantly fix whatever is wrong. At the same time, you can learn strategies and techniques to better support your child. Although it's nearly impossible for a parent not to worry, worrying is not the thing that will help. Rather, it's your love, effort, and steady presence that will make the difference.

Here are a few steps I encourage you to take, based on my clinical experience and the experiences of the parents I interviewed.

Step 1: Gather Information

If you are concerned about your child's mood, attitude, behavior, interactions with others, or orientation to reality, you should trust your instincts and gather more information. While what concerns you could just signal a passing phase in normal development, it could also signal that your child needs guidance or help that they aren't already getting. That doesn't necessarily mean they have a mental health condition. Children come with different temperaments, traits, personalities, learning styles, abilities, and deficits. They respond differently to emotional, relational, or environmental stresses and develop differently at different rates. What you are noticing may be a sign that they are struggling with a developmental challenge, a learning difference, an emotion they can't name and don't know what to do with, discomfort with a changed sense of their identity, or challenges in navigating peer relationships. They may be responding to hormonal changes or to the very real difficulties they witness or experience in an unjust and imperfect world. Growing up is rarely easy for anyone.

Changes in bodies, hormones, brain maturation, and the social process of finding a peer group is only a partial list of the normal changes happening during adolescence. Teens are judged on everything from their knowledge of physics to their looks to their job or college acceptances. It is a stressful time in life, and the pandemic isolation made it all harder.

One of the fundamental developmental tasks of an adolescent is to establish an identity of their own, separate from you—and finding an identity is a challenge at a time when so many other things are changing. Rebellion, experimentation, defiance, sarcasm, and eye-rolling are some common, often unconscious strategies teens use to announce their separateness from you; these can be worrisome, trying, even infuriating at times. Many adolescents guard their privacy and save most intimate communication for their peers. Whether they are struggling with the normal challenges of adolescence or with a mental health concern, they may still be ambivalent about letting you know, no matter how good your relationship with your child is.

It's important to remember that even though your teen may at times seem invested in pushing you away, they are just doing what they are developmentally supposed to be doing—if not always in a graceful manner. They still very much need your love and support. They still need you to set and keep the boundaries they're testing. And they still need you to keep reaching out to let them know you're still there, no matter what—and especially if you suspect they're troubled by something or see behavior changes that concern you.

Developing an identity can include learning about—and sometimes being confused by—one's gender identity and sexual orientation. While many families and communities are accepting, some are not. Adolescents also sometimes firm up shaky identities by shaming, bullying, or excluding people they perceive as "other," thus adding to the mental health risk for those excluded. But there is help available through the Trevor Project, a nonprofit devoted to suicide prevention that provides crisis resources specifically for LGBTQ+ youth. It is available 24/7 and is free across the United States, and they have plans to expand internationally. They also provide online text and chat support, accessible at their website.

Stress brings out vulnerabilities, and adolescence is stressful. Certain mental health symptoms or diagnoses may first appear in the teen years, including anxiety, persistent sadness or major depression, ADHD, OCD, self-harm behaviors, eating disorders, and substance use. Some of these conditions have neurobiological and genetic bases; others arise as counterproductive ways of dealing with stresses and/or emotional conflicts. As alarming as this information may be, it's important to remember that many teens live with mental health conditions; many find their way to care; and many continue to function and move forward in their lives. It is hard to watch our kids struggle, but their experiences may also endow them with greater self-awareness and emotional maturity, inform creative or vocational endeavors, and lead to a compassion for others that will ultimately enrich their lives.

Parents very often struggle with the question of what normal teen behavior is, and what is a manifestation of a mental health condition. I am asked this question often, and it is a big topic, so I asked my colleague Christine Crawford, a child and adolescent psychiatrist like me, to speak to that in chapter 17.

I love working with adolescents. It is a kinetic stage of life—alive with key questions on identity and relationships, symptom management, and integrating the possibility of a mental health condition into an identity. I've learned that for teens, diagnosis is also developmental; not fixed but iterative. But even when the nature of their mental health struggles looks a bit fuzzier than we might like, there are interventions that will nevertheless work and help. Coping tools, cognitive behavioral ideas, family involvement, and communication are all effective in helping teens heal and thrive.

One way to begin to get information and learn from other parents is to enroll in the NAMI Basics Education Program. This is a free program for parents and other caregivers of children and adolescents with mental health symptoms, whether there has been a formal diagnosis or not. NAMI Basics is taught by two trained individuals who are also caregivers of children with mental health challenges—people who have been there—and consists of six two-and-a-half-hour classes packed with information, discussions, and skills exercises. It's specifically designed to help participants gain a better understanding of the challenges mental health conditions are creating for your child—and your family—and to provide guidance in how you can best support your child.

NAMI Basics can help you begin to assess:

- The impact mental health conditions can have on your entire family
- Different types of mental health care professionals and available treatment options and therapies

- An overview of the public mental health care, school and juvenile justice systems, and resources to help you navigate these systems
- How to advocate for your child's rights at school and in health care settings
- How to prepare for and respond to crisis situations (self-harm, suicide attempts, etc.)
- The importance of taking care of yourself (the caregiver)

NAMI Basics works. Formal research has shown it to be helpful and effective for those who participate. The program is also offered in an online format that allows parents or caregivers to take the entire course at their own pace, in their own homes and as their life allows. A Spanish version is also available, called Bases y Fundamentos de NAMI.

Step 2: Talk Directly to Your Child or Teen

To know what's going on with your child, and to help them, you should begin by talking to them directly about your concerns and engage them in an open discussion about what they are experiencing. Whatever your child's age, I believe it is critical to keep the conversation going. Remind your child that you are open to listening to and supporting them, even about topics they sense are charged, or ones they fear. Be prepared for this conversation not to occur when you are ready, and not to go as you planned. Your child may not respond to your first approach or may deny that anything is wrong except that you are being intrusive or annoying. Two months later, when you are on a work deadline, your child may approach you: "Can we talk about my sadness? It's getting pretty bad." The love you have devoted to your child since before they were born, and your openness and receptiveness to what they have to say, will pay off. Even if the conversation begins at the most inconvenient time for you, even if it is about something you don't want to hear or something your child feels is shameful, the important thing is that the conversation is happening. Your child knows that whatever they are dealing with, they're not alone. This is a priceless moment of parenting.

If your child is an adolescent, their natural developmental desire to separate from you and form a distinct sense of themselves may make them reluctant to share their mental health experience with their family. Keeping the conversation going is a priority, but it may be harder than it sounds. If your child isn't open to the conversation, and your concern grows, read William Miller's introduction to Motivational Interviewing (MI) in chapter 17. MI is a technique he designed to engage people who are ambivalent about discussing their own concerns about themselves. Remember, if there is something about your child's mood or behavior that concerns you, it is likely concerning them, too. The key to having the conversation may be in how you approach it.

Once you realize that your child is experiencing a behavioral, emotional, learning, or mental health issue, more will be required of you. You will have to figure out how best to gather information, find help, manage your (and your child's) stress and anxiety, and advocate for your child in the world. Added challenges include dealing with the ramifications of meeting your child's needs in your life and your family's life. As if parenting and/or working wasn't hard enough already, your child's difficulties can affect other relationships in the family, stir up powerful feelings, and spark conflicts. Equal parts self-compassion, support, and grit is what I prescribe for parents facing these unknowns.

You may feel alone with your concerns and your feelings, but you aren't. Help is available, even if at times it feels impossible to find or access. You will gain more clarity about your child's issues. Kids and teens have many strengths. They grow and develop, and very often they get better. They are natural learners and can learn how to manage their experiences with practice. The difficulties they're having now may ultimately inform—or reveal—gifts and talents. They will find community, and so will you.

For parents, kids, teens, and professionals alike, openness and curiosity are valuable attributes in sorting hard questions. The question of what is going on with a child or teen who is struggling can be a hard one to answer with certainty, but an open mind and an iterative approach can help. Because kids and teens are developing and moving through developmental stages, the picture is, even more so than with adults, a feature film and not a snapshot. It is common for a kid's or teen's emotional and behavioral presentation to change over years or even locations (e.g., at home versus at school).

One woman I interviewed told me that, as a teen, her interaction with her parents surprised her, and meant a great deal to her. Pooja Mehta is a twenty-six-year-old mental health and suicide prevention advocate. Her work is inspired by her lived experience, which she also taps to inform policy on Capitol Hill and beyond. As a teenager, Pooja initially felt shame about her mental health experiences and kept them to herself. She told me that in her South Asian community, mental health was rarely discussed. But staying silent became too much to bear:

When I was fourteen, I had my first panic attack. I'm literally sitting on my back porch and my heart starts racing and I start hearing these voices in my head and I'm freaking out. I'm like, "Oh, oh my God, what is happening?" Because the only time I had ever seen this, hearing voices that aren't real, was like in horror movies. I'm thinking, "There is something seriously wrong with you." And I didn't know what to do. And so, I went to a park near my house and had a full-on breakdown and then came home and pretended like nothing happened. And I kept doing that for a year.

I would have voices in my head just reinforcing negative self-talk. It manifested like it was coming from an outside source. It felt like the universe or God or whatever was telling me that I'm worthless, I'm useless, nobody loves me, you should hurt yourself, you should kill yourself. I wrote down what I was thinking in a notebook. I hid that notebook between my box spring in my mattress, but, of course, my mother found it. And she calls me to the back porch one day. She and my dad are sitting there. My mom is holding the notebook and . . . I'm so scared. I'm mentally preparing myself to be told, "You need to be put somewhere and kept there, you're dangerous, this, that, whatever."

Fortunately, that did not happen. Pooja went on to share her parents' response:

My parents sat me down and they explained to me that this is a chemical imbalance. Both my parents are pharmacists, and my dad was like, "Antidepressants are the number one selling drug on the market." They really just normalized it for me. They made me feel like, this is not how it's supposed to be, but we're going to figure out how to get you to the point where you're okay.

Pooja has gone on to be an advocate for mental health awareness and openness in multiple settings. Not everyone finds a diary, but with some luck there will be an opportunity to engage with your teen around the critical topic of mental health. Teens do understandably guard their privacy, but it is critical to engage them in every step of the process of learning how to manage their mental health symptoms. There are many ways you can help them beyond seeking formal treatment or intervention. For example, if your child has issues with impulse control, martial arts are great and often my first recommendation. Creative arts—visual, musical, dramatic, or literary—are wonderful ways for kids and teens to express and share feelings, and sometimes to discover identity or find community. Exercise helps relieve anxiety; sports can give kids a sense of belonging and skills useful well beyond the field of play. Finding some activity your child enjoys, and is good at, is a helpful confidence builder. These are helpful interventions that can also build skills, character, and confidence, forge community, and enrich your child's life for decades to come. There is no reason they cannot coexist with professional support, should professional support also prove to be important.

If you have decided, based on concerns about problems in functioning or severity of symptoms, that your child needs further assessment, then let's look at some avenues for obtaining one.

Step 3: Get an Assessment

Getting an assessment by a mental health professional is a formal way to benefit from the knowledge of someone who has been trained in making sense of youth and young adult mental health. If appropriate and necessary, they can help you put together a collaborative intervention or treatment plan.

I know it isn't always easy to get kids to attend an initial meeting. "Let's go see a psychiatrist" may not strike joy into their hearts. When I saw kids of all ages in private practice, I would tell the parents their job was to get their child to come see me once. After that it was on me to engage and connect with the kid, so they'd be willing to return a second time. It turns out, kids love to be heard.

The routes to finding help for youth can be even more complex than they are for adults given the central role of schools and an opaque and overburdened child mental health system. In many cases, parents must consistently advocate to find solutions to put together the many puzzles of the child mental health service world.

The increase in pandemic-related distress has also strained under-resourced mental health care service providers. The rising demand has greatly increased caseloads and the stress of their work. There are many good people capable of helping your child, but getting an appointment can be a significant hurdle. For example, you would be very lucky to find a child and adolescent psychiatrist or psychologist in private practice that accepts both new patients and your insurance. There is a profound shortage of child and adolescent psychiatrists—only a quarter of the number that is needed, per multiple reports. In addition, these providers are especially underrepresented in minority and rural communities.

Pediatricians and nurses pick up much of the slack, but this shortage can leave them overextended.

Often, the best place to begin is with your pediatrician, family doctor, or clinical nurse specialist. These professionals have training in child and adolescent development and can often address many basic mental health questions, including helping you sort typical childhood behavior from behaviors or symptoms that may require assessment. Some practices have direct links to social workers or psychologists to help with assessment and triage. Many pediatricians have long-term relationships with families, and this can normalize initial conversations about a subject people find hard to talk about. Pediatricians are unsung heroes in the mental health world for this population.

If you have private insurance, you may or may not find an in-network mental health professional in your provider directory to do an assessment. Unfortunately, these listings are just that, listings; they do not usually specify what the provider's focus is, or whether they do mental health evaluations for kids and teens, which can result in a lot of fruitless phone calls and frustration. If you can't find an appropriate covered provider, you may have to advocate for your child with your insurance company. If there are no in-network providers, the insurer may have to pay for one who is out of network but will likely need to be prodded to do so. The insurer may or may not assist you in finding a qualified out-of-network provider who also agrees to the insurer's payment terms and documentation requirements.

I encourage parents to build a paper trail documenting your efforts to find a provider, and your interactions with the insurer; this is a heavily regulated industry, and this is the language insurers speak. Document your calls and interactions with network providers, your calls to the insurer, and your requests for help with out-of-network providers. Ask for names and include dates. If your insurer does not direct you to a covered provider but then denies your request for coverage for someone out of network, follow the insurer's appeal process and respond to every appeal letter they send you. Every state has a regulatory agency looking over care in health insurance plans often called something like the Division of Insurance. If your first efforts fail, copy the regulatory agency in your paper trail. This might be the last thing you want to deal with, but it could pay off.

Community health clinics and mental health centers also often have resources to help families attain a mental health assessment for your child or adolescent. These centers too are often overburdened with demand, especially since the onset of the pandemic, so there may be a wait. The pandemic helped to foster the use of teletherapy (real-time video sessions), which has been shown to be as effective as in-person care and more accessible for many. Teletherapy is another silver lining of the pandemic—it works, and for many it increases access and convenience.

In seeking mental health care for your child or adolescent, look for providers who demonstrate empathy and who your teen might connect with. Ideally, it will be a person who also seems skilled in finding collaborative ways to also engage you and your family. Medications can in some cases be useful tools, and knowing and attending to potential side effects is important. Complete independent information on the risks and benefits of particular medications is available on NAMI's website.

A serious mental illness diagnosis like bipolar disorder or schizophrenia may make everything more difficult for your child and for you, at least initially. It may be unclear the ways in which the illness will affect your child's life—you may have questions such as how, how much, and for how long. Not knowing whether your kid will be okay is scary. It is very important for you to find support for yourself.

A prognosis that is uncertain, and a future that is hard to see, add anxiety and ambiguity to a diagnosis both for you and your child. Personally, I cringe when professionals make authoritative prognostic pronouncements about how someone with a mental illness is going to fare in life. I have had many dozens of people at NAMI over the years tell me that their doctor said they would never do this or never do that, and, of course, it turned out not to be true. People can be resilient, find strengths, and often do well over time.

Keep in mind, too, that you are sometimes more expert than the experts. Angelina Hudson is a fifty-two-year-old Black mother of three young adults and a nonprofit leader who now serves NAMI Greater Houston as executive director. She told me she grew up with a dad with untreated bipolar disorder. Two of her children—now adults—had diagnoses of ADHD and, later, bipolar disorder; and her third child was diagnosed with autism. Angelina shared with me what she learned at NAMI Basics that helped her ignore a doctor's very pessimistic prognosis about the future of one of her sons, who was then four years old, and to act like the expert on her child that she was:

> When the doctor said, "What do you want for your son?" I said, "I don't know. He's four. Football, get married, go to college?" He said, "Your son will never do any of that. Your son is on the bottom 2 percent of the population." These were his words. My husband was sitting in the corner just sobbing uncontrollably. And I said, "You know what?" He said, "What?" I said, "I need two things." He said, "What do you need?" I said, "I need my keys and my purse. Where are they? We are getting up out of here. We don't need you. We don't need any of this."
>
> He said my son wasn't going to talk. He wasn't going to learn like other kids learn, and that was true, but he did learn to talk, and he's smart. The NAMI Basics class told me, "You're the expert." But, if they hadn't already put that in me, I would have folded like a piece of paper with that doctor.

Angelina found another way to gather resources and advocate for her son's care through the school systems in her area:

> I went to several schools, and I was pretending that I was moving to all of these really nice affluent neighborhoods so I could get more information, because the neighborhood where we lived, they had no information. I would go to these other neighborhoods, and I would say, "My son, he's not developing. If we were to purchase a home here, what would you do? How would you accept my child into your school?" and those special ed

chairs would then give me a tour of the facility. They would show me what curriculum they used, and I wrote that down. Then I went back to my home school, and when they said, "What do you want?" I said, "I want this. I want this curriculum. I want this device. I don't want a speech therapist from here. I want a speech therapist with these credentials." I got that information from these tours.

Betsey O'Brien of South Carolina is a sixty-seven-year-old mother of two children, one of whom lives with a diagnosis of schizoaffective disorder and autism spectrum disorder. In our conversation, she talked about the importance of persistence and optimism when advocating for her son. "I always tell people when you're working with the schools, with professionals, be the pleasant pest. Just try to get what you need, but in a kind and caring way."

After many hospitalizations and unsuccessful trials of several medications, Betsey advocated for her son to try clozapine, the only FDA-approved medicine for treatment-resistant schizophrenia. Her son's provider was hesitant to prescribe it, but Betsey's insistence that the request be formally added to his record for next time made all the difference when they inevitably returned:

> I typed on one sheet all the times he was hospitalized from age seven up to the last one; how old he was, how long he was there, so they could see that he was a frequent flier. He's going to be back. "Oh, we see that you had asked for clozapine the last time you were here," and it was in the record. The rest is history. Since then, his outpatient psychiatrist has just been amazed at my son's success.

To give you an idea of the kind of people you will learn from if you take the course, Betsey is now a teacher for NAMI Basics.

Professionals can be wonderful, but I wish I could find a way to mandate that they keep those kinds of prognostic declarations to themselves. For example, a teen with a new diagnosis of bipolar disorder may be told that they need to take their meds forever. Forever is a long time, and medicines have important side effects, especially when you are seventeen. For professional and human reasons, it can be hard to simply say, "I don't know how your teen will do, but I will be here along the journey." But if a mental health care provider says that to you, know that you are likely in good hands. Parents must hold the uncertainty along with their teen. It is a lot to bear, which is why support is so important.

• • •

If your child is having trouble in school, either in academic performance or social behavior, you will want to obtain what is called a neuropsychological assessment. Learning challenges, or learning disabilities, are not mental health conditions, but they do also often affect mental health. Children who are struggling in school likely don't know what they are struggling with or why, but they do perceive that they are somehow not in sync with their peers, or not doing what adults seem to expect them to do. They may feel frustrated or angry or sad, act out, or withdraw. Their struggles affect every aspect of life, not just their schoolwork.

The most common assessment tools are given by school professionals or private psychologists. These assessments provide a picture of whether learning issues, executive function or attention issues, or emotional concerns are affecting a child's ability to thrive academically and socially in a classroom environment. They do this by examining the discrete skills and abilities required for learning generally, and by illuminating which ones in particular a child may be struggling with, including whether a child's emotions or difficulties with attention are contributing to difficulties with learning. Based on these tests, a neuropsychologist will make recommendations about interventions or accommodations that may help a child continue to learn and thrive.

Neuropsychological testing may or may not be provided by the school itself; moreover, you may or may not trust the school's interpretation of the assessment. Private testing can be expensive and is not necessarily covered by health insurance. "Learning issues," and in-born neurological differences, are not considered to be health or mental health concerns, so evaluations for them are not considered covered expenses. To get an insurer to pay for some, or all, of an evaluation, the issue must be framed as a medical or mental health concern. Even then, getting coverage can involve a battle with the insurer. You can sometimes access neuropsychological testing for reduced rates, or on a sliding scale, through the psychology department of universities or hospitals in your area.

What you learn from a neuropsychological or mental health assessment may help you get a sense of what your child seems to be struggling with, but it may not answer every question. Openness and curiosity are valuable attributes in sorting through the pieces of information you gather. Coming to understand and diagnose what is going on very often involves an iterative approach, over time. Because kids are developing and moving through developmental stages, a snapshot taken at one moment in time may be hard to interpret; but put the individual frames together and the movie tells a bigger story.

Mental health issues that first manifest when kids are young may stay with them as they mature and can morph into other diagnoses. To the extent that symptoms are related to delays or difficulties in normal development, they can also fade as kids grow, master developmental challenges, and figure out how to surmount or compensate for differences or deficits. Professionals can have a hard time drawing diagnostic lines for kids and teens, and sometimes different clinicians diagnose the same symptoms differently. An individual's diagnoses may also change over time, to the frustration of all. Many parents I've spoken to reported that getting different or changing diagnoses for their children at a time when they were desperate for answers and effective help was a confusing and at times demoralizing experience.

Another challenge is that there is significantly less research focused on young people. But despite these many negatives, as a psychiatrist working with youth and families, I have seen many young people get better. Regardless of the diagnosis, as they developed neurologically, emotionally, and socially, or developed greater awareness of their mental health condition and learned strategies to manage it, there was a natural flow toward health. My work with families often reminded me of the power of a loving foundation in kids' ability to surmount wired-in challenges and learn the skills they need to thrive socially and academically. Knowing that your child needs help and intervening early significantly increases the odds for a good outcome. It's important to remember that you don't need absolute clarity in order to help your child. Many techniques, interventions, and family strategies work across multiple diagnoses.

Once you and your child know they are struggling with a mental health condition that interferes with their ability or willingness to attend school or to learn, or that has led to self-harming or dangerously defiant or illegal behavior, it may become necessary to engage with the school to develop a plan that makes sense. As is the case with everything related to mental health, school resources differ from district to district and state to state.

Step 4: Access and Leverage School Resources

When a child has a learning difference or disability related to that condition, you will have to work with their school and school district to get your child the services and supports they need.

The availability of resources varies greatly by school district and by state. The NAMI Basics program devotes one of its six classes entirely to navigating school and state mental health systems. It explains and helps you understand what your child is entitled to from the school system in your state and the different types of educational accommodations that are available but not always easily accessible. Public schools are required by federal law to provide children a free and "appropriate" public education, and that extends to students with learning or behavioral health challenges. The two primary laws that impact children with special needs are the Individuals with Disabilities Education Act, or IDEA, and Section 504 of the Rehabilitation Act. It can be confusing and overwhelming to understand these, so I encourage you to learn more in the NAMI Basics program.

You can request that your child's school meet with you and evaluate your child for the need for special services and accommodations that will allow them to have a better learning experience at school—which decreases the overall frustration that your child may be experiencing. It may be something as simple as permission to have a longer time to complete tests or other assignments, or something more involved, such as a full evaluation to determine if the challenges are severe enough that an Individual Education Plan (IEP) is required. It's important to know that NAMI and other similar organizations can help you navigate this path to support you as you advocate for your child. The first step is understanding that you are your child's best champion, and to do that effectively you have to be able to understand what's involved.

Parents often need additional mental health information and tools to work with schools as well as with their own children. Educators, psychologists, and mental health professionals all speak somewhat different languages, and the parent often must interpret and integrate these worlds to get their child the services and accommodations they need. Monique Owens, a fifty-four-year-old African American Christian mom of six adult children and grandmom of eight, found that she didn't have a way to articulate her son's needs to his school until she found NAMI Basics, which helped her learn how to advocate with the school system for his 504 plan. She figured out how to read neuropsychological testing on her own. As she told me:

> If I didn't have NAMI Basics information, it would've been much more challenging to get help for my child. I felt I needed to be a diligent parent. Since I didn't want doctors talking over my head, and I didn't want advocates talking for me as if I wasn't there, I had him tested and read the entire report (along with a dictionary, of course) because I had to educate myself on what my child was going through. It was important to his development that I embraced the tools that NAMI teaches.

One of them is to advocate for support, so I incorporated the help of his teachers because he qualified for a 504 plan. I had to educate them about his capabilities and limitations in addition to whatever his mental challenges were. The major obstacle was that the school system only acknowledged the ADHD diagnosis. They wouldn't address his other learning disabilities. So, unfortunately, they were only partially giving him what he needed to be successful in his academics.

. . .

Middle schools and high schools differ in terms of their sensitivity to mental health concerns and in the resources and support they offer. A well-functioning school culture and resources can help students identify mental health symptoms and provide guidance in how to seek help if needed. When schools offer counseling support and a welcoming environment, it can change lives. That was certainly the case for two people I talked to.

Haley Amering, who described her success with DBT for borderline personality disorder in chapter 4, remembered feeling that there was something not quite right about how she felt around the time she went to middle school:

> I noticed when I was around ten, eleven years old, that there was something going on with my mental health. I just didn't have the terminology and wasn't able to articulate it. I would say I really started piecing everything together—that it was a mental health issue—when I was around twelve. The way I can describe it is that there was less energy and excitement. Time was moving really slow, but then not moving at all. I was just aware that I didn't feel as happy and bubbly as I once did when I was a younger kid, even though I was still very young.

It wasn't until she started middle school, the sixth grade, that the school's counseling services did outreach. Haley recalled:

They helped me become more aware that I could go to a trusted adult that worked at the school, and that I could talk about whatever I was going through, because middle school is not the most inviting time for children.

Every grade had a guidance counselor. I was lucky enough to meet mine early on in my middle school career. That was a huge protective factor and it saved me from going through a lot worse things because I had that support and outlet. I would say that what helped me realize more clearly that there was something going on with me was the outreach that my school had at the time and the staff that they had surrounding mental health.

It is common for students not to be able to identify or name their own experience of mental illness, but when they keep that experience to themselves it can present a safety risk, especially given the disturbing rise in the frequency of teen suicide. Being able to name the experience can be an essential first step in the process of expressing one's feelings and seeking help. I talked with one woman who realized that she had a particular mental health condition through a school presentation.

Diana Chao is a Buyi Chinese American immigrant in her early twenties living outside Los Angeles. She is the founder of the largest global mental health nonprofit for youth, called Letters to Strangers, and reports she lives with bipolar disorder. Diana told me that early on in her mental health journey, her school's suicide prevention programming was key in helping her identify her experience and ultimately seek help:

I think it got to the point in high school where I started to seriously consider self-harm and suicide, and I was like, "That doesn't necessarily seem like it should be happening." And I remember, we had this one school rally where they brought in a psychologist to talk about suicide prevention and stuff, and he was mentioning these symptoms, and I was like, "Yeah, wait, I do that." And then that's when I started to realize maybe there is something going on.

Haley and Diana were fortunate. While schools in general are becoming more aware of the need to cultivate awareness of mental health concerns among both students and faculty, they can and may be interested in doing more. Schools that do not have this capacity can utilize a free NAMI program—Ending the Silence (ETS)—if they want to proactively approach mental health from a first-person perspective in their health curriculum. You, or your teen, may want to encourage their school to host it.

ETS is a fifty-minute presentation about what mental health symptoms look like in youth. It's designed for middle and high school students but is also available in a different version for families and for school staff. Now NAMI's fastest growing program to date, ETS is presented by a parent/caregiver and a young adult who not only provide basic information, but also share their personal experiences of mental illness with students. One of the hallmarks of the presentation is letting students know when it is not okay to keep a secret. It emphasizes how important it is for them to notice what is going on with their friends, and to help them begin to get the help they need.

I spoke to someone who could have used the program when he was a student with emerging mental health and substance use issues and has found purpose as an adult in presenting it to others. Mike Smith, a thirty-seven-year-old who lives in Wisconsin, told me he has presented Ending the Silence to every single school in his local school district— over two hundred presentations in all. He helped many students discuss and understand mental illness, and teachers have welcomed him to come for repeat visits. "I get a lot of silly questions about what bands I like, or what books I like to read," Mike told me. "Once you get a couple of those out of the way, then they really start to open up." He described what he feels, talking to teens:

> I think the greatest feeling is when someone comes up to me after class and wants to talk; needs to talk, really. They need to talk and feel comfortable enough to talk to me. That is an amazing feeling. And because

I've gotten to know a lot of the teachers in the county, I hear from them after my presentation, "Oh, we had a student come in who said she's been struggling with this for a long time, and now she's willing to go get help." And before my presentation she wasn't asking for help.

He remembered specific moments where he heard from teens themselves about making an impact:

I don't remember the first time it happened, but it happens almost weekly. I'll go to a grocery store or McDonald's, and someone will say, "Hey, I know you. You came into my sophomore year health class." Or "My brother told me about you, he had you in his class." Other people tell me how what I had to say impacted them or a friend. I've heard, "I had a friend who had a lot of anxiety problems and wasn't sure what to do, and after we saw your presentation, she went and talked to the school guidance counselor." It's amazing.

Brenda Hilligoss, an Illinois parent of a son who had mental health challenges, is one of the people who helped develop NAMI Ending the Silence. She explained to me how her experience as a parent informed her approach in the curriculum design:

Because my son was a freshman in high school, too, I knew exactly who the target audience was and what they would respond to; and to be interesting, not authoritative. In class, there would be so many hands up—kids asking questions or sharing their personal stories like, "I just got out of an inpatient for OCD" or "my brother has so and so"—that we could not get through them all.

We took advantage of the infrastructure already in the schools, and at the end of the presentation we introduced kids to the school social worker or directed them to the counseling center. "Hi, I'm Joe Smith. I'm a counselor. I'm right down the hall." Often, their offices would be flooded, they would have a line out the door.

Brenda went on to recall a powerful moment early on:

We were at a high school and a teacher handed me a letter. "Dear NAMI, I just want you to know I saw your presentation about mental illness, and it made me think of my brother. And so, after the presentation I went home and talked to my mom, and we went and got him help." I still keep that letter.

More and more schools are seeing the need to add a mental health module to health class. To learn how to introduce Ending the Silence in your school district, contact the NAMI in your community or state.

Step 5: Care for Yourself

Being a parent of a child with a mental health condition can be worrisome, sad, frustrating, infuriating, and stressful. It is inevitably exhausting. Getting better care for your child—being a treatment advocate in a system that is overworked and understaffed—is only one of the many roles you may have to fill.

You know that the best thing you can do for your child is to create an open, accepting, stress-free environment, but that is probably going to remain an ideal that few can reach. There may be some days that look like that, and I hope you can recall them in harder times. Parents often have different opinions about what to do, and different ways of managing this stress. This can create conflict in a marriage or within the family. I have sat with many parents where the wife has a rich support network, and the husband speaks only to her. This won't usually help with family dynamics. I have encouraged many fathers to get support outside their marriage to add a pressure-relief valve.

The parents I interviewed told me they also had to learn to take care of themselves to go the distance for their families. Telling an overwhelmed parent during a crisis to take time for themselves can seem like just another ridiculous task to do in an overfilled day. Perhaps when the crisis has abated this perspective can be of use: You are worthy of time and self-care.

Some parents told me they found meaning in advocacy for mental health causes, but for others it is important to do other things that matter, such as pursuing their own interests, nurturing their own career, maintaining their own friendships, and being there for other people that they love. Many found that taking care of themselves provided a healthy separation from their kids. They learned that being unhealthy won't help get your kid on the road to health, and a choice to truncate or limit your own life won't help your child learn how to live a fulfilling life of their own.

The Resources section (page 389) lists many places to look for information as you begin your journey as a parent of a child with developmental, behavioral, or mental health challenges. You can start by reading about collaborative and engaging approaches to dealing with an urgent behavior issue, before or in the absence of a particular diagnosis, such as *The Explosive Child* by Ross Greene; or find books that are helpful if you have a particular presumptive diagnosis like ADHD or anxiety. Some books and workbooks are directed to teens and offer techniques for learning how to manage their experience themselves, which is optimal.

Helping a Young Adult

When a child turns eighteen, the equation can change substantially. For some adult teens, legal autonomy doesn't change much: the mental health conversation continues as before, and they welcome parents into their care as appropriate. For others, autonomy and legal rights change what parents can and cannot do, and what information they can and can't access. Young adults may move away from home to college with legal authority over their own medical records, and confidentiality laws can knock parents out of the information loop. Some kids may withhold information from parents and are now within their rights to do so. Unfortunately, their newfound legal autonomy coincides with years that have risk for mental health and addiction issues. This transition when a child turns eighteen, which may render parents unable to communicate with providers or institutions even to provide information that could inform treatment planning, or to participate in that planning, often comes as a surprise. If your teen is in care, the transition from teen to adult care in mental health practices or systems can be full of dropped handoffs. This adds another level of burden, confusion, and frustration and can feel like starting over again. Chapter 13 includes some guidance on managing the legal rules of communication for college students.

Young Adults in College

Many adult teens go to work after high school; we discuss workplace culture in chapter 10. Many go to college, an environment which offers different challenges in mental health. Colleges vary greatly in their ability to provide assessment and care for their students. It can be hard to assess a college's capacity from the outside in the frenzy of applications to multiple schools, but once your adult teen is admitted, it will be useful to know what the chosen school does and does not offer, and then to engage in planning based on your child's needs.

There are many conditions that appear in the years before, during, and right after the college years. Problems that may develop in the teen/young adult years include anxiety disorders, major depression, bipolar disorder, OCD, eating disorders, psychosis spectrum issues (including schizophrenia), borderline personality disorder (this may present with emotional dysregulation and self-harm behaviors), and substance use disorder. This phase of life carries risk. Keeping the conversation as open as possible is key as your child goes away and the college effectively becomes your child's guardian. I am not an advocate of "helicopter parenting," but I believe issues of safety and mental health are important to share openly, to facilitate collaborative problem-solving. Some students may get the help they need at their university's counseling center. Some schools do not have this capacity, which requires more problem-solving between parents, adult teens, school authorities in some cases, and often with insurance companies.

Miana Bryant is a twenty-five-year-old African American woman who is currently pursuing a master's degree at Howard University School of Social Work and working as a registered behavioral health technician. In our interview, she described the onset of her depressive symptoms:

> I had just left Maryland and moved to North Carolina to go to school. It was my first time being away from my family ever in my life. Then, my second year of college, my high school relationship ended abruptly. That's what started it; I thought it was just a reaction to a breakup and me taking it hard. After the first month, once I noticed that I still had no desire to do anything, very easily being able to cry—at that point, I started to feel like maybe it was about something else. Even then, I still kind of just brushed it off. Now, once we got to the third month, that's when I realized that, okay, there's something more going on here. The catalyst that made me realize I needed to go speak to someone was that I sat in my dorm room for a week. I didn't go to class. I didn't go to see friends. I sat in my bed for a week with the blinds closed watching *Criminal Minds* from season one all the way through, and all I ate was M&Ms. By the end of that week, I kind of realized, something is going on here.

Miana went on to share how she found help through her school:

> I went to the student health center on campus. Once my doctor ruled out any physical ailments, she recommended and referred me to a psychiatrist. I told him how I was feeling, how I'd been locked in my room for a week. And he immediately diagnosed me with major depressive disorder and general anxiety disorder. Then I was put on an antidepressant. And that began my journey on diagnosis and medication.

Reflecting on this experience, she shared two pieces of advice for other college students:

Number one would be, don't believe your dismissive thoughts: "It's not that big of a deal; it's not something that you should bring up to people; it's not that important." It is that important. It is that big of a deal. And trust yourself, your true self. Trust in the person that you feel is being lost in the fog.

And number two, I know it's not easy for everyone. I was at a college with mental health resources—where it was relatively easy. But you can log on to Google and take a self-diagnosis test. Talk to somebody, like your doctor. Bring it up to somebody because you never know who's able to help. You would never know what opportunities or what resources somebody has access to that may be able to honestly help you.

Miana started a mental health club called the Mental Elephant at her college. She named it to convey the message that mental health is often the elephant in the room and that students need to talk about it and support each other.

Early Intervention for New Onset Psychosis

The symptoms of psychosis—seeing or hearing things, fixed false beliefs, excessive suspicions, paranoia—are scary, both for the person experiencing them and for their parents. These symptoms often first appear in young adulthood. Psychosis is itself a symptom, not a diagnosis. There are many possible causes, from being drug induced (e.g., marijuana, PCP, steroids), to bipolar disorder, to schizophrenia and other conditions. It can take time to sort out what is causing these symptoms.

A relatively new, game-changing model of care has been successfully developed specifically for the early presentation of psychosis in the last decade. The model, called Coordinated Specialty Care (CSC), can be found in just under three-hundred programs across the country.

This creative model, also called NAVIGATE for First Episode of Psychosis (FEP), was invented in Australia and is now being adopted in the

United States. This model is strengths-based, goal-oriented, and actively engages the family. I volunteered at a clinic offering this program for five years and saw how well it worked and what a major development it is over old models of care. It was inspiring to help young adults get back on track in their own lives.

For Ky Quickbane and his family, a CSC program was largely luck. Ky, who we met earlier, told me he first experienced psychosis and depression when he came home during a break from college. Ky received strengths-based, compassionate care in his CSC program:

I will credit my psychiatrist at the first episode service. I heard her say, "Our job as psychiatrists with patients who are experiencing psychosis is not to judge." If somebody says there is a danger, say there is a dinosaur coming to eat me, their job is not to be like, "That definitely isn't happening," and confront the patient and that kind of thing. Their job as a mental health professional is trying to figure out what that dinosaur represents to that person. Why is their body going into hypervigilance? As I was asked the right questions by a psychiatrist, by a counselor, those prompts and guidance helped me to have difficult conversations about my identity and my mental health experience.

Ky now works as a peer counselor and advocate. He is working to make the mental health conversation easier both in his daily work and by participating in this book. Matcheri Keshavan discusses this early psychosis treatment model in chapter 18.

Recovery Is Possible

As dire as it can seem when your child is struggling, the odds are that things can and will get better. Josh Santana is a twenty-five-year-old youth community music educator and a real estate agent in Boston whom we met in chapter 4. In his "life-story-so-far," he illuminated the possibility of recovery, how a young person with a complicated mental health history can become a high-functioning adult living a fulfilling and admirable life:

> I got removed from mainstream preschool because I assaulted a teacher during a behavioral outburst. I was four years old and wasn't permitted to return to mainstream kindergarten unless my mom agreed to have me psychologically evaluated and have a paraprofessional stay with me throughout my entire kindergarten year as well. From five years old and on, I was heavily medicated, and a lot of those initial years were a blur.
>
> Very early on I realized that not only did I have all these really challenging behavioral issues, but I was also very cognitively advanced for my age. In early middle school I discovered how much I was excelling academically, having earned perfect scores on different standardized tests for Massachusetts, including in English and Math. But around the time I was twelve years old in the sixth grade, I started developing severe behavioral issues again. I would have disturbing outbursts in the middle of class, often yelling loudly in an attempt to release internal angst. Imagine being so advanced that your academic grades were always A's, but you never made it on the honor roll because your conduct grades were always F's. That's what my time in middle school was like. The dichotomy between my gifted cognitive functioning and my often disparaged, disruptive behavior took a huge toll on me mentally and stinted my formation of my identity.

Josh went on to share that he struggled with managing his depression in high school because he didn't have the proper coping mechanisms. But with time, he started learning some new skills:

> Some of the things that I've learned after harnessing my mental illness is that not everything has to be perfect. If I got a C on a particular assignment, it wasn't the end of the world. I learned to accept the quality of work that I was able to produce at any given time, even with all the other

things I had going on during that same time. I learned to trust that I did have the ability to be as highly academically achieving as I wanted to be, even though the grading structure of schooling isn't accommodating to people with mental illness and how it affects the work they do. I learned that instead of letting my mental illness make me suffer in school by giving assignments either all or nothing, I could accept my best effort at any given time. I learned to use each assignment as a baby step to reaching my goal of earning a college degree.

Now, after twenty years, he told me:

I've learned how to advocate for myself and how to be comfortable finding and asking for support. I've also learned that advocating for others is important to me. I'm currently able to do this by participating in community groups like the Me2/Orchestra [a classical musical organization for people with mental illness]. I want to teach people how to find support, advocate for themselves, and implement strategies to add to their ever-growing mental illness management toolbox.

Josh's story illustrates how important it is to look at the movie of his life and not the snapshot of him in preschool or middle school. He learned and developed tools to make a difference for himself. This kind of first-person perspective is what we will develop in Part II.

PART II

The Recovery Journey: Evidence from Lived Experience

EIGHT

Themes of Recovery: Lessons from First-Person Experience

How do people define recovery for themselves? What are the enduring approaches and strategies that help people sustain recovery over time? In my interviews for this book, I asked those who have lived with a mental health condition how they approached these questions. Many have been living with mental illness for years, or even decades, and have had time to reflect on what made a difference for them in transcending their symptoms—whether hearing voices, substance use, severe mood symptoms, self-harm, or suicide attempts—to create fulfilling lives. They wanted to share their first-person expertise and hard-won lessons in the hope that you or a loved one will find them useful.

I believe that you can learn from what helped someone else and, at the same time, acknowledge that one person's experience is not everyone's experience. What worked for the people in this chapter may not work so well for you. To discuss what helps people in their recovery is also not to deny that many people who live with mental health conditions don't have such positive outcomes. In Part III, family members share their experiences of coping with the problems that arise when a loved one cannot see that they are ill, living with someone who deals with overwhelming symptoms, and dealing with the loss of a loved one by suicide.

The stories in this chapter are not, however, unrepresentative. Many people do well over time. In multiple studies of people with diverse diagnoses, people report that their quality of life has gotten better as they age. For a young person with severe, confusing, and overwhelming symptoms, it may be reassuring to know that the full-length feature film of their life with a mental health condition is likely to be more upbeat and positive than a snapshot would be. Recovery is possible, but the stories are largely untold.

There is no one right way, or single path, to recovery. While everyone I interviewed had a unique perspective, some consistent themes emerged from their stories. These recovery themes aren't focused on the tactical tools like medication, peer support, psychotherapy, or engagement in a spiritual or faith community employed in the first stages of the journey that we discussed in chapter 4. Instead, they have to do with broader, philosophical approaches to living that develop through use of those tactical tools—through reflection, spiritual and emotional growth, and the attainment of greater self-awareness. "Both/and" thinking—leveraging wisdom and tools both from and beyond conventional mental health care—continues, with more *both*s and more *and*s.

After having the privilege of hearing so many people's different lived experiences of recovery, I chose to frame them in the light of a few broad themes that consistently came up. They include acceptance, a journey orientation, self-determination, developing belief in oneself, belief in something bigger (faith), looking inward to be present, and looking outward for community and purpose.

Acceptance

Many people describe acceptance as a critical and challenging element of recovery. Like recovery itself, acceptance is a process—something that happens in increments over time. How difficult that process is, and how long it takes, is different for each person, but it is rarely fast or easy for anyone. It is hard to let go of our idea or image of who we are, and the kind of life we expected or wanted to have, and embrace the reality that we have a mental health condition; that we may have challenges to meet and burdens to bear that we didn't ask for; that we may not be entirely in control of our mind or of what path we take in life; that we can't change our genes or erase a traumatic event or force ourselves to be "over it." This can be a major threshold people struggle to cross, and in the course of recovery, you may have to cross it again and again—when a treatment doesn't work, when symptoms reoccur, when pain returns, or when a mental health condition impacts progress in work or relationships with friends or family. The problematic prejudice surrounding mental health conditions is also a significant obstacle to acceptance.

But our interviewees also recognized the paradox that acceptance is very often a prerequisite for change. That "dialectic" is the foundational insight at the center of Dialectical Behavior Therapy (DBT), created by Marsha Linehan, which guides participants toward "radical acceptance." It is also a core tenet of 12-step programs, in which meetings often open or close with a recitation of Reinhold Neibuhr's "Serenity Prayer": "God grant me the serenity to accept the things I cannot change. . . . "

We can work our way through and beyond painful feelings—whether they arise from a mental health condition we wish we didn't have, or any other reality we are powerless to change through force of will—only if we acknowledge them and accept the reality that created them. Only by accepting reality, do we (again, paradoxically) achieve some detachment or separation from it; this frees up our energy and opens up the possibility for change, including a change in the way we see and understand ourselves.

Kurt Mihelish of Montana has been a volunteer for Meals on Wheels for many years. He has a community, a family, and a best friend who shares his passion for finding treasures in pawn shops. He told me he also has come to know that even with good treatment, he will still hear voices; and that he will continue to deal with other people's discomfort about his illness. In his view:

> If you can deal with the stigma, and you can accept the facts and realize, "I'm going to be like this for the rest of my life," you can move forward and find some happiness. You don't have to be a CEO of Google to consider yourself recovered. Just find some little things in life, some happiness, and some people around you that are cool with you. You don't have to conquer the world.

Kurt has transcended negative social attitudes by accepting them. He described his experience of being interviewed for this book as liberating. To be open about his lived experience is another step on his path toward recovery.

Robert Cubby, the police officer we met earlier who spoke about his PTSD, now works to train others in the law enforcement community to deal with trauma. He also sees acceptance of a new reality as one key to moving forward. He explained that that message isn't always easy for others to hear:

> What is recovery? Being able to resume. You're not going to get back the life you had. But you can resume a life that's acceptable to you; you can function every day in comfort and do everyday tasks without things springing up and hitting you. I keep hearing time and again: "I want my life back the way it was." It's never going to happen. You're never going to be the person you once were. That is the death of that version of yourself— and that's really hard to accept. And some of them refuse. They don't want to hear that, and they lock into what they want to do. And they need to make that breakthrough. Recovery is making that breakthrough.

As we saw in chapter 6, there are new and creative approaches and interventions for handling the aftermath of traumatic experiences.

Robert's point is that once you accept that your life has changed as a result of the trauma you experienced, you can find those ways out.

Journey, Not Destination

Mental health conditions are rarely short-term events. There are no cures. The illnesses can wax and wane, and serious symptoms may recur or be ever present. Many people have found a way to turn the long-term nature of their condition into a strength, by adopting the perspective that recovery is an ongoing journey of learning.

Liam Winters is a white man in his twenties and a former NAMI employee living in Arlington, Virginia. He spoke about how both he and members of his family live with serious mental illness. Liam has already learned to reevaluate what recovery means, and that his condition is best seen through a long-term lens:

> It's important to see it as not a linear process where "I had this difficult time in my life and then I just got better." It might be great for a lot of people to see someone who struggled and got to the other side, but I think a lack of discussion about the nuances can be harmful to people like me, who feel well, and then feel bad, and then well again, and keep going through that cycle.
>
> I think if I'm doing better over time with my mental health condition and with being happy—viewing it not on a month-by-month basis but over the long term—that would be recovery. And that's something I've also gained—just that perspective. Even when I'm really depressed now, I know it's like, "Something's happening in my brain. I can't really control it. I'll feel better soon."

Christine Yu Moutier is a half-Asian, half-white psychiatrist and the chief medical officer of the American Foundation for Suicide Prevention. Christine, now in her fifties, lives in New York and is married with two young adult children. Mental health advocacy and suicide prevention is her life's work, stemming from personal lived experience and multiple losses to suicide in her professional life. A leader in promoting access to mental health services and openness in the medical community, she is very open about her own experience of taking a year off medical school on a mental health leave. "I'd say recovery is an ongoing process of healing and discovering and practicing new strategies to thrive," she told me. Christine went on to say:

> I don't really see it as a linear or "one and done" construct. Some people do reach certain goals and milestones in their recovery that are very significant and important. But in my own life, it's been phases of change and growth. And it requires a lot of humility to be strong enough to face it, to face the feedback and the truth about what vulnerabilities are still present, and what I still need to do to keep managing them.

Dante Murry of Kentucky is a forty-nine-year-old African American who is recently married and the father of three and stepfather to his wife's three children. He works as a teacher, facilitating multiple support groups for NAMI. Dante, who told me he lives with schizoaffective disorder, described recovery as a journey that is both individual and cyclical:

> Recovery for me is person-centric, because each person's coping skills are different. It's holistic. For me, speaking from my lived experience of how recovery helped me, it's cyclical. It's like a wheel—a life wheel. In one phase, you might be at one part of the spectrum. And next thing you know, the situation changes. And the thing is, you might not be at a low, you might be on a high. It just depends. Recovery is an ongoing process.

Self-Determination

In many of my interviews, people reported that deciding for themselves what they want—having recovery goals that are self-defined and self-determined—was an essential aspect of recovery more generally.

Kristina Saffran of California is the twenty-nine-year-old cofounder and CEO of Equip Health, a company that provides virtual treatment for eating disorders, and the cofounder of Project HEAL, a nonprofit that works to ensure everyone with an eating disorder has the opportunities and resources to heal. She told me that since recovering from anorexia, which started when she was a teenager, she's made it her life's mission to ensure that everyone has access to treatment that works. In reference to her own recovery, she told me:

My brain used to be entirely consumed with food, weight, and calories. There was no space for anything else. For example, I would panic before going out to dinner, scanning the menu to make sure there was something I could eat, and cancel plans with friends if something wasn't on the "safe" list. Now, when I make plans with friends, I don't care where we eat, but am focused on the company and conversation. My life is so much bigger, and I'm not going to sacrifice my values to fit a certain size or see a certain number on the scale.

Haley Comerford, who shared in chapter 5 how she became addicted to OxyContin in her teens to self-medicate her anxiety, told me she has successfully stayed sober by setting goals for her recovery that are both simple and profound. "My goals are to stay clean and to die clean," she told me. "As morbid as that sounds, I think that's the goal, to not die from something like heroin overdose or suicide, but to die clean."

Self-determination isn't just about setting goals; it's about deciding who you are and what your relationship is to your own mental health condition and recovery. Many people find that over time, their mental health experience evolves from being a dominant force in their lives to one that, though still important, is less central. This process does not have to take decades.

Laura Fritz, a TikTok creator in her twenties from North Carolina, is a stay-at-home mother of two who has also experienced an evolution in her sense of herself as a person living with bipolar disorder. I found

Laura after she made a video for Mental Health Awareness Week describing her own experience with bipolar disorder to her followers. She finds that her growing family is helping her place her mental health journey in perspective:

> In the beginning, I felt like having bipolar disorder was a huge part of my identity, something that I would think about constantly. I would think, "What is this group of people going to think if they find out?" Or I associated just the illness and the diagnosis with who I was. Now I feel that, while it still is a major part of me, there's so many other things that come first. It's become just something that I have to manage.
>
> The most helpful things for me are the medicine and the support. For me, I need medication. Finding the right medications changed my life. My parents and my husband are my greatest support systems. Even though they can't fully understand, they empathize with me, and they just have a lot of compassion for my situation.
>
> People on TikTok, they see me as Lena's mom, or just Laura, someone who creates fun videos. One of my worries putting out that video was, "Is this going to be my label now?" But I don't think it is. Recovery to me is getting back to being yourself. Like when you go through a mental health crisis, it's like you almost lose part of yourself, and you struggle, and you doubt and suffer. Then with recovery, it's like you're getting back to who you were before, or even better than you were before.

Believing in Yourself

Multiple people told me that as mental health conditions cause changes in emotions, thinking, perceptions and/or behavior, they can make it hard to believe in yourself. Many discussed the process of developing trust in and love for yourself as vitally important in their recovery journey. They each found a different way to get there.

Emma Winters, a twenty-five-year-old white woman who lives in New York City and works as communications manager for a nonprofit, was diagnosed with bipolar I when she was in college. She described the on-set of her condition this way:

> It's not overnight. It takes a long time. To me, I think the most important part of recovery, maybe besides medication, was just really learning to trust myself again; to trust the decisions that I made for myself as a young adult. I always was very self-aware, but especially after the manic episode, it became more like self-doubt: "I don't know if I should take this job because it might be too stressful." Or "I don't know if I should live by myself because maybe I'm too vulnerable for that." I think recovery for me is getting to the point where I really feel like I know what's best for me, and that I can take care of myself, not in a lonely way where I don't reach out for support, but in a way where I feel confident in my own choices.

For Nancy-Lee Mauger, self-love evolved as her views about mental illness itself evolved. She told me, "The day you realize you can love yourself, that for me is recovery. That's when I was able to stop believing that I couldn't be fixed. Nobody can fix you; you have to fix yourself. The minute that I could say, 'Hey, this is what I am, this is my physical body, this is my emotional mind, all of these things, I still love myself.' I'm fifty-eight years old and I think maybe just last year I started to love myself."

Trevor McCauley, who we met earlier, noted that gaining trust in his own ability to take care of himself involved acquiring the kind of perspective that comes only over time. When I asked him what recovery meant, he responded:

> In one word, it's *growth*. When you're first diagnosed, your problems are "What the heck am I going to do when I wake up in the morning?" Growth means here are different problems and challenges. And the way I look at it is, if you don't pass the test the first time, the first year, the first month, you're going to get another one sooner or later, and you're going

to have to learn how to pass the test. But you'll always be given another opportunity. How I view growth is you eventually pass the test, and you move on to a new test. There are so many situations that I am presented with today, that ten years ago I would have just walked out that door.

Belief in Something Bigger: Faith and Spirituality

Many find that having a set of philosophical principles to live by, a spiritual practice, or a religious faith is critical to mental health recovery. Some had a strong spiritual or faith orientation prior to the onset of their mental health condition, and some developed it afterward.

Spirituality and religion have been important to Elisa Norman her whole life. An African American single mother of two who grew up in southwest Atlanta, Elisa told me her experience of mental illness began at twenty-five after the birth of her son, when for the first time she experienced delusions and heard voices from God. These symptoms, and their religious content, added complexity to her understanding of faith:

> At one time, I was going to the hospital and telling everybody that Jesus was coming. And they were like, "Yeah, okay. Yeah, right. Whatever." But when I get to church, and I hear the pastor say, "Well, Jesus is coming," it's like, "Well, why are *you* not in the hospital?"

Elisa told me it took her until her most recent hospitalization to fully sort out her illness experience and her spiritual self, and to resolve the dilemma she'd been wrestling with for eighteen years:

> I realized that even when I'm taking my medication on a regular basis, every now and again I still hear God; and that might just be my spiritual side. I could be a very spiritual woman also living with bipolar/schizoaffective disorder. At one point, my thing was, "I need to tell everybody." And then I realized, wait a minute. Some of that stuff might be just for me. It's like when a superhero gets their superpowers. In the beginning, they don't

know how to use them. I call my spirituality my superpower, but I had to go to the hospital to learn how to navigate through it.

Elisa has integrated her spiritual superpower with the real knowledge that she also has an illness, and that she can manage this illness to have a full life with her faith intact.

Michael Hauck of Connecticut developed a faith perspective during his experience of managing a long-term mental health condition:

The only way one can really overcome mental illness is to get to know yourself. I immerse myself in thought and prayer. Contemplation, mindfulness, and a desire to know you need a higher power or God, if you will. It's part of who I am. I love to be contemplative and get to know myself.

I have a deep desire to express myself, what I've been through, and what I can do to bring strength to other people who are struggling; just letting them know that they're not alone and they can get through this. I would just hold their hands and let them know I've been to the exact place that they're at, and that it's very dark, but light always wins. I would tell them, "Love brings the healing. You're on a journey, and you're going to make it through this. Your heart will know the most glorious, splendid gift of God. Trust yourself. Just trust yourself."

Janet Berkowitz, who we met in chapter 4, has lived with suicidality and bipolar disorder for decades. Now her mission is to work to support other people who have these challenges. Here is how she explained it to me:

I do believe that all of us are here for a divine purpose. All of our purposes look different. Just because I live with a mental health condition does not mean that I can't fulfill the purpose that I have for my life. My partner, Phil, taught me to see recovery as being in a place in which you accept whatever mental condition you're living with and whatever experience you're having in the moment. It's more than acceptance. It's remembering that who you are is pure love.

Kenya "The Visionaire" Phillips, of Georgia, is a forty-six-year-old African American widow and single mother. She is also a woman of faith who, as she describes it, "embraces her village while living, eating, and breathing a lifestyle of recovery and resiliency." In her professional life, she is a writer and the manager of two of NAMI's national ongoing support groups. Kenya told me that she lives with bipolar disorder and found a way to reconcile her decision to take medication and her faith in God:

Faith connects to mental health so heavily. I'm Christian. I'm a 100 percent believer. I come from seven generations—all the way back to the plantation—of Methodist ministers. I'm in ministry myself, but what I struggled with was the issue of, do I take medication? I struggled with it because it seemed so unnatural. I felt it was a force outside of the norm. . . . I can take a Tylenol for that one moment—that's not ongoing—but when I was told I might have to take medication the rest of my life, I struggled with that. Because it meant to me, okay, my mind is no longer mine.

However, over time, I started to look at stuff differently, meaning that, if I'm a believer, then why wouldn't there be people out there who are serving in their vocational call to help me get better? Just like I'm a writer, and my writing is meant to offer prophetic healing that can help someone else feel better. My lens shifted; the way I perceived things shifted. In the process, I became more accountable to my well-being.

Staying Present

Many of us struggle to stay present in a world full of distractions. Yet the theme of being present and participating in life came up in many of the conversations on recovery. Philip A. Lederer, a community health center physician, musician, and educator living in Massachusetts concurred, but he sees the relationship between being present and recovery through the lens of his passion. He told me:

It's mindfulness. It's being present in the moment. Our life is a melody that we're playing on the fiddle. It's going all over the place. We're traveling around and crashing. Recovery, to me, is if you still have the melody. You pop all your strings, and your bow wears out, there's no more melody. But as long as you can keep playing that melody, it's pretty good.

Looking Outward: Recovery with and for Others

People look not only inward but also outward as they think about recovery. Recovery with others—and for others—can be transformative. Many people clearly acknowledge the role of community in recovery, and of both receiving from and giving to others.

Jeanne Porter, of Arizona, told me how following her experience with postpartum depression in the mid-1960s, she helped to start a support group, an initiative that made her an early pioneer of peer support. This group later morphed into NAMI Montana. For Jeanne, the importance of connection is also integrated with her faith:

> Recovery helps us understand that we're all in this together. That we're meant to reach out to one another. I'm kind of a "Jesus person," so I believe in reaching out to other people. And I feel like I have helped people understand that we are special regardless of whether we have trouble with our mental health. We're worth a lot to one another and to the world. Love one another. This is who we're meant to be, don't you think?

Carole Furr, a fifty-one-year-old white, married accountant who plays the French horn and lives in Vermont, told me she suffers from anxiety and mood disorders and has noticed the value of giving to others as part of the recovery process. This idea, which is integral to the 12-step model of recovery, is one that the mental health community is learning. As Carole said to me, "There are stages of it and one of the stages that's important is giving back; is passing it on to other people. I think in AA, they say that if we don't pass it on, we lose it. That is maybe a piece that the conventional mental health establishment doesn't have yet."

For Chastity Murry, a forty-seven-year-old teacher and facilitator of NAMI support groups who lives in Kentucky with her husband, Dante, and their children, building positive connections with others and diligently caring for herself are critical parts of recovery:

> My definition of recovery is being able to help others; to inspire others to do good things, and to inspire myself to help others. First, it's about taking care of myself: medications, therapy, trauma therapy, working on coping skills every day—those things are what keep me grounded. And what's inspired me is helping others. My daughter is going to school to be a dental assistant. I feel so honored and so blessed that I can actually help her get to that point. Even though I've got mental health issues, I actually helped her.

· · ·

There are many ways to define and sustain a recovery. This chapter captures only a sampling of perspectives, representing only some of the common themes on how people sustain themselves living with a long-term mental health condition. The most important point is that many do. There are many challenges and few direct routes, but recovery is possible.

NINE

The Power of Peers and Community

J ust as the experience of a mental illness is unique to each individual, so is the path to recovery. But that doesn't mean you walk that path alone. During my interviews for this book, the factors people cited most often as central to recovery were a connection with peers, support from a community, and the ability to give back to others. By peers, I mean people with lived experience who can offer support and education and serve as guides for recovery. These peer connections can be with an individual or a group; they can happen informally or with people formally trained to serve as peer counselors or peer specialists; and they can happen online or in person, in a variety of settings. There is growing research evidence that peer support helps people get better, a fact that will continue to shape services and influence mental health practitioners and institutions. When peers are formally certified and paid as peer specialists, they bring a unique perspective to the workforce.

More critically, peer connection and community support serve as one solution to the major issues of social isolation and loneliness faced by millions around the globe, regardless of whether they have a mental health condition. As many people learned during the Covid-19 pandemic, a lack of social connection can be distressing and have serious consequences for both physical and mental health. Researchers examined multiple studies and concluded that loneliness, social isolation, or both, were associated with an increased risk for coronary heart disease and stroke equivalent to the risks posed by smoking and obesity. Humans are social creatures, with a universal need to feel understood and connected. Yet many do not.

People who live with mental illnesses face even greater risks of loneliness and its consequences—another reason the peer support movement is so essential. Some mental health conditions—particularly in the acute phase of the illness process—specifically reduce social drive and/or impair social skills. Major depression and schizophrenia, for example, can lead to reduced social drive and contact, especially when symptoms are heightened. Panic disorder often leads to agoraphobia—not wanting to leave the house—and social anxiety disorder specifically impacts the ability to be with people. The paranoia often associated with psychosis can make people understandably afraid of others. Manic and addictive behavior can undermine social relationships, hurt people, and may cause major rifts in families. People with mental illnesses often face prejudice and feel shame, which poses another hurdle to forming and sustaining relationships.

But the problem of loneliness for people with mental health conditions is often more structural than it is clinical. There is a national trend to close state hospitals and group homes and promote (a still inadequate amount) of subsidized Section 8 apartments or single residency occupancy (SRO) housing. This disinvestment means that those who are able to find housing, even those few who live in proximity to potential peers, are left without the structure or opportunities to connect that a group program would once have provided. I heard this comment often in my community mental health days: People made connections in congregate settings, and loneliness was the biggest issue they faced in independent living. They still wanted to live independently in most cases, but the problem of developing a social world became paramount. Housing and employment discrimination significantly narrow two major avenues for connection—the home and workplace. The prison system is another place people living with a mental illness may end up in lieu of a hospital or group home, where solitary confinement—the ultimate form of structural isolation—is overused to manage people who are experiencing symptoms despite the fact that isolation is well known to cause, or exacerbate, mental health problems.

At the same time, people with lived experience now have many more ways to find connection and community in our society. The peer movement has never been stronger or more vocal. In this chapter, I'll introduce a few examples of remarkable communities that are designed to be inclusive and welcoming; detail the rise of the role of peer specialists; and discuss steady improvement in people's attitudes toward mental health challenges.

Sharing Your Story

There is a great healing power in sharing first-person experience. More and more people in recovery have discovered that power as they listened to others, and then felt empowered to share their own experiences. The people in this book are a part of a growing movement. More celebrities, athletes, and politicians have come forward publicly to share their experiences with mental health conditions in just the last few years than ever before. The culture is changing, and people can feel this change.

Some people have elected to become mental health peer support resources for others, whether in informal settings or by becoming trained peer support specialists. This can happen behind closed doors or in a more public setting. There is no best way.

When Clifford Beers published his autobiography, *A Mind That Found Itself*, in 1908, he was among the first people to share their story of mental illness and recovery publicly. He wrote of his own experience: "As I penetrated and conquered the mysteries of that dark side of my life, it no longer held any terror for me." He was an early first-person experience expert and paved a path for others to follow. His book and his advocacy began an organization now called Mental Health America, which has taken the lead on helping to create standards for certifying peer support specialists. More than a hundred years later, this strategy of sharing continues to empower people.

One of NAMI's most critical internal advisory groups is the Peer Leadership Council (PLC). This group, composed of peer representatives from all over the country, was founded to connect NAMI's work directly with the communities we serve. Jeremiah Rainville of Rhode Island, current chair of the PLC, has been involved with NAMI for half his life. He is also a certified community support professional (CCSP), a certified peer recovery specialist (CPRS), a certified community health worker, and peer program manager at NAMI Rhode Island.

In our interview, Jeremiah reflected on the value of peer work at large, his role in the council, and the chosen family he found through NAMI after experiencing trauma from both his biological and adoptive families:

> Peer work really helped me, because when you go to a hospital, sometimes it's more helpful to talk to your peers than the actual staff. Peer support is amazing, and becoming part of the PLC was an eye-opener; that it wasn't just what I could do in Rhode Island, but what I could do to make sure peers are heard across the United States.
>
> I do think NAMI is like a family. I've actually been living with a family that I met through NAMI, and I've been here four or five years now. For me, that's an accomplishment, that I was able to connect with a family. Sometimes I tell myself, "I really don't like people." But I really do like people. I've just been around a lot of bad people and it's tough to find the good ones.

Sharing Anonymously

While some people become comfortable sharing their lived experience of mental health conditions openly and publicly, others may feel more comfortable sharing exclusively with peers. Peer communities of this kind already exist worldwide, many of them modeled along the lines of the substance use recovery fellowships, AA and NA (Narcotics Anonymous). Anonymous groups specifically for people with mental health conditions include Emotions Anonymous, Double Trouble in Recovery (addiction and mental illness), and Suicide Anonymous.

For Janet Berkowitz, who in chapter 4 described the theater workshop she created called Suicide Denied, anonymity helped in her recovery journey:

> I did not want to talk about suicide in my day program because they were sending people to the hospital when anybody talked about it. So, I had to start my own thing. At Suicide Anonymous we often get people who are close to the edge. We can't report them, because it's anonymous, but we will stay with them after the meeting and support them as peers. In my twelve years, I have found it to be the most helpful way to stay recovered.

If anonymity is important to you, there is likely a community you can access that honors that approach.

Intentional Communities

An intentional community is designed from its outset to be welcoming to people with lived experience and to promote connection. Examples range from intentional communities affiliated with NAMI and club-houses, to pop-up bakeries and community orchestras. This is a growing movement toward inclusive and accepting communities, and you are more likely now than ever before to find one that is a fit for you.

NAMI-Affiliated Peer Communities
Of the many NAMI programs, there are several that directly engage the community of people with lived experience. (There is also a large peer community of families at NAMI that we'll discuss in Part III.) NAMI has multiple peer-focused courses and support groups, including NAMI Peer-to-Peer, NAMI Connections groups, and In Our Own Voice

(IOOV), where two people in recovery tell their story to audiences at businesses, hospitals, colleges, and elsewhere, an experience that has great impact both on the people who speak and on their listeners.

For many years after its founding, NAMI focused its education and support efforts on families. A watershed moment came in 2000 with the launch of the Peer-to-Peer Recovery Education Course, the outgrowth of a program first developed and piloted by Kathryn Cohan McNulty, a sixty-six-year-old mother and grandmother who lives with her husband, Jim, in the northwestern corner of Rhode Island. Kathryn graduated with a BS in behavioral science and came to the mental health field first as a provider. But her knowledge of the medical model and years of graduate-level fieldwork were also informed by personal experience of serious mental illness and involvement in peer activities. She brought it all together by developing the Peer-to-Peer course. She told me how it began:

> My husband ran a support group and I used to go to it faithfully, with other people who were living with the same things that I was, the social and psychiatric problems, the brain problems, the financial problems. I had two small children at that time, and I wasn't doing the dishes, and someone was like, "Oh, you could use paper plates." And oh my God, that changed our lives forever. And that was one of a thousand lightbulb moments that occurred during my time in that group.

Kathryn knew peers had a lot to teach one another. As she thought about the model that would become the course, she recognized the value of a scripted, structured approach. She thought it would work because as she recalled, "People with mental illness, typically we have executive function problems, memory problems, staying on task/focus issues—not all the time but at various times. So, a script overcomes all this if people are trained to use the script to teach others." She also knew that making the Peer-to-Peer course part of NAMI would be a process, given their longtime focus on programming exclusively for families. Fortunately, the course was well received, and the integration of the peer voice was strengthened within NAMI as a result.

Nikki Rashes of Illinois, a wife, stepmom, grandma, and mental health advocate, who shared about accepting her own diagnosis of bipolar disorder after learning about family history, found that NAMI In Our Own Voice provided a space where she could share her experiences in a way that was both healing and empowering:

When I went through the training, that was my first experience being in a room with people who I knew had mental health conditions. These were people who understood it and could talk about it. I remember sitting in the hotel room that night at the training and everybody joking about their experiences in the hospital and where they had been. It was kind of that dark humor that people outside wouldn't understand. And it was like, "Wow, I found my family here. People get it."

And then I did my first presentation at one of NAMI Metro's general meetings. My voice shook through the entire thing. It was liberating, an empowering feeling. But at the moment, it was absolutely terrifying and made me feel so vulnerable. People came up to me afterward, and especially family members told me, "You gave us hope," or "We hope our child can reach the point you're at." It was just heartwarming. And I think that's where the empowerment came in, knowing I could make a difference to somebody.

For Kimberly Comer, it was mandated that she attend an IOOV presentation as part of her release after years of incarceration and hospitalization. It was there she found hope. She spoke to me of the power of being a participant in NAMI's peer-led programs:

I went because that was the only way I was going to get discharged. And to my surprise, that group was life changing. Because at the age of forty-eight, they were going to discharge me to go live in my car. With no plan. I had no life. Nothing to go back to. I'd destroyed everything, again, and had no energy to put it back together. I knew when they let me leave with those prescriptions, that I was going to take my life. That was my plan.

Somebody had a different plan, because that group I was required to go to was where I was introduced to NAMI, which helped me go from treatment-focused to recovery-focused. The young lady that shared her story about recovery, she had a diagnosis very similar to mine. She was married, had a home, children. She was going to school for social work. She had a life, and for the first time in my life, I had hope.

Clubhouses

While NAMI is one good way to find a peer community, there are many others. One is a physical place that exists in many countries and most American cities: the clubhouse.

The first clubhouse was created in the early 1940s, when a group of people who were inpatients at a New York state psychiatric hospital began to meet for mutual support. A self-help group of that kind, inside a psychiatric facility, was highly unusual if not entirely nonexistent at that time. Participants were interested in continuing to meet outside the hospital after they were released. Michael Obolensky, a former patient, and Elizabeth Schermerhorn, a former hospital volunteer, led the first official "outpatient" meeting of their group, which they named WANA (We Are Not Alone). They later changed their name to Fountain House, after supporters helped them purchase a building in Manhattan distinguished by the small fountain outside. As they created a growing community, they chose to call themselves members, not patients or clients, as they had been called at the state hospital.

WANA and Fountain House are the origin story of the modern international clubhouse movement. Today, such clubhouses are open to anyone with a serious mental illness and can be found in over thirty countries and at more than three hundred sites. The clubhouse model is an environment expressly designed to combat the social isolation that people living with mental illnesses often face. Clubhouses offer connection, free membership, support, employment opportunities, and an invaluable peer-based community. I was impressed when visiting one clubhouse in Boston, where members regularly send cards to people who have been out of touch to remind them that they are part of a community and to let them know they are missed.

Christina Sparrock, a fifty-four-year-old Black woman living in New York City, spoke to me about the acceptance she feels in her clubhouse community:

> Once I became a member of Fountain House, they found me a support system to help me with any issues that I may have. I love just being myself and not pretending to be well all the time as I had to do in other environments. I think it's more about building relationships, meeting people where they're at. Whether it's when they're well, becoming unwell, or in a crisis. I think it's important to build that rapport and trust with individuals. It's about empowering peers. In many programs, policies are created top-down, from management. I always say, "No, no, no. It has to be from peer up. It's about us." Right? And we know how best to engage with other people who look, walk, talk, and act like us. We speak the same language.

The clubhouse concept has been adapted and has inspired other ways to suit the needs of particular communities. Rosemary Ketchum, an elected official, mental health advocate, former NAMI employee, and proud trans woman in Wheeling, West Virginia, helped to spearhead the creation of a drop-in center in her local NAMI office:

> The drop-in center really came out of the idea that many of the folks who we were serving had housing insecurity and were not connected to doctors, and they needed a safe place to be outside of their camps or shelters. That blossomed into more structured advocacy, and a nine-to-five, five-days-a-week center. Rather than just being a place for people to hang out, it became a place where people can talk about their lived experience and share their perspectives. And then we would have various groups and

professionals come in to help and make referrals to various health care resources in the city.

It became a staple in a very short amount of time because most of the other services our homeless or vulnerable communities would receive were incredibly transactional. It was, if you need something to eat, you go, you grab it, you leave, you go someplace else. And that's it, because through no fault of their own, many of the organizations were based on efficiency: the more folks we can serve the better. NAMI's approach was just dramatically different. It was: Please stay. Please take up our time. We want you to be here with us. And that was a shift for the folks we were serving—that we weren't trying to kick them out after lunch, and we asked them to stay.

Creativity in Common

NAMI, the clubhouse model, and other groups, such as the Depression and Bipolar Support Alliance (DBSA) and Mental Health America, are some of the older and more recognized peer-led support groups and spaces. But people around the country are also using creative arts already commonly employed in service of recovery—art, theater, music, baking, and more—to gather like-minded people with and without mental health conditions in supportive spaces where all are welcome.

For example, the Me2/Orchestra was created in Burlington, Vermont, in 2011 by Caroline Whiddon, who remains executive director, and conductor Ronald Braunstein. The orchestra, which now has affiliates in Boston and Manchester, New Hampshire, bills itself as "the world's only classical music organization created for individuals with mental illnesses and the people who support them." It is a peer community that has had an enormous impact on the musicians who have joined it, including writer and flutist Susie Seligson, who described it as "a whole orchestra of people who were moved to be there for that reason, and then they made beautiful music. It's magical."

The Orchestra was also magical for French horn player Nancy-Lee Mauger, who spoke of the courage she saw in those around her: "If you're struggling with mental illness, if you don't have courage, you must find it somewhere. You show up to these concerts, and you watch your fellow members open their hearts to people and tell their stories, and it gives you a little bit more courage. Even if you can't do it yet, you're eventually going to believe that you're okay."

Conductor Ronald Braunstein had the experience of becoming a beneficiary of the open and welcoming community he'd helped to create. "When he was depressed, I had to practically drag him to the rehearsal," Caroline Whiddon recalled. Ronald remembered a pivotal moment:

> I just instinctively went to the middle of the room, and I said to the players, I'm in the middle of a depression. Can you help me get through this rehearsal? There was such a feeling of like, "of course." I mean, what other conductor could publicly share in a rehearsal something as stigmatized as mental illness and not be thrown out? That was really something else. And they stuck with me.

Pop-Up Baking Communities for Depression Awareness

In 2013, Emma Thomas came up with an idea both to raise depression awareness and raise funds for a mental health charity in the UK. She called her brainchild the Depressed Cake Shop and invited people to come bake together and sell their confections. It quickly caught on, inspiring over two hundred pop-up events around the globe and evolving into a virtual, intentional, peer community that facilitates local and flexible involvement by its members, local bakers who want to join the mission. DCS brings together community and the idea of behavioral activation—doing things that elicit positive feelings.

Valerie Van Galder, a woman living in California who works in the film business, serves as president of Depressed Cake Shop Foundation. She spoke in our interview about the solace she found in this peer community:

> I had been caring for my father for five years, as he was experiencing severe mental health issues, when I discovered that baking and decorating cakes

helped me manage my mental health, which was beginning to suffer. A woman in LA posted that she wanted to do a Depressed Cake Shop and I decided to partner with her. I had a feeling that this project was going to give me solace, but it turned out to be more than that—it was one of the best nights of my life. The experience was exactly what our world needs: people in community eating together, sharing their experiences, and raising money to support those working in the mental health space. It was beautiful.

She recalled that word spread through social media efforts, and shops started popping up around the world. As a 501c3, all their funds are donated to the local charities, and they provide communities with a branded fundraising apparatus. Valerie went on to say:

Most of us never imagined that mental health was something we would ever share so openly. Almost every day I get a note from someone who has discovered that baking really can be therapeutic. It is really a magical organization. Anyone who's ever organized a shop is changed by the experience. I can tell you with certainty it changed me, and I actually believe it may have saved me.

Sascha Biesi, the chef and baker we met earlier, hosts events and shared how the Depressed Cake Shop provided a strong sense of hope and community:

As I became open about telling my story, and was going on the news, people were coming in just wanting to talk about their own losses or their own kid or friend or family member. It was really a cool experience because, through that, I really felt like it was okay, what I've been through. It all made sense in that moment. We turned our entire bakery into a Depressed Cake Shop for the whole month. There were plaques hanging on the walls with inspirational quotes and messages like, "You are not your mental illness," and "You are beautiful." We had artists hang art that was relevant. We had a little jar with a note pad so people could leave or take notes of hope. You knew you were somewhere different when you walked in, because we have this big window painted with the quote, "As long as there is cake, there is hope, and there's always cake." That was when people really started to let their guard down and connect with us on a much deeper level. I decided that if I can accomplish everything that I've accomplished while dealing with a mental health issue, I can provide people with hope. Instead of hiding mental illness, being ashamed of it, and thinking people will judge me for it, I decided to flip the narrative.

The Rise of Peer Specialists

Peer connection happens organically, but it has been increasingly valued as a paid professional service.

Clarence Jordan is a Black man from Tennessee who works for Beacon Health Options, a behavioral health company. He is an advocate, veteran, and father. He spoke to me about the inclusivity of peer support in recovery and the early days of the peer movement in Tennessee:

My mentor Michael uses language like that—"We." It's always inclusive. And it lit a fire underneath me. I want to be inclusive when I talk about recovery, because we are going through this together. I began as a peer counselor, and I ran into a bit of difficulty with that. I was told I needed to quit the job. And I said, "Well, why?" And they said, "Well, it's a conflict. You're a patient. You can't be providing treatment for someone else who is also a patient." And I thought, well, that's not true. Nonetheless, I was directed to resign from the position.

Michael wasn't going to accept that. I told him, "I'm a patient. And I can't work providing support for other patients." He said, "That's bullshit, Clarence. I do it every day. I run this place."

It wasn't long after that the Tennessee mental health consumer association came calling. They wanted another board member and wanted to know if I wanted to serve on their board. I said sure. It was during those early years that we put together a very enlightened department of mental health and substance use. That's essentially how the peer movement here in Tennessee began.

Clarence shares more of his story and explains how you can begin the process of becoming a peer advocate in chapter 17.

The peer movement may only recently have been given a name, but it is not new. People have long found peer communities helpful. When he was in the hospital, Lloyd Hale found many ways to connect with peers. Later, he became a peer specialist himself. He reflected on his early experience benefitting from peer support, and on his own role as a peer specialist:

> We would gather all the patients and staff together, and we would discuss issues we would love to see changed to better our experience in the state hospital. Or we would use that time to talk about things that were going extremely well. Even though the peer support title hadn't been invented, the best help that I received was peer support in the hospital. When I became a peer specialist, I never saw myself as knowing more than the people I was helping. I saw myself as learning from them just as much as they were learning from me. I never looked at my recovery and thought, "I arrived and I'm here." It was an exchange for me.

The mental health field was slow to recognize that peers can make a huge difference as professionals helping others in therapeutic settings. Not only do they supplement a strained workforce; they offer something medical professionals often cannot. Their experience needs to be valued— and compensated. Georgia was the first state to fund certified peer specialists (CPS) through its Medicaid panel. Many other states have followed suit, and advocates across the country are working to expand payment for peer services.

Brenda Adams of Kansas developed mental health symptoms and described how she used her experience of needing help after giving it to become a professional peer specialist:

After seven years of working with the state hospital, I lost my job, I crashed. When I went back to the mental health center, the same individuals that I worked with before helped me out. I saw peers that I worked with at the state hospital, and they were very, very kind to me.

Being a certified peer specialist, you help the next person navigate through the mental health system and get what they need, and get the right supports and resources. We want to be viewed as professionals as well. I do a lot. I'm in the area where I see people I know from years ago, and if I can help them, I will. If I have a few minutes to listen, I will. If I have a couple of dollars and they're hungry, I will offer it.

Tera Carter, a forty-six-year-old Black woman, is a certified peer specialist and mother of three living in Atlanta. She works for Georgia's mobile crisis team and is now the alumni coordinator at Skyland Trail mental health treatment facility. She is the second responder along with a clinician on 988 crisis calls and provides the compassionate perspective only a peer can offer. Tera told me:

I use my judgment as it relates to me sharing my experiences. Like, say we're assessing someone, and they have a mood disorder, and they say, "I'm never going to be able to get better." That's when I step in and say, "Oh no, no. You can get better." Then I tell them my experience, and they're like, "Are you serious?" To which I say, "I'm very serious. I've been in crisis; I've lost just about everything and had to rebuild; I've had to find the right medications."

She added, "It really gives people hope. It gives them hope to be able to see that it is possible to do better. But I also make sure that I share that it requires work, it requires commitment, and it requires consistency. You have to hang in there."

Many find this mission compelling in its potential to change the system. Patrick Kaufmann of Michigan described how and why he was inspired to become a peer specialist:

I thought, "Wow, you got the perfect job. You get to hang out with people, tell them about your recovery, get them excited, and get paid for it." So I started by volunteering in places, doing whatever I could. That was magic, to suddenly feel like I had something of value to offer. Also, I think I was angry with the mental health system. This was a way to create some positive change out of my experience; to be involved with the system but have a positive influence on it.

George Kaufmann, Patrick's father, a seventy-nine-year-old retiree living in central California, shared with me a memorable moment in Patrick's mental health journey: "One of the things that Patrick said one time was, 'I used to look back on those first ten years and think it was a lost decade, but now I realize those were the qualifications for my job.'"

Another person whose work helping others gives him purpose is Ray Lay. Ray is a formerly homeless, honorably discharged US Marine who told me he lives with a dual diagnosis of schizoaffective disorder and substance use issues. One of my favorite interview moments with Ray was his description of what peer work means to him:

I get compensated, but it ain't about money. It's the satisfaction of working with my fellow vets and watching them change their life. That's a payment that you can't go in your pocket and give. You got to go in your heart and give that. And a lot of them have paid me like that: the satisfaction of helping to train others to become peer support specialists. There were many, many days I used to say, "Why me? Why am I hearing these voices, why?" For many days, I did not accept my condition. I wholeheartedly embrace it now. The service and the purpose, they work hand in hand because, through the service, I found my purpose. And also, I believe that's one of the biggest ways of how I have been able to maintain both my stability and my sobriety. It's a medicine that I don't have to take the top off.

• • •

My good friend Mike Kahn—a psychiatrist who loves his family, teaching, learning, and baseball trivia; who, in other words, is a peer of mine—asked me over lunch one day what I learned from the many interviews I conducted for the book. The answer I gave was simple and clear: the power of peers. In all our training, studying with some brilliant researchers and clinicians, we hadn't learned this basic truth of how people can make a difference for each other.

As Ray Lay so beautifully articulated, purpose and peers are a medicine you don't have to uncap. The Resources section for this chapter offers some ideas on where you may find a community that offers you this critical medicine, with no side effects.

TEN

Culture and Identity: Barriers and Opportunities

The topic of different cultural approaches to mental health and illness, and what that means when it comes to getting help, came up in many of the conversations I had for this book. In addition to racial and ethnic identity, culture also contains many other dimensions that interact. Every setting in which people have some shared identity or reason for coming together has a culture. For example, sexual orientation and gender identity intersect with race or ethnic identity; economic class intersects with religious identity. Workplaces have a culture that can impact employees and mental health access.

Culture can present barriers to care—for example, when mental health care workers don't speak the same language as their clients or have biases (conscious or unconscious) about people of different faiths or races. We already saw in chapter 5 how the cultures of addiction recovery and mental health recovery can clash, though they are becoming more integrated over time. Culture can also provide sources of strength and healing, such as a strong sense of community, that help people stay well and feel connected.

Many of the people I interviewed for this book were born or raised outside the United States or at least influenced by a culture and heritage other than those born and raised in the States. I learned a lot from them about how they experienced their cultural identity, religion, or workplace and how that had an impact on their mental health journey. Culture can evolve. Many people told me they felt things were changing for the better when it comes to their interactions with mental health practitioners and institutions, which gave me hope that we are making some progress in the field.

While culture is not limited to race and ethnicity, it is important to address the unique hurdles and challenges people of color experience in navigating a health care system designed by and for white people. My conversation with Tracy Green, an African American woman from Texas who grew up in the South under difficult conditions, illustrated how the larger American media culture broadly and the culture of psychiatry specifically were unwelcoming for one person who needed help.

Tracy's childhood and adolescence were plagued by poverty, alcoholism, domestic violence, and sexual abuse. As an adult diagnosed with mental illness, she found herself in another kind of difficult environment—a psychiatric hospital in Texas:

> I was diagnosed with major depression and also dissociative identity disorder (DID). And all I knew, and all people would refer to, was *Sybil*, and: "Black people don't get DID." There is no one else that I can compare myself to. It took the movie *Frankie & Alice* for me to finally say, "Okay. Okay. So I'm not the only Black person." I know that was [a] fictionalization of a real person. Halle Berry played the part. It was twenty years into my diagnosis before I got to see somebody that looked like me, that I could relate to. Do you how crazy that is? It was another level of validation. Believe it or not, even in the hospitals . . . after four or five hospitalizations, I was the only Black person and had a nurse, the only other Black person I saw, say, "What are you doing here? We don't come to the hospital."

Tracy experienced neither representation nor a welcoming, culturally sensitive inpatient environment. And the lack of trust, stemming from institutional racism, that Black hospital staff members shared with her is further evidence of a failure of psychiatric culture.

Medical and Psychiatric Racism

Before I share more first-person experiences, I want to frame the conversations with some basic information about the reckoning within the medical and mental health professions on their history of racism, which is, belatedly, just beginning.

There are many examples of abuse of people of color that have flowed from racism in the medical and mental health fields. One notorious example is the Tuskegee experiment. The US Public Health Service withheld treatment from Black patients with syphilis in order to study the untreated course of the disease. This infamous experiment represented a profound breach of trust by national authorities and by the medical profession. Astonishingly, this study didn't end until 1972, and its negative impact on trust continues today. I heard this understandable suspicion when Covid-19 vaccines were introduced and people of color with personal or family experience of medical abuse asked me whether the medicine, and the people administering it, could really be trusted.

Professional responses to the problem of systemic racism have been very slow to materialize. The American Medical Association waited more than one hundred years to formally apologize to Black doctors for excluding them from their organization. In 2021, after the murder of George Floyd, virtually every professional society related to mental health came out with a public apology about their role in supporting systemic racism. The American Psychiatric Association notes the risk today of misdiagnosis of people of color by white doctors, and it describes in its apology the many examples of its own failures and its long-standing participation in systemic racism. In their 2021 apology, the American Psychological Association cited many of their own failures as well. That same year, the National Association of Social Workers (NASW), the organization representing the most common type of practitioner found in the mental health field, also acknowledged they have been complicit in racist practices. These organizations have established work groups to address these issues, and you can access information about their work and statements of their findings through their respective websites. But for many who have lived with the consequences of this racism or had to form their own professional associations because they were excluded or ignored, these recent statements and related action plans have been criticized as too little and too late.

This history has had, and continues to have, important consequences for people of color, among them delayed access to fewer, sometimes inadequate, and often culturally insensitive services, resulting in poorer outcomes in mental health care and health care. Rising youth suicide rates for youth from underserved populations (for example, among Black and trans youth) are one likely by-product of this cultural failure, though there is much more to learn on risk and protective factors for young people.

In this chapter, people share their experiences of mental health and illness through the lenses of race, ethnicity, gender, sexual orientation, and some other cultural factors like religion and the workplace. While the people interviewed for this book are all currently living in the United States, many originally came from or were strongly influenced by cultures of other nations, including Japan, China, India, Nepal, Germany, Ecuador, and Spain.

As noted, the mental health care professions still have a lot of work to do to ensure they can deliver equitable and culturally informed mental health care to all. Our blindness, conscious and unconscious biases, and failure to develop a sufficiently diverse and cross-cultural workforce have been problematic, but hopefully we are improving. How do various groups of people think about mental health and illness, and about seeking help or treatment for mental health conditions? What does culture contribute to encouraging or discouraging people to seek help or cultivate peer support? I was impressed at how similarly people approached mental illness across many parts of the world, as well as by some particular and specific cultural differences.

I'll start with a person who had different cultural experiences within her own family. Corinne Foxx, who we met earlier, told me that while both sides of her family worked to support her to get the help she needed, their approaches differed:

> I'm biracial, so I have an African American family and a German American family. I feel like when I first told my African American side that I had anxiety and panic, their gut instinct was, "Well, we don't talk about that. We've all had those feelings too and just don't go public with it." They thought all these terrible things would happen if I revealed that. I went public anyway, and, instead, I found so much love and positivity. That has opened up communication within my own family, too, about their own struggles.
>
> It wasn't the same on my mother's side of my family, which is white. I went to my mom first, and though she had never reached out to a mental health professional before, she was super open to it. She went to my appointments with me; she dropped me off. She saw that I was struggling. My mother's side of the family was a lot more receptive to talking about what they were going through, too.
>
> Overall, I did feel like there was a bigger fear on the African American side of my family to talk about their pain. I assume that it's a learned behavior of protection, from being oppressed in so many different ways and not wanting to reveal one more thing that could hold you down. So, I can empathize with them. And when it got to the point that I didn't want to go to school, I couldn't function, I think a parent does everything they can to help their child. Then my dad was super receptive as well.

Within what might look like one culture to outsiders, there can be many nuances. Jonathan Ordonez, a twenty-four-year-old, cisgender, gay Latino man from Trenton, New Jersey, described the difference in how the two sides of his family approached mental health:

> I'm blessed with my family. My maternal uncle had very serious depression. It got to a point where he was having suicidal ideations. And that

side of the family was very understanding because they had to quickly learn that he has no choice over whether he's feeling depressed or not. My mom's side of the family is from Spain, and I think they're more open to talking about mental illness. My dad is Ecuadorian, and that side tends to have a very difficult time understanding depression.

Despite the many different cultures of my interviewees, there were many commonalities in their stories. But there are also distinctive differences, even within families of similar cultures. That's why professionals need to work with each person on their own terms, without preconceptions about their culture or identity.

Sukhmani Kaur Bal's experience of South Asian culture affected her perception of her own mental illness. A twenty-eight-year-old Punjabi-Sikh woman from Berkeley, California, Sukhmani told me how she initially struggled against the cultural framework that shaped her family's understanding of mental health challenges:

I remember being in the library one day at school, and I just happened to be flipping through this book, and it listed the symptoms of depression. I was like, "Oh my god, that's me." As an eleven-year-old, how do you start processing the fact that you have a mental illness, especially when your only exposure to people with mental illnesses is like *Law & Order: SVU*, where people who were different were "crazy," "evil," or "scary"? I thought, I must be evil or scary.

I brought it up to my parents and there was this incredible resistance from them that anything could be wrong. I remember very clearly them saying, like, "These are white people diseases. These are problems that white people have; they're not problems that Indian people have. You just need to work harder. You need to study and focus on school." Like it would just go away. Indian culture is very heavily focused on status within the community. Anything that detracts from that status needs to be corrected, and that correction comes at any cost.

Kumi Macdonald is an Asian and Christian woman living in recovery from depression and anxiety and supporting family members who also have mental health conditions. A wife and mother of three, she was born in Japan and raised in California. Kumi described the cultural expectations around discussing mental health that she grew up with:

I remember telling my mom, "Mom, I think there's something wrong with me." And she said, "You're going to be all right. If you can verbalize that, you'll be fine." And that was kind of how our family resolved things. In Asian culture, we have to always have this "Suck it up. Be tough because we're fighters" attitude. I think coming out of the war, people had to survive to build up their economy and build back their culture. And then being an immigrant, we thought, "No, we have to be strong. We can't show weakness. Keep going."

This fighting spirit is what is in a lot of Asian Americans, and also a shame of saying we're weak or vulnerable, which is really looked down on. And so oftentimes my parents would be like, "Come on. Suck it up. You can do it. We can do it." And that's how our family survived the move, and all of our day-to-day struggles. Part of the culture is this high level of perfectionism.

I was interested in how similar Kumi's experience of her culture's approach to mental health was to that of longtime NAMI benefactor Jutta Kohn of Connecticut, who is of German descent. Jutta felt her culture's approach contributed to the delay in her getting help for her son. She recalled:

When I think back, there were so many telltale signs that our son was struggling, but growing up in Germany, you just get up and you move. Finding sympathy for a child being behaviorally off wasn't in my DNA, nor in my mother's. When my mother had cancer and was in a hospital, there was a young man who was there for a psychiatric illness. That's when it struck my mother, "Oh, my God. This is real." It was the first time she really understood that this isn't just a matter of "Come on, get going." It's a matter of: There's something wrong.

Jutta's mother, the "tough German," finally saw that there was something there.

Gender, Sexuality, and Intersectional Identities

Culture is continually evolving in many dimensions, including how we conceptualize gender, sexuality, and the roles of both in our identity. Thus, gender roles and sexual identity also affect the mental health journey. For example, we know that women seek help more than men. Men also have higher rates of death by suicide. Members of the LGBTQ+ community, especially transgender and nonbinary folks, experience certain hardships at a higher rate, including homelessness, eating disorders, substance use, and suicidality. The adverse impact of these factors can be compounded when the person is also experiencing stress as a consequence of racism, socio-economic class, or a problematic living environment. The Trevor Project offers a variety of resources on suicide prevention for the LGBTQ+ population.

Several interviewees I spoke with reflected on the role gender and sexuality have played in their mental health journey, either as barriers to overcome in getting help, or as protective factors that helped them find a supportive and accepting community.

NAMI Ambassador Brad Gage is a writer, host, and comedian who currently produces a video series aimed at finding better models of masculinity. He shared his experience as a straight, white, Midwestern guy overcoming the stereotype that seeking help is a weakness:

My most important journey has been gaining the understanding that I have been socialized in a particular way: seeing emotions as weakness and seeing the idea of asking for help as weakness. In many men's or boys' minds, weakness is the antithesis of manhood. But the more help I've asked for, the better my life has gotten. I grew up learning from key figures in film and TV and from my father. I saw myself as, "the more masculine you are, the less help you need, and the more you're able to bottle up your emotions, the stronger you are." But it's not always great if there's things going on in your life that would be helpful to share. Going to therapy, it can be a punchline. There's a stigma there. Now I think the culture is absolutely improving. The Rock goes to therapy, and who's more masculine than him?

The "toxic masculinity," as it has come to be called, that Brad describes is not exclusive to Midwestern American culture. Jonathan Ordonez also discussed his experience of "machismo" within his Latino family, and how it relates to toxic masculinity and mental health:

I've seen that Latin American countries are very big on machismo, which is toxic masculinity in Spanish. It is just this idea that men must act a certain way. Men aren't allowed to express emotion; they're not allowed to be depressed. It's kind of expected for the woman to be emotional, and for them to be sad. I relate it back to the period when there was a diagnosis of hysteria they'd give to women. A lot of times, that's what men, and even other women, will equate it to—they won't say it's mental illness—they'll say, "She's crazy." And I think a lot of that has to do with stigma, but also it intertwines with the language. Older generations of Latinos, especially, don't have the language to say, "Let's talk about mental illness," or "I'm willing to listen to you."

Jonathan's best friend and partner in mental health advocacy, Roselin Dueñas, is a young, first-generation American, Hispanic, queer woman. She described two other language barriers:

Language is definitely a barrier I have encountered in my mental health journey. Sometimes I don't know how to express myself to my family properly because I don't know the right words in Spanish. When I would

want to bring my mom to therapy to hear me out, I would be stuck trans-
lating, as my therapist didn't speak Spanish. This would lessen the experience for me and defeat the purpose of having a third party involved, as I
felt my sessions were not as helpful as they should have been.

Despite the barriers, Roselin has still encouraged her mother to open
up and talk more freely with her, with the acknowledgment and understanding that mental health wasn't talked about in her generation:

> Culture has a big influence on why people don't speak about their mental
> health. I know from what my mom has told me; she's opened up a lot
> about her own issues with me—we actually have so many common
> struggles—but she never spoke up about it with others. She told me, "My
> mom wouldn't give us a safe space for us to talk about it. So, I didn't know
> how to." Knowing this, I try to be more understanding of her difficulties
> in accepting my mental health conditions. I know it's difficult for her to
> be here and understand, but she is trying, which I appreciate.

Language, however, is just one barrier to care inherent in the lack of
diversity among mental health care providers. Kristina Saffran, introduced earlier, is working to change the cultural conversation around
who eating disorders affect. Her mission, which guides the company
she established and the eating disorder recovery programs they offer, is
inspired by her recognition that many people with eating disorders and
their families feel excluded by the current culture of treatment. She
explained:

> About 40 percent of folks with eating disorders are men, much more than
> folks recognize. I think, unfortunately, a lot of the ways that we've con-
> ceptualized eating disorders, the language we use around wanting to be
> thinner, not loving your body, it presents differently in men. Oftentimes,
> men want to be more muscular, become obsessed with the gym, things of
> that nature. It's obviously going to present differently.

But unfortunately, if you Google eating disorders, I would bet 90 percent of the websites you're going to find are clearly geared toward women, which sends a strong message to men of "I'm not wanted here." And frankly, it's bigger than men. It's anybody who doesn't fit the stereotype of a young, white, thin, cisgender girl. If you're trans, if you're Black, if you're older, if you're in a larger body, they go to these websites and they're like, "I don't see myself. I can't have an eating disorder."

We've been intentional about changing the cultural conversation and showcasing the diversity of eating disorders at Equip. We make sure that our company and providers reflect the true diversity of those who struggle: We have males, people of all races and ethnicities, transgender and nonbinary folks, and people in larger bodies. In our marketing, we use illustrations that showcase that diversity, in addition to neutral colors and testimonials from those outside the stereotype.

A mental health care provider sensitive to issues of intersectional identity was critical to Ky Quickbane. Ky shared with me how a first-episode psychosis program, with a provider who accepted and celebrated him for his trans identity, helped him to accept himself and become well enough to begin his journey as a peer specialist:

I had, for all my life, suppressed the more masculine aspects of myself. And I don't in any way think tangible evidence is required for people to be transgender; however, if somebody wants to express their gender, it's important. I think the problem came as I started to question my perception of myself, my circumstances, how my parents never really let me be fully who I was supposed to be.

When I was younger, there were no trans men in the media, ever. I had no examples that it was okay to be a more masculine-assigned-female-at-birth person. So, a high level of stress came from my perception that there was something in me that I could not change for the sake of my parents, or for other people. I started to go haywire.

As Ky's mental health continued to deteriorate, his mother enrolled him in a first episode psychosis program:

> The first episode psychosis program gave me a support system to not only be seen, but to embrace the parts of myself that I had suppressed for so long. My experience as a trans person is absolutely interlaid with the mental health system and how a person gets treated. Because I'm not only somebody who sometimes hears voices and sees things that aren't there; there are other aspects of my life that other people are not going to have experience with, as well, and that is okay. But as I met more people in the mental health system, as I was asked the right questions by a psychiatrist, by a counselor, those prompts and guidance helped me learn how to have difficult conversations.
>
> I was just like, "Please, for the love of God, recognize me for the parts of myself that want to be alive and that want to be recognized and expressed." Because for so much of my life, I had been beating myself up; I didn't know that there was any other way. And I'm just fortunate enough to have had people there to—when I start taking too many steps toward the cliff—grab my shoulders, and just lightly touch me, and not ask, "What's wrong with you?" but "What happened to you?"
>
> What I am now is somebody who *wants* to be here, and not just to communicate and to celebrate and to experience all the lovely things in life that I couldn't see before. My role, my thread in the tapestry of human connectedness, is to help people realize that there are resources and reasons to stick around, because we don't always have the road map.

The intersectional nature of cultural barriers to mental health urges us, once again, to treat the individual as a whole person, acknowledging all the parts of their identity that have contributed to where they are in their mental health journey. Whether your gender, sexuality, or other identity has served as a barrier or as a protective factor, it is a piece of your story that should be recognized, affirmed, and factored into the care you receive.

Broadening Definitions of Culture

Wherever people gather in groups, they may form specific cultural views on mental health. Anywhere there is culture, there can be cultural barriers around a topic, such as mental illness, that's prone to provoke shame. I'll discuss a few key arenas relevant to how people interface with mental health—in the workplace and in faith communities.

Workplace Culture

The workplace is another dimension with which people in groups think and talk about mental health conditions. Some organizations offer support and are proactive; some are still ignoring their employees' mental health. During the pandemic, I saw a great surge in the number of companies and organizations interested in attending to their employees' mental health, though each work environment had its own approach. Leadership at work is a critical variable that creates the culture people work in.

One person I spoke with had two very different experiences with work culture. Wendy Ascione-Juska, a white woman in her midforties from Michigan who has bipolar disorder, told me her first employer did not help her or work with her in any way. Later, she found a workplace that was fully supportive:

> I had been at a nonprofit for a couple of years, and I was in a manic state. I left and went home to Michigan for a couple weeks, came back to work, and was immediately put on probation. I was told I can't bring my personal life into work. My schedule was restricted and my work was closely monitored.
>
> I didn't ask for a particular accommodation for my mental health condition because I didn't know what kind of accommodation I needed. It was thrown back at me: "You've got this issue, and you need to separate that from your work situation." I understand that philosophy, but, in reality, when you're struggling with something like bipolar, it does impact

your work in some ways. There needs to be some sort of understanding. They pulled me in one day and said, "We just don't think you're able to do it, and we're letting you go." I was very angry. I thought, "This is really unfair."

When I had my second manic episode a year later, I was working at the University of Michigan, and it was a completely different work experience. They wanted me to get well. They knew that I was sick, and that I needed to take some time to regroup. They let me take a few weeks. The first day back, I was just answering emails and taking it easy. The dean of the school said, "We just want her well," and that was the same thing my supervisor said to me: "We want you well."

In chapter 17, attorney Ron Honberg discusses the Americans with Disability Act and how to ask for accommodations in the workplace.

Religious Communities

In previous chapters, we've heard some people share how religion and faith communities have made a positive difference in their recovery journey. That community can be strong and healing. There is a group called NAMI FaithNet, for example, which gathers people of all faiths to create support for people who are interested in the role of spirituality in recovering with a mental health condition. Other people spoke about experiences where organized religion had discouraged people from accepting their own challenges, or from seeking help for themselves or for family members in ways other than the practice of faith. Of course, there is a difference between a religion, per se, and the congregations, groups, faith leaders, or imperfect human beings who gather to share or observe it. It's not the religion itself, but rather the particular religious community that may be more or less supportive.

Angela Brisbin, a forty-seven-year-old mother of three who lives in Missouri, is an administrator for an online clozapine support group and a full-time college student working to become a psychiatric nurse practitioner. Angela, who is also actively involved with NAMI of Greater

Kansas City, has an adult son, Michael, who was diagnosed with schizophrenia at age nineteen. She recalled in our interview how she lost precious time in seeking an assessment or care for Michael because of a lack of mental health awareness and training in her church:

> He had some major changes happen; rash behavior. He lost interest in school; he didn't want to hang out with his friends. He was having prodromal (early stage) schizophrenia symptoms, so he would stay up late for hours. We thought initially that it had something to do with rebellion and teenage stuff. I did speak to the youth pastor about it. He did not understand mental illness either. He thought it was just rebellion and anger.
>
> It would have helped if the pastors would have said, "He needs to see a doctor," because I looked to them for guidance. I was bitter about it, after everything. We might not have wasted a whole year or two years. I believe that prayer is helpful, and God is in control here. But I believe that God created science, and I believe that we're supposed to utilize the medication. It's there for a reason. And I wish that we would have been directed by our pastors early, at some point, and not just been told to pray. I think they need the education. Because what they're doing now is actually hurting people.

Cultural barriers can prevent individuals and communities from developing an integrated perspective on mental health, which in turn leads to delays in treatment. Early treatment is a good idea in virtually all instances. Fortunately, Angela helped Michael, now twenty-four years old and a college student, get good care. He now serves on the board of directors for NAMI of Greater Kansas City and runs a NAMI young adult support group. He plans to be a social worker after his graduation and work in the mental health field.

Culture Changers and Evolution

Cultural perceptions of mental health and illness are not fixed. I couldn't have written this book and found 130 people willing to publicly share their mental health experiences a decade ago. I heard many hopeful notes in these interviews on how different groups or people were coming to think and talk about mental health and illness in a more open way.

Diane Banks of Texas is a fifty-six-year-old Black doctoral student working on her dissertation. She is a proud mental health advocate who wants to see others in the Black community and other underrepresented communities reach a state of mental wellness. Diane told me of the importance of her faith, saying, "I know that had it not been for my faith, I wouldn't have had the fortitude to push through." She went on to share how a new understanding of mental health conditions is just beginning to transform attitudes among Black churchgoers:

I grew up the granddaughter of a pastor, so in our house, we didn't talk about mental health. It was always, "Girl, just pray. Everything's going to be okay." In the past two years, in the church that I belong to now, I was so grateful when I heard the pastor talk about mental health from the pulpit. Hearing that message from the pulpit made me feel that I was not alone. And it doesn't really happen much in my community, in the Black community.

A lot of times, pastors and personnel are not equipped to deal with the topic of mental health. A good friend of mine, he's a pastor now, said, "Many times pastors don't know how to deal with this stuff. I don't know if I'm going to make somebody's situation worse, so I just set it to the side," but he affirmed that our Black churches need help as it relates to mental health.

All churches need it, but mainly our Black churches need it because we have a history of not addressing the mental health aspect. Mental health has for too long been thought of as rooted in the devil, or the family just doesn't want shame, so we're going to hide it. One thing that has consistently been brought up was that we've lost a lot in the Black community even before the pandemic, not only in the congregation, but we lost a lot of clergy to suicide over these past years. This has a huge impact on mental health in our Black community, which is why I and some of our church leaders are working hard to bridge all these churches together and bring NAMI in.

Joseph Feaster Jr. is a Black man and an attorney who grew up in East Elmhurst, New York, and came to Boston in 1967 to attend Northeastern University and its law school in 1972. His son, Joseph D. Feaster III, died by suicide in August 2010. Joseph discussed how he, a mental health advocate, is received in the Black faith community and in historically Black colleges when he talks about mental health and illness:

> I think there's now more receptivity within the Black church on mental health. What I try to do with my ministry is to point out to them that their faith counseling may not be sufficient in order to address mental illness. So, I have to help them balance both of those things; a preacher's feeling that they can pray people into recovery, and also recognizing that that is not always what a person will need, particularly one who is afflicted with mental illness.

Lorenzo Lewis of Arkansas is working to create an alternative place for community members to get the kind of mental health support that their church may not yet provide. He is the founder of the Confess Project, which aims to build a culture of mental health for Black boys, men, and their families through a movement reimagining barbershops as safe spaces and barbers as mental health first responders.

Lorenzo found community and support at his aunt's barbershop as a boy, and he realized that the crisis in access and conversation about mental health for Black men in particular could be addressed through barbershops. Lorenzo told me how the Confess Project came to be, and explained why he views education as a pivotal resource for his community:

> I worked in the behavioral health system. That's where I recognized the disparity in mental health for Black people. And obviously, I'd seen it in

myself, after going through some challenges. That's when I recognized that the Confess Project could be started. It is truthfully about showing people that you can overcome, that you don't have to be a product of your environment, that you can use your experiences for purpose, and help bring change to your community.

A huge component of the lack of mental health care in our community has to do with how we were raised and how we view things—our perspective on how families engage wellness and treatment, and how we may view strength as having a religious component or that it means figuring things out ourselves. I think a lot of the resistance or disinterest is learned historical behavior, instilled from day one. Secondary to that is a lack of familiarity and education. The most important thing is that the idea of mental health treatment does not connect to them—they do not understand it, and then they cannot connect because of the lack of education.

On how the barbershop interplays with the Black church specifically, Lorenzo said:

The barbershop and the Black church are very connected. A lot of deacons, pastors, and church members go to barbershops. But there is a comfort in barbershops that does not exist in church. Churches just don't have the same infrastructure barbershops can have. The barbershop is a bridge. It's where anything can exist. We like to say, "Everything can hang out."

When you think about mental health, part of the barbershop is being in the most unapologetic space as possible. We got to have people really feel that they can lean in and say how they feel. In the barbershop, because of that context, that's why I know we can change the world, and particularly change our community, in the way that we respond with mental health services. Our job is to say we're going to educate people, we're going to build community, we're going to provide resources and opportunities. We're going to create a movement and an ecosystem where they can thrive.

The Culture of Mental Health Care

Given the differences among cultures in their approach to mental health and illness, and the complexity and intersectionality within them, are there ways to create better connections between different cultures and the culture of the professional mental health community itself? Several people talked about experiences that illuminate some potential pathways where the mental health profession can evolve, and people of marginalized and underserved cultures can find a better "fit" with mental health professionals.

Some people I spoke with found that having a provider who shared some aspects of their culture was very helpful to them. Christina Sparrock of New York City felt having a provider who was also Black made a difference:

> I was feeling the anxiety in my throat. I was having palpitations and I couldn't figure out why and my blood pressure was fluctuating. What I liked about my psychiatrist was that he was an African American male, and so we were able to talk about the racism in America. We were able to drill down about what was really going on in my life and why I was being activated or triggered. We talked about my childhood, about how race played into my education at school, at my public school, how race played into the media and the news, and my perception of myself, how race played into my workforce experience. Not feeling equal, adequate, or worthy. And I was like, damn, racism is a big deal and it contributed to the deterioration of my mental health.

Sukhmani Kaur Bal also found the understanding she needed in the form of a person from her culture who could also work with her family:

> I was really fortunate because I had a PCP that really advocated for me. And I got therapy, but the issue with therapy was that I was holding a lot back, because I didn't know if I was their only Indian patient, and I didn't want to be some sort of specimen representative of the entire subcontinent.

And this was right after 9/11 happened. I remember thinking, "I don't want them to think my parents are bad people, because of 9/11." I was very worried about the perception of things because at the time, people that look like us were being killed. It was this really scary time.

Because I held so much back and because it wasn't effective therapy, it eventually led to my suicidality at age fifteen. I had planned my attempt, and I ended up in the hospital for a couple weeks. There I met this really phenomenal doctor, who I still talk to. He's sweet, and he is an Indian man. That was a turning point in my treatment because I had an Indian provider talking to my Indian parents, and in a language that they could understand. Their shared history is what got me on medication for the first time in my life. It was that shared history that got me into therapy that was more effective. It was that shared history that really built that trust that I needed to flourish.

On the other hand, when a mental health provider makes assumptions about a patient based on a simplistic or stereotypical view of their culture, rather than seeking to understand the unique individual, it can lead to failures that break trust. Diana Chao explained to me how the nuances of family culture, and having immigrant parents, led to an empathic failure with a mental health provider when she sought help for her mental health:

For physical health, there wasn't as much cultural stigma involved. If I was talking about my psychological issues, I would have to explain my family background and my cultural background. I wanted to make it clear that I don't blame my family for what happened. I recognize that they were in a system that they themselves did not understand how to get out of. There was one therapy session I had with a new therapist. And after I told her my story, she said, "So you're like this probably because your parents are tiger parents." And I was like, "That's the entire opposite of my point."

Sometimes people will start to blame my culture, my family. And I always just say, "My family and my background have indeed created a lot of pain and fear for me, but they've also created a lot of resilience and support, and they've taught me a lot about my own strengths and how to be proud of the way I look, even though I was teased every single day for the way I spoke and the way my name sounded." So, I just wanted to emphasize that, because I don't want people to walk away and just think, "Asians, that's how they are." Because it's more nuanced, and oftentimes more beautiful than that.

Critically, some people find help even when they don't have a cultural match with their provider. Cathy Guild knows firsthand that the traditional beliefs and ways of the past do not have to control your future. Cathy did find help—from male and female therapists of different sexual orientations who she liked—but she's "never had a person of color." However, Cathy's open nature and broad perspective helped her overcome this potential barrier to care. She has a good message for mental health providers to hear about the importance of developing cultural humility to help someone who has a different experience and background than they do: "I'm always open to a therapist until they say something that closes me off to them."

For Kristina Saffran, inclusion requires more than just visual representation. She described how her company is taking steps to fill the gaps:

While we talk about how eating disorders affect a wide swath of individuals, training has been so inaccessible that the field has ended up looking just like me. There's no diversity in those who are treating folks with eating disorders, so we've been able to go out to the communities that we know are affected and bring in mentors and providers who can match the lived experiences of who we're trying to help, above and beyond the experience of an eating disorder.

For example, the trans community experiences eating disorders at four times the rate of the cisgender community, so we have a number of trans mentors and parents who parented kids who were transitioning at the same time that they had their eating disorders. We have family mentors from across the socio-economic spectrum, including those who've lived in food insecurity while helping their loved one to recover. And we've had mentors in larger bodies who've helped families unpack their own weight stigma in order to help their loved one fully heal.

Kristina's focus on the intersectionality of health care—the idea that all the different parts of a person's identity contribute to how they're able to access care and the quality of care they get—also centers on treating the whole person. She explained that her company is "on a mission to ensure that everyone has access to treatment that works and leads to full and lasting recovery. We designed treatment to be fully virtual so that in addition to access, folks can bring their entire village to help them recover, and also build a life worth living to drown out the eating disorder."

Kevin Dedner serves as founder and CEO of Washington, DC–based Hurdle Health, which provides culturally intentional teletherapy to eliminate barriers that make it harder for people of color to get mental health care. He told me about his personal journey into care, and how hard it was for him to find someone who understood his larger cultural experience as a Black man:

At our company, we are deliberate with our words. For example, while the phrase "culturally competent" has been acceptable language the last twenty years in mental health and general health, when you unpack the language, it intuits an arrogant assumption that a therapist or doctor can become competent in someone's racialized experience in the world through a class or by some studious effort. It leaves no room for continuous learning. At Hurdle, I have banned the term "cultural competency." Instead, we begin by exercising "cultural intentionality," we practice "cultural humility," and ultimately strive for "cultural responsiveness" in therapy.

Kevin went on to share that the key was the clinician's attitude:

When I tell my story to a therapist, do they believe me? Or do they look at me like a deer in headlights? Or worse yet, are they dismissive of my experience? Research tells us that 50 percent of ethnic minorities terminate therapy prematurely. We must follow statistics like this with a compassionate, objective inquiry—why are BIPOC more inclined to terminate prematurely? At Hurdle, our clinical research reveals that oftentimes it's because the therapist is either dismissive of a client's racialized experience or is bringing their own biases to the counseling session, ultimately creating unintended microaggressions in what should be a safe place.

I was fortunate. I did not become a statistic because I eventually found a therapist who was using the technique that we now train our therapists in. He was asking me questions in a way that validated my story and what I was experiencing as a Black man in America. He acknowledged my experiences as truth.

I asked Kevin if having a diverse mental health workforce is the key, and how that might help people of color in their care journey. He responded:

In health care, we do see better outcomes when people look like one another. It is intellectually dishonest to assume that race alone is the driving factor in creating care models that are relevant to BIPOC when you understand the vast differential between the number of people who are seeking care, and the number of mental health providers. There just simply aren't enough therapists to meet the current demand. This is especially true for BIPOC where we have seen increasing rates of treatment-seeking behavior since the death of George Floyd. To meet the growing mental health needs of minorities, we must rethink the flawed system. The way that therapists are trained to think about therapy is from our learnings in supporting middle-class white people, whose experience is very different than people of color. We cannot simply rely on BIPOC therapists to treat BIPOC. The need is too great. Ultimately, we must scale the type of culturally intentional training that Hurdle provides its therapists. Cultural humility training must become ubiquitous in mental health care, something required of *all* therapists.

Given that we are generations away from having a sufficiently diverse workforce, Kevin is working to grow a workforce that is culturally humble, responsive, and intentional. A professional with that kind of training could improve the mental health care experience for clients of all races, ethnicities, religions, genders, and sexual orientations in the years to come.

For this book, I interviewed only 130 people, meaning there are many more cultural perspectives on mental health and illness that are not represented here. My hope is that the conversations I share will begin to convey something about how mental health and illness, and mental health care, are experienced in different cultures. These perspectives increased my interest in this important and complex area, and I hope they do for you as well.

ELEVEN

Becoming an Advocate

N o one sets out hoping to become an expert on the experience of mental illness. But once you are, you have a lot to offer others. You can make your experience meaningful by reaching out to people newer to the process of recovery, engaging with "big picture issues" like the social marginalization of people with mental health conditions, or advocating for the availability and quality of mental health services. You know firsthand what is missing and what isn't working in our broken mental health care system; how people have and haven't supported you; and what relationships, therapies, activities, environments, and experiences have had significant positive impact on your recovery. By becoming an advocate, whether in the personal, public, or legal spheres, you give your lived experience new meaning. Most likely, your advocacy will help enhance, enrich, and sustain your recovery.

Advocacy has become a powerful mission for many of the people I interviewed, and Nick Emeigh, who we met earlier, is one of them. Nick attempted suicide for the first time at age twenty-three, after his mother died. He struggled with addiction, episodes of psychosis, and recurring suicidality. He has been hospitalized multiple times and spent years trying to find an effective treatment regimen. He was even threatened with jail after an overdose attempt. As he struggled to navigate the health care system, Nick felt responsible for the stress his illness put on his family. He felt he would not get better.

Nick sought purpose, but he felt lost. While living in a substance use recovery house, a friend recommended he tell his story for NAMI Ending the Silence (ETS), a program that organizes presentations on living with mental health conditions and recovery to high schoolers. Initially, he was skeptical. At that point, recovery for him meant the ability to conceal everything he had felt and experienced, which was something he couldn't do and didn't think he'd be able to do anytime soon. Nick told me:

> The day I decided that I was going to tell my story for NAMI was the day I came home from an intensive outpatient program, and a guy had died by suicide in our bathroom. And I realized that that was probably going to happen to me, too, if I didn't do something. I needed to do something.

His engagement grew from there. Starting with ETS, Nick found that by telling his story, he could be exactly who he was *and* have a powerful impact on people. He embarked on a journey that would change his understanding of recovery and turn him into an advocate.

During our conversation, Nick recalled the time he invented NAMI Man, the black-and-green-clad NAMI superhero who has come to embody NAMI's attitude about living with mental health conditions:

> We had a NAMI Walk every year, and Debbie—the executive director of NAMI Bucks County—said, "We don't have a mental health superhero." I said, "People in recovery are *all* mental health superheroes." I survived three suicide attempts. And even though I wasn't happy when I woke up from some of them, I felt pretty powerful that I'd survived. I said, "You know what? I'm in recovery; I'll be a superhero. I'll be NAMI Man." It just so happens that "NAMI MAN" is an anagram, and it stuck.

When Horsham Clinic, a behavioral health facility where Nick had once been a patient, invited him to read a story to their kids, he thought, "Why don't I come as NAMI Man and read to the kids?" And so, NAMI

Man was invited to come visit the children's unit. He recalled thinking, "Honest to God, I did not know that kids quite that young were hospitalized." Nick detailed his first encounter:

> I was shocked walking in there. The techs and the nurses warned me that some of these kids are not going to be into this, and that they have behavioral issues. And I said, "Yeah, well, me too. The whole point of me being here is that that's who I am." I walk in and some of the kids are like, "Who is this dude?"
>
> I said, "I'm your mental health superhero. You read comic books and stuff, and you watch cartoons, and you know Superman and Batman and all that stuff? Well, what do they do?" The kids answered, "They save the day and kill bad guys and stuff." They asked, "Do you kill bad guys?" I said, "No, I don't hurt anybody. I crush the stigma," and they're like, what is that?
>
> I asked, "Do you like being in here? Do you like being in the hospital?"
>
> "No, we don't know why we're here. This sucks."

Nick remembered telling them:

> A lot of the reason that you don't know why you're here, and what mental health is, and that no one ever talks about it, is stigma. When I was in the hospital, my parents weren't happy that I was there, and they never talked about it to anybody, and we never talked about it. And my life would have been a little bit easier if we did. So, I crushed the stigma, so that it's easier for us to talk about this stuff.
>
> There was one kid I remember, who asked me: "Are you a *real* superhero?" I said, "I'm your superhero." I told him I'd been through tough times too. I told him, "Superheroes are real people too. Did you know that?" He said no. So, I took off my mask, and I said, "My name is Nick. And I work for a place called NAMI. The reason I turned into a superhero is because I was in this hospital. I was a patient here and I got the help

that I needed. So technically, you're a superhero too, since you're here getting the help you need. And I want you to help people one day, too, when you get through this."

That was the first time I really thought, "My God, I could have killed myself. Like I really could have killed myself." And driving home that day, I remember that was one of the first times I thought, "Not only do I not *want* to die, but I am also *afraid* to die now." I kept thinking of all the things I could do with NAMI Man and how many kids are going to be in these facilities that I could go and visit.

For Nick, and for many others, advocacy played a key part in a years-long struggle to make peace with, and find meaning in, their lived experience. By helping others, Nick has also sustained his own recovery. By creating a new identity as a superhero, he has taken ownership of how he sees himself.

Self-Advocacy: Overcoming Obstacles

For most people living with a mental health condition, advocacy begins in advocating for themselves: They encounter some frustrating obstacle to treatment, services, or recovery that seems unnecessary, unjust, nonsensical, or incomprehensible, and they find themselves working to surmount it. They may recognize somewhere along the way that the obstacle is systemic but not unchangeable. And as they begin to speak up for change that would serve their recovery, they discover that the act of speaking up itself serves their recovery. When we can use our own experiences to change our circumstances, we regain power over our own lives.

Lloyd Hale, introduced in chapter 4, experienced early in his journey negative side effects from clozapine, a medication he took to manage psychosis. This led him to do something he was fearful of: have an honest talk with the doctor who had recommended the medicine. He recalled:

Some of the side effects were heavy drooling and drowsiness. I was choking on saliva at night, and I had to say something. Have you ever been in an experience where you want to be quiet about something, but something pokes you so hard that you got to say something?

It was my introduction to advocacy. I said to my doctor, "Hey, I want to comply, I want to be part of my recovery, and my treatment, but this is hard. What can we do so that I can be well, but I can continue along my journey, taking my medication and stuff like that?" So, we began immediately to identify ways to reduce the drooling and help with some of the sedation. Even the hardships were beneficial, as I learned how to advocate for myself.

As a result of this conversation, Lloyd was able to problem-solve with his doctor and had fewer side effects. Realizing he could advocate to be an active participant in his own treatment plan made a positive shift in Lloyd's relationship to treatment, and his treatment plan became a true collaboration between him and his care team.

Cathy Guild, who we met in chapter 5, began her journey by having to overcome her family's aversion to her getting mental health treatment at all—even in the wake of a devastating traumatic experience: She was sexually assaulted at age sixteen, and her mother denied her request to see a therapist. "She said, 'Go to your room. You are crazy. I don't have crazy children,'" Cathy told me. "That was her thinking: 'Something is wrong with you. Keep it inside. Work it out. You are not strong.'"

Cathy didn't get help until many years later, after she lost custody of her children in the wake of her drug use. But when she did, the experience was transformational. She told me: "I began to see a therapist and learned I can talk to someone without being punished. They told me I am not crazy. That I'm not alone. Other people go through this. Who knew there could be a plan to help you feel and get better? It was amazing." Now Cathy works in a health setting. She came to understand where trauma had led her, and how many other Black women were subject to traumas of various kinds:

My biggest thing in doing this interview is wanting women who feel like—when you start using drugs—there is nothing else that you can do: There is. When you feel that you can't be anything, or can't accomplish anything, you can. Everything starts with a goal, and changing your goals will change your life, and having a therapist to help you and say: "What can we do with that?" and "There's a reason behind this," is amazing.

I love my babies, and I felt like no one would take care of them the way that I would. I want Black women to know they can get their kids back, and you can quote me on that. Don't ever feel that you cannot get your children back, achieve greatness, and be whoever you want to be. You can.

Advocating for Better Research

Advocacy is a critical need in the mental health services. The treatment tools we have are also often inadequate, so advocating for better research is also crucial.

Wendy Ascione-Juska, who we met earlier, learned that the largest long-term research study of people with bipolar disorder, called the Heinz C. Prechter Bipolar Research Program, was being run at the University of Michigan. Like many people, she joined it, eager to help others:

> I've been a part of the study for a long time. It's low-impact for me, but high-impact for what it can do to help others. I'm not doing it for the money. It's been helpful just to learn. I go on the website to see what studies have been done based off it. This is my condition, and people can potentially learn a lot from this study. That was my motivation for participating.

Public Advocacy: Opening the Conversation and Creating Resources

Once people learn how to advocate for their own wellness and goals within the context of treatment, many are driven to share what they have learned and open wider conversations around the shame, prejudice, or discrimination they faced on their journey to getting help. The ability to share at different points in your journey opens the door to community building with others who may have had similar struggles but follow a different path to recovery.

Diana Chao, who we met earlier, found healing by becoming her own pen pal. When she realized that writing letters helped her process her thoughts and feelings in a constructive and personal way, she wondered if others might feel the same. This reflex to share, to help, and to welcome others into a community of care evolved into what's now the largest mental health organization for youth in the world. She told me:

> I'd decided I needed to dedicate myself to healing, and I was trying dif-ferent techniques that people had suggested, like journaling, meditation, things like that. But when I was trying to journal because of the depressive episodes I was having, sometimes I would go down a very negative spiral and I had no feedback system to control that.
>
> So, I started writing these letters to strangers, or whoever. And what I realized was that having this imaginary recipient forced me to be more thoughtful about the feelings I was putting down. It forced me to articu-late to myself what exactly I was feeling. Also, you don't really want to just leave it at the cliffhanger. So, I felt like I had to come up with some sort of way to tie things up, like a letter does. Even if I didn't have a resolution to an issue I was writing about, I still had to reflect on, "Well, are there options that I could pursue for a resolution to occur?" And that started to make me realize my own voice.

Diana began to wonder whether what she'd learned, and what was working for her, could help other people as well. In her sophomore year, she started a student club at her high school called Letters to Strangers. It began with small lunch meetings but soon snowballed. There are now more than one hundred branches of Letters to Strangers in over twenty countries, as well as counseling centers for youth in Liberia and Zimba-bwe. There are twelve city chapters in India alone that host huge events every year. Diana estimates that the organization, and the free resources it makes available, has reached more than 100,000 people. She believes that one of the most important aspects of Letters to Strangers is that it focuses on intersectionality:

> When I first started to do this work, and the reason why I decided to go public with my story after I graduated from high school, was because I didn't see anyone who looked like me, from the sort of cultural backgrounds that affected my wellness journey. I wanted to emphasize these different elements and how they can impact your well-being.

Miana Bryant, the Howard University grad student introduced in chapter 7, works in Prince George's County as a registered behavioral technician. When she was an undergrad in 2017, Miana started a supportive group chat with friends experiencing symptoms of depression. The group—the Mental Elephant—created a welcoming space for college students to speak openly about their symptoms in a less formal setting than a traditional university counseling center. Much like Letters to Strangers, the group snowballed unexpectedly:

> The Mental Elephant started after I received my diagnosis. I kept talking to my friend, and I realized that a lot of my friends had the same symptoms and a lot of the same issues. I started a group chat, and it kept getting bigger, so we decided to have a meetup on my college campus. A lightbulb went off in my mind: I can start a campus organization.
>
> Originally, when I pitched it to my school, they told me no, because the campus already had a counseling center and a student health care center, so they didn't really see the point in an organization based on mental health. But I kept going with things. I also kept receiving warnings from the school to stop holding events on campus. When it was time for organization registration again, and they saw a) that I wasn't stopping, and b) the momentum of our mental health organization, they agreed to let me officially create the Mental Elephant.

Some people, like Bethany Yeiser of Ohio, focus not just on providing peer support for people with a particular mental health condition, but on reaching out to inform and enlighten the public. Bethany founded the CURESZ (Comprehensive Understanding via Research and Education into Schizophrenia) Foundation with Henry Nasrallah, a professor of psychiatry at the University of Cincinnati. Their goal was to frame schizophrenia as a treatable condition not unlike diabetes or heart disease:

> The CURESZ Foundation was Dr. Nasrallah's idea and we established it together. He wanted to provide patients and their families with advocacy and education about cutting-edge and underutilized treatments for schizophrenia that they may never had heard about, and which may help them return to their baseline. CURESZ presents schizophrenia as a treatable brain disorder; a neuroplasticity and neurochemical neurological illness. We have created CURESZ clubs, and one of their most important focuses is to help college students get out this word that when it comes to depression, anxiety, or schizophrenia—we're talking about medical brain conditions.
>
> There should be no hesitancy in getting help for any physical problem, including one's brain disorder. When I was first diagnosed with schizophrenia, I thought that I'd be locked away somewhere. I had no clue that it was treatable or that it was a brain disorder.
>
> We also have a mentoring program with about twenty mentors serving about sixty mentees. We have a monthly Monday meeting called "Ask the Doctor," where six families register in advance and log on for ninety minutes to hear answers to their many questions about the biology and treatment of serious mental illness in their families. In addition, we have a monthly Sunday night meeting slot that's an open meeting for patients' families to get advice from individuals who have recovered.

Becoming a public advocate may seem intimidating or unattainable, but even the largest advocacy organizations started somewhere, usually with a small group of people who decided they wanted to see change and started working to make it happen.

The Culture Changers

Many focus their advocacy on the root of the challenges within their community. A single person can often be a catalyst in their community just by living their full and honest truth, demonstrating that recovery is possible; that mental health is vital; and that community is key in maintaining it.

Kenya Phillips, who we met earlier, published a book of poetry, *Word Play Series 1 Winter: Emotional Spasms*, which was inspired by her experience of living with bipolar disorder. By speaking her truth openly and honestly, Kenya allowed others to realize they can pursue the same without compromising their spirituality or beliefs. Kenya's story also shows that artistic or literary self-expression can be a form of advocacy:

> I grew up in a United Methodist church—very conservative and predominately African American. Talking about mental health was taboo—that wasn't said, but that nonverbal communication was happening. A couple of years later, I run into some of these same people in the community and they be like: "Kenya, thank you so much for being free in your truth." For that purpose, and that purpose alone, I'm unapologetic about it. We have organizations within the church to support mental health, and we talk freely about it, and we bring it back home.
>
> If you're silent, you're aiding the problem. We must be free. I'm free and speaking about it. It doesn't matter where I'm at. I'm: "This is what it is." Yes, it's liberating. I just love being free in this space.

Christine Yu Moutier made mental health advocacy and suicide prevention her life's work after her own lived experience as well as multiple losses to suicide in her professional life. Christine shared earlier that she had to take a medical leave of absence from medical school because she was dealing with suicidal thoughts and an eating disorder. She later became the dean of students at that same medical school. Knowing what she did about the pressures that students are under, and with her new authority, she wanted to make mental health something it was safe to talk about. Christine decided to share her experience with the students:

> The week I became dean, I asked my supervisor if it was okay to tell my story to the students. Because the students had said, "You have to be part of a town hall and come and engage with us and tell us who you are." I wasn't sure. Am I really allowed to talk about personal experiences, especially involving struggle? And so, I wrote it out. And I ran it by my boss. And she said, "Yes, you should talk about it. Share it." Sharing my own story of vulnerability, healing through the support of others and with treatment, and finding solidarity with so many others has been profoundly transformative for me.

Now as the medical director of American Foundation for Suicide Prevention, Christine is leading a movement to humanize medical education toward mental health support nationwide. This change is also happening on the ground in medical schools, driven by both faculty leaders like Christine and students whose own lived experiences have inspired them to pursue a career of service.

Pranita Mainali is a thirty-two-year-old from Nepal who is the mother of a toddler and currently a resident psychiatrist. Her experience with mental illness in her own family inspired her to choose the profession of mental health advocate:

> I was very optimistic that whoever was treating my mom would be able to help her in some way, but I was not satisfied because I could see her not getting better. I wanted to know, why is my family not like a normal family, why is my mom not like a normal mom?
>
> My reason for becoming a psychiatrist was because of my own experience. I think my experience made me more mature than I should have

been at that time. And nobody was there to help me, nobody was there to guide me. So I came all the way from Nepal trying to help my mother, and also trying to pursue my dream at the same time. I think not only do I relate to somebody who has mental illness, but also I relate to someone whose loved one is going through the same. This connection, that's the reason I love psychiatry, because I understand. I know how it feels.

I told Pranita that our stories were similar—that I had also gone into psychiatry to better understand what happened to my father, and to help others who faced similar struggles. She responded:

I think the core of the story could always be the same, that is, love for your loved one. During my residency interviews, when somebody would ask me why I was interested in psychiatry, I'd tell them my story. I don't think there could be any more of a motivational factor than your desire to help somebody when you have seen your own family member go through the same.

Pranita is on her way to becoming an excellent doctor, and she told me her mother is doing well. Many medical students could benefit from learning more about lived experience. NAMI has a program called NAMI Provider, which offers three key perspectives of lived experience—that of a person with mental illness, that of a family member, and also that of a health care professional who is either a family member or has a mental illness themselves. NAMI Provider was developed to provide health care professionals insights into the lived experience of the people they were caring for, but has also proven to be effective for medical students.

Des Moines University (DMU) School of Osteopathic Medicine was the first school to integrate NAMI Provider into their curriculum. Peggy Huppert, the executive director of NAMI Iowa, is a white, married sixty-three-year-old with three adult children and two grandchildren. She told me about the growth of the NAMI Provider program in the medical school here:

We need to do more for our students to differentiate them in the very competitive residency process. We know that family doctors prescribe 80 percent of psychotropic drugs, and 80 percent of DMU students go into family medicine, so what can we do to make them more equipped to be better providers of mental health care as family docs? The first year, the NAMI Provider program was optional. We had forty-five students take it. Then they decided that they wanted to make it mandatory, so we've now been doing it for three years.

James Chambliss, a thirty-four-year-old white psychiatry resident in Des Moines, took the NAMI Provider course and reported it made a difference in how he sees people who live with mental health conditions:

The part I like best about the program is that it creates the opportunity to interact with medical students and shape the way in which they may practice as providers. I like the way the course is structured to provide the perspective of an individual who struggles with mental health, as well as a family member of an individual who struggles with mental health. As providers, we see patients for a snapshot of their life and at times when they are not at their best. Viewing patients in these moments of acute crisis can shape our viewpoints. I like how the program works to expand that perspective and create an understanding that these moments are challenging for the patient too. Patients with mental health struggles can be seen in any specialty, and may be quite challenging, but they are still trying their best and still deserve thorough evaluation and help.

Kimberly Comer of Florida, who we met in chapter 6, told me how critical it is that medical providers offer hope to people. She knows this firsthand:

I worked in the medical field for fifteen years before I started my wellness journey and what I know of that system, and many systems, is that when you work in it for too long, and all you see are people that are unwell, people who are breaking the law, you lose hope. You don't know that people do recover. People do learn what they need to know to be able to live their healthiest quality of life. But the most important thing that anyone can provide them is hope. That's the piece I always tell them. You may be the first person to provide them hope and a resource for recovery. Don't blow it.

Advocating for Services: The Personal Is Political

Once people have empowered themselves to speak out in favor of positive change in their communities, many become engaged in advocating for more enlightened, effective, and socially just policies and legislation in the wider world.

Sixteen-year-old Kaitlyn Tollefson is a high school junior who began advocating for mental health care access after she noticed the problem of student suicides in her school district. She lives in Colorado, where she works with organizations and school clubs to destigmatize mental health care through leadership, service, and policy change. After starting a school project on ways to reduce stress for students, Kaitlyn turned her attention to advocating for policy change:

There are so many people struggling, and it's not talked about enough. Mental health goes under the covers, and it inspired me to start working at advocacy. In ninth grade, I was able to join a program called Young Invincibles. I applied when I was fifteen, almost sixteen. They take people ages sixteen to thirty-four. It's a group of young adults who help, work, and strategize on how to make a change for the better, and how to advocate for the public at the state level.

She went on to explain how she got connected with the bill:

We were able to choose a capstone project—what bill we wanted to work on—and I saw the mental health bill, and I thought: "That's exactly what

I have been trying to do." And so, I ended up testifying in the Colorado House first, and then the Senate. . . . And both chambers passed it with unanimous votes, which was amazing. It's House Bill 21-1068, and it's a mental health and wellness bill to get insurance to cover one annual mental health and wellness checkup in the state of Colorado. Before this bill was passed in 2021, insurance was not required to cover a mental health and wellness visit separate from a regular visit. They were trying to count your regular annual checkup at the doctor's office as your mental health and wellness checkup, which is not the same. Physicians don't have the time to cover all the stuff that they could do with mental health. So, it's a cool bill. It allows more people to get access.

Telling stories based on first-person experience is a powerful tool in changing the hearts and minds of those in political power. Eric Smith of San Antonio shared his vulnerabilities with legislators in multiple states in the process of advocating for what is called Assisted Outpatient Treatment (AOT). This means using civil courts and treatment teams to help people with severe mental illness on an outpatient basis if they have struggled with (or against) voluntary care—perhaps due to anosognosia, as was the case for Eric—and may pose a danger to themselves or to the community. He told me that his lived experience was valued by lawmakers:

I believe the lawmakers were willing to learn. There was a lot of open-mindedness—not just politician doublespeak, but very substantive and meaningful statements, and questions at times. I wanted to be thoughtful enough to express that there were also people from the lived experience population who were just as vehemently against AOT as I was for it, and that I was listening to them. Wherever there's opposition, when people feel strongly one way or another, I listen, thoughtfully.

Not only does Eric's lived experience give him an important perspective that should be critical in the creation of policy, but he is also respectful of the lived experience of others, even when they disagree with him.

To me, this illustrated one of the core strengths of peer advocacy: respect for the diverse experiences and opinions of others. Eric advocates so that others might understand his experience:

> I really hope people understand that for me, the most forceful and coercive thing that I have ever experienced is not inpatient hospitalization. It is not being jailed. It is not Assisted Outpatient Treatment. The most forceful and coercive thing I have ever experienced was when my own severe mental illness went untreated or undertreated.

Eric credits AOT for helping free him from that coercive and forceful cycle, and he wants people to understand that it can help others like it did him. After being placed in AOT in Texas, Eric went from being a high school dropout and diagnosed with severe mental illness to graduating magna cum laude with a degree in psychology followed by a master's degree in social work. He is now a nationally recognized public advocate for AOT, testifying in legislatures across the country.

First-person advocacy is a superpower that is as effective as it is authentic, and we will need this type of advocacy for a very long time. It changes minds and helps write laws. It was first-person advocacy that led to the creation of the federal mental health parity law, the 988 Crisis Response line, the early psychosis infrastructure, and many other changes.

You may also find yourself advocating in other ways. For example, you can sponsor a newcomer in a 12-step program or lobby for more affordable housing in your town. If you want to learn how to become a mental health advocate and share your story to help yourself, to move the conversation forward in your community, or to create services or laws, the NAMI Smarts for Advocacy program can get you started. For a list of more options and organizations, see the Resources section.

PART III

Family Matters

TWELVE

Family Connection and Communication

Having a mental health condition, or loving someone who has a mental health condition, challenges relationships. It is a high-stress, high-stakes situation, and very few families, if any, are instantly adept at handling and communicating about it. When no one knows what to do or what to say, people are likely to do or say the "wrong" things, provoking conflict; or they might avoid communication altogether, which could fracture connection. If that's what is happening in your family, please know that you are not alone, and that things can get better. In my decades at NAMI, and in my clinical work in multiple settings, I have seen many families find ways to discuss hard topics, make difficult decisions, heal ruptures, and move their relationships forward using empathy, self-care, boundary-setting, and concrete skills.

In my own life, my family missed many opportunities to discuss what was right in front of us. Our shame kept us silent and isolated us from one another. When my father, while manic, cut the grass on our front lawn in bizarre patterns for all to see, it was a public reminder of what we were failing to discuss inside our home. My reaction was to get up early and re-mow the lawn in neat rows before school. Although an honest conversation would have been much more productive, I was desperate to cling to some thread of order and dignity.

Ever since our failed communication efforts, I have been interested in people who figured out how to address issues effectively and deepen relationships while one or more family members lives with a mental health condition. In this chapter, we will meet people—parents and their children, siblings, spouses, and the chosen family of close friends—who have improved their communication and connection with one another when faced with mental illness.

I met many families that did so much better than we did. One was the Donahoe family. John Donahoe, a sixty-seven-year-old white architect and musician in the Nashville area, told me about the initial apprehension he and his wife Nancy felt when treatment providers recommended ECT (electroconvulsive therapy, more colloquially known as shock treatment) for their son Alex's mental health symptoms. John recalled:

> After Alex was hospitalized, the psychiatrist told us that he was catatonic— he wasn't eating and was shuffling when he walked. The psychiatrist said, "We don't think your boy is getting any better, and we think we should try ECT." That's when we thought about *One Flew Over the Cuckoo's Nest*, and oh my god, just imagining . . .

Nancy, a retired nurse, described how they sought more information and ultimately decided to move forward with treatment:

> John asked the psychiatrist, on a scale of one to ten, how bad was Alex? He said "ten." Initially we'd said, "Absolutely not," but we looked at each other and said, "Let's learn about this ECT thing." John's brother, who's a doctor, said, "If he's catatonic, you need to do this. If it were my son, I would do it." We said okay. After a series of treatments, Alex called John and left him a voicemail telling him that he loved him. He was getting better. To me, ECT was miraculous. He's a different kid. He's better, in my opinion, than he has been for a long time.

Talking about concerns, gathering information, and making informed decisions is the best path.

NAMI Family-to-Family

John and Nancy Donahoe learned to open their minds and talk to each other about a difficult subject that provoked strong feelings. But talking directly about difficult subjects to a loved one with a mental health condition can be even more challenging. And if the loved one is an adult child, old parent-child dynamics can add an extra dimension of difficulty. However, you can learn new approaches that not only improve communication but also strengthen relationships. A NAMI Family-to-Family class is one good place to get support and information, as well as to begin learning those new skills.

NAMI Family-to-Family is a free eight-session course for family members of someone with a mental illness. It provides information to promote understanding of mental health conditions, fosters improved communication, and provides tools for advocacy. The course is offered either online or in person and is taught by other experienced family members who have become trained facilitators. Research studies have shown that the course increases hope and empowerment for those who take it.

NAMI Family-to-Family was created by Joyce Burland, a psychologist who experienced firsthand how mental health care professionals blamed families and saw a need for families to support and teach each other. Joyce watched as her own family was blamed for her sister's schizophrenia, and when her own daughter became ill a generation later, not much had changed. "Family members were being attacked by the profession and blamed for their adult child's illness," she told me. "They were given no resources. If it were any other illness there would be some source of concern, or even compassion, right? And there was not a bit of it."

In the late 1990s, with the help of many Vermont families, Joyce created a curriculum for family members of people with serious mental illnesses to teach other families. People found the classes so helpful that demand to enroll in them quickly exceeded capacity. Joyce developed the model of Family-to-Family through what she calls a trauma and resilience lens, reflecting her insight that a serious illness in a loved one is often experienced as a traumatic event, and that dealing with it draws on deep reserves of resilience and strength. "I learned from my own family being shattered, that we had the strength to pull together and do something for those of us who had mental illness," Joyce told me. "We had found a resilience that allowed us to do this. So, when the professionals would say you can't have families teaching, I'd say, yes, we can." In fact, it's precisely because the teachers have personal experience that the Family-to-Family course has had such a positive impact for hundreds of thousands of families.

Joyce also emphasized the importance of self-care; that family members are doing the best thing for their loved one, and for their family, when they prioritize attending to their own well-being. "This was what I understood deeply," she said. "The family member thinks, since they're not the sick one, they don't deserve this kind of support. But this is long-term illness. So, we want to be sure that you remain strong and resilient because you are a lifetime caretaker."

Professionals today would be very unlikely to treat families in the way that inspired Joyce to develop Family-to-Family. But the needs for support and education remain critical. In these next five chapters, people also share what they have learned. Every family is unique, yet the tools and approaches that have worked for some of them may be of use to you.

Improving Intergenerational Relationships: Parents and Adult Children

James Ramirez is a parent I interviewed who benefited from the new approaches to communication with their adult children. He's a sixty-five-year-old father of four and a retired power generation specialist living in Oregon who now serves as a trainer for several NAMI service programs.

When he took the Family-to-Family class to better understand his son's experience with mental illness, one of the things he learned was that he had to let go of his own vision of what his son's life would be. Being an engineer and architect, he found a unique way to communicate that to his son:

> I decided to share with my son what NAMI has done for me through Family-to-Family. The only thing I could think of to use was an Etch-a-Sketch. I took this Etch-a-Sketch, and I began to do this drawing as a metaphor for my perception of what I'd planned our life as a family to be. So, I drew this road, with buildings, cars, and trees, and you could see in the distance, this example of what things would look like for us at the end of this golden path. I sat down with my son and said, "This is what I perceived your life to be. All this stuff I planned: that you have a wife, you have a son, and here's the road that I planned for us all to be upon." I shook the Etch-a-Sketch and my drawing disappeared. I said, "Now, *you* draw for *me*. What is your life going to be?"

James's acceptance of his son's independence, he told me, was a foundation for an improved relationship.

Acceptance was also a key for George Kaufmann of California. He told me in our interview that he had to accept that his son Patrick would have to find his own way to recovery:

> The hardest thing, especially for parents, is to let go and let our kids have their own struggles. It's not helpful to try to fix the problem, and that's what we try to do as parents. We want to make it easier for our kids. We don't realize that we're not doing them any favors by doing that. In fact, all we're doing is pushing them further away. It's not helpful to focus on their mental illness, being the hovering parent. In fact, it's disempowering. It's important for us not to determine goals for somebody else.
>
> I think one of the factors in Patrick's recovery was that it was all up to him. Everyone has to have their own aims in life, and Patrick, we learned, didn't need any help from us to make those decisions.

Patrick has been my greatest teacher when it comes to understanding mental illness. I was able to finally shut up and listen to him, and hear him, and not be judgmental about what I was hearing. It was a slow process for me, but one I'm glad happened.

George made the point that letting go of efforts to determine his son's path isn't something he does perfectly every day:

The interesting thing is that when everything's going fine, I can keep my composure and my balance. When we're under stress, we tend to revert to the way we used to be. Maybe it's a part of human nature, I don't know. I do know my life has been drastically enriched by having mental illness in my family. Because it gave me a perspective that I had never had before.

Patrick Kaufmann, who now works as a peer specialist in Michigan, spoke of how his parents' shifted perspective gave him the space he needed to find his own way:

The idea of letting go is important, because if somebody's drowning and you're in a boat, and you jump in to save them, you end up drowning each other. So, feeling like my parents were jumping in with me, and they were going to drown with me, didn't help anything. Knowing that they were okay made a difference; not feeling like every decision I made was going to affect them so deeply. Because it was painful to feel like somebody was that invested in you, and you didn't feel able to care enough for yourself to make them happy. When they stopped trying to rescue me, it made me feel like they believed I could do it.

Babu George Mathew is a South Asian American dad in his late sixties living in the foothills of Colorado and serving as the board president of NAMI Colorado. Babu told me his only daughter lives with clinical depression and anxiety, and their relationship had long been strained, until Babu discovered a new freedom to express himself in Family-to-Family:

> Family-to-Family is a sanctuary. We come there just as we are, as broken as we are, and we share the stories. We have the freedom to talk, we have the freedom to cry if we need. It has been such a powerful experience.
>
> We always say that being vulnerable is not a weakness, it's a strength. I have seen men coming and breaking down there, and that provides relief and healing. It took me real strength to come to that point back in 2010, as a South Asian macho man, to say sorry to my own daughter, and I have experienced healing in that.
>
> My daughter is a huge influence for me. It's because of her strength that I'm here. It is sometimes our children that change us.

Communication can be essential to taking the first big step. Sheryl and Richard Smith, both retired teachers in Wisconsin, found Family-to-Family very helpful. Yet clear and persistent communication was needed to help Richard attend. Richard told me:

> Sheryl is the hero in this particular situation. She dragged me kicking and screaming into NAMI. It was hard for me to accept the fact that our son Michael had a mental illness. I didn't want that for him.

For Sheryl, teaching Family-to-Family became a highlight of her career:

> I taught school for forty years, and I have never felt such fulfillment in teaching as I have in teaching Family-to-Family, because people come in desperate need of the class, and most of them leave with so much.

Sheryl and Richard now teach Family-to-Family together.

Sierra Grandy, who we met earlier, spoke to me about how her family came to understand that mental illness is a topic that can be discussed openly. Sierra and her family also learned specific skills to support each other more effectively:

> My family's great. However, they're just average, real Minnesotans. They don't have the resources or knowledge to know exactly what's happening with my mental health. They were doing the best they could, but sometimes I didn't get what I needed.
>
> They utilized some of NAMI's online resources during the Covid-19 pandemic. Before I was the black sheep in the family. Now everything's open. I don't feel any shame about mental illness when I'm talking to my family about it.
>
> The biggest thing that's helped as we've grown is setting boundaries. So, if I call or my mom calls, whichever, we will automatically be like, "Are you looking for advice or are you looking to have somebody listen to you?" We'll acknowledge right away what the intention of the call is about. We had to fall on our face enough times to know how to do that.

Anita Herron is a middle-aged white woman who grew up in a military family and currently works for NAMI. She is an adoptive and birth mother with three adult children who have mental health conditions. Anita spoke to me about how NAMI Homefront, a support program for veterans and their families, helped her gain insights and skills that allowed her to rebuild a relationship with her father, who served in the Vietnam War:

> When I started studying NAMI Homefront, I was very pleased when we had wives and sisters of Vietnam veterans joining the classes. Wow. These are people my parents' age. I was so excited. And I would listen to them and understand the hatred that their Vietnam veteran held inside. I was ready to sever the relationship with my dad at the time. He had said some horrible things to me growing up. And I listened to the people at NAMI Homefront, and I said, "Here we go diagnosing people, but . . . my dad has PTSD from Vietnam."

So Anita studied it and said, "I'm going to take the things that I've learned in Homefront, and I'm going to use them to build this relationship." She continued:

What I learned is understanding and acceptance that my dad might not understand that he has PTSD. One day, I talked to him in the kitchen, and I said, "Hey, Dad, NAMI has this program called NAMI Homefront. And I manage it and teach it."

He said, "I don't want to hear about this psycho-mumble-jumble bullshit." I said, "Okay." Well, about an hour later, he's standing in the kitchen just looking down. He said, "I was thinking about that psycho-mumble-jumble bullshit you were talking about. I think I might be depressed. You talked about that PTSD bullshit that I keep hearing about from these people in Iraq and these young guys, and they don't know how to handle this and that. We called it shell shock." Bingo. He does understand PTSD—as shell shock. And without telling me, he told me that he recognizes that he has this.

I was a mouthy teenager. When my dad would spew hate at me, my first instinct was to spew it back. Now I can stop and say, "Well, Dad, that wasn't very nice. I think this or that." And he will actually apologize now, or he will say, "Well, what do you mean?" And he will have a conversation with me.

Between Siblings

Sibling relationships are important and often overlooked. For many people, their siblings know them the longest, and sometimes the best, of anyone in their life. Here, siblings in their twenties (the Winters family) and in their sixties (the Berkowitz family) discuss what they have learned in their lives facing mental health conditions together.

Liam Winters is a former NAMI employee living in Arlington, Virginia. He was distressed when his sister Emma was hospitalized for mental health issues, something he had been through himself about a year prior:

I got a call from my mom, and she said, "I just want you to know, don't freak out, but Emma's been hospitalized in an inpatient facility." That was one of the scariest and saddest moments of my life. I didn't know what I could do. I've always wrestled with how much of my own experience to share when I know it's important that she has her own experiences and learns on her own. I don't want to generalize my experiences to her. I went to an inpatient setting when I was twenty. Then I was twenty-two when my mom called me with that news about Emma.

For Emma, who works for a nonprofit in New York City, Liam's support—and support from her other siblings—was a defining part of her recovery:

Liam was totally supportive, especially right when I came out of the hospital. He was always calling me and sending me Spotify playlists. He was just really trying to help me and giving me advice. Sometimes, we're different, so the advice didn't land, but it meant so much that he was reaching out to me. At that point, I felt afraid, and I didn't want to feel alone. There was a while where I heard from him almost every day. I also called my older brother in the hospital, and it was good to talk to him because he's very practical. He said, "Look how well Liam's doing. You can be like that too. You'll take care of yourself. You will."

Now Liam, in turn, can benefit from Emma's support both as a sibling, and as a peer:

I've gotten to the point where I am very receptive to feedback from others, particularly Emma, who also lives with bipolar disorder. She's able to notice that in me, and also get it and not judge me. I think for us it was important, and will continue to be important, that we laugh about it. We have a great, very messed-up sense of humor. Because we've both been through it, we totally get that about each other. And it's great to have that feedback loop.

We've already met Janet Berkowitz, the peer specialist in New Jersey who struggled with suicidality and now designs and facilitates creative workshops focused on suicide prevention and bullying. Janet's sister, Cynthia, is a child and adolescent psychiatrist in Massachusetts, a mother of two, stepmother of three, and grandmother of seven. It took Janet and Cynthia decades to learn to navigate the many aspects of their relationship. During Janet's manic episodes, she told me she "couldn't hear it" when Cynthia encouraged her to get help. But she also worried about the stress of her illness on their relationship:

There was a point where I started telling myself, my sister is a psychiatrist, and I want to be careful not to blur the lines of sisterhood and make her my therapist in any way. I needed to honor the fact that she was a doctor in mental health, and I'm a consumer. I didn't want to cross that boundary. I knew Cynthia loved me; I knew what she was going through with it. I also worried that when Mom and Dad died, she would feel like she needed to watch over me, and I wanted to be careful that that didn't become too much pressure. That's why I worked so hard to get so much help on my own.

Cynthia had to learn how to set boundaries, too—not just for Janet, but for herself:

I have to avoid being Janet's psychiatrist. I had to really accept the limits of my powers.

We're polite to each other in our family. You never hang up on anybody on the phone. There was a point where Janet was calling me constantly, wanting to convince me to participate in an emotional growth training she had done. And finally, having been coached, I said, "You know, I can't talk about this anymore. If you keep asking me this, I have to hang up." Janet told me that it was a turning point for her because she realized, "Hey, I have to knock it off because my sister isn't going to do this." I set a good boundary that helped a great deal.

Janet and Cynthia have developed a deep friendship. "I see it as a long, slow, gradual story—a forty-year story of dealing with this," Cynthia told me. "People keep evolving over time and things can get difficult, but it's good to have a perspective that things can get better and change."

Cynthia has incorporated the lessons she learned in her relationship with her sister into her clinical work. She noticed that a lot of families are very opposed to bringing siblings in for family groups, not wanting the siblings to be burdened. But she feels that that's a mistake. "Remember the sibling," she advises, adding that "there's a need to hear siblings, what they're going through, what their questions are, and to talk it through. There is a risk that the sibling could be affected, and you need to talk about that risk and how to manage it."

Family by Choice

Some people define their family as people they deeply connect with, even if they are not related by blood. This takes many forms. For Roselin Dueñas and Jonathan Ordonez—two people who share a deep bond through their shared culture and sexual identity—choosing each other as family made a huge difference in their recovery.

Roselin, a first-generation Hispanic American and queer woman, felt that Jonathan and his family provided acceptance and support that were vital especially when her family relationships were strained due to their difficulties accepting her sexuality:

> I would say we are a family to each other; that he is a brother to me. In 2019, I checked myself into a hospital and he was the one that drove me there and dealt with it all. I remember he was very worried about me, and I'm sorry I put him through that. I was just pushing everyone away, and I wouldn't answer his calls. And he's like, "What's wrong? Why are you ignoring us?" And then he said, "You'll have to get a restraining order if you want me to leave you alone. I'm not giving up on you."

This was a very emotional experience for me, as he had more faith in me than I did in myself at the time, and I could tell how loved and appreciated I was. I also love his family. Especially his mom, who is very accepting, which meant so much to me because my mom still struggles with accepting my sexuality. To find another motherly figure was just life changing. Overall, Jonny and his loved ones are my chosen family that I am lucky to have with me.

For Jonathan, a cisgender, gay Latino man, his friendship with Roselin gave him an increased sense of empathy and openness about mental illness:

Our friendship has taught me to be more empathetic. I've always been an empathetic person, and I consider myself a people person. But through Ros, I've learned a lot about having friends who are very open about mental illness in a way that I don't have with my other friendships. There's an openness we have.

Couples and Partnerships

Some couples make it work whether one or both of them, or their child, has a mental health condition. They do so with specific skills: boundaries, problem-solving, acceptance, and love. For Cathleen Payne, a sixty-one-year-old woman who told me she has lived with borderline personality disorder for over fifty years, a major turning point in her relationship with her husband, Jim, was when he took a class called Family Connections, taught by the National Education Alliance for Borderline Personality Disorder (NEA-BPD). She recalled:

I talk about my life before my husband, Jim, took the Family Connections course, just chaos and pain, and my life after, when he was learning skills in a world where there is something you can do to help manage the pain. If Jim hadn't taken that course, I don't know if I'd be here today. It was transformational in our lives to know that you could actually get treatment and manage your symptoms. Jim got better at responding to my stabbing emotional pain, and this helped me overcome my resistance to the thought of having BPD, and I began to look into specialized treatment like DBT.

Jim agrees that the Family Connections course marked a turning point for their marriage, but that change didn't come easily:

I literally felt at sea at that point. For the first third of the course, I hardly even said a word. I was just so stunned by everything. I had a love-hate relationship with the course and learning about BPD. And then at the end, I couldn't stop. I took the training so I could lead it, just to continue to be involved and develop skills from that course, including DBT-based skills.

After I took the Family Connections course, we began to adjust in fundamental ways. And all the marital therapy that we went through helped too. Then I could better help her during an incident, realizing it's not about me.

Family Connections was a turning point, but some of the skills involved in navigating their relationship through the stormy periods of Cathleen's BPD took the couple years to develop. Cathleen shared one skill that was particularly helpful:

Over the years, as my incidents began to decrease from many times a day to several times a week, we started to develop a skill. I would say, "I can listen to your feelings about my incident for a short period of time, Jim. Usually not for a long time because I start getting dysregulated again. But I can listen to you for about sixty seconds." So, I said, "We can call this a 'sixty.'" And gradually, I was able to listen longer than sixty seconds, but we still call it a "sixty."

To help us cope with BPD in our relationship, we sometimes think of ourselves as a couple of porcupines. He sometimes feels my quills, and I sometimes feel his. The quills are there, but there's more to us than our quills. We also have softer, caring sides. We even like to collect pairs of stuffed toy porcupines to remind us of this. I now have a *Porcupine Love* blog for sharing my experiences, tips, and tools for couples where a partner has BPD or other emotion dysregulation.

Ronald Braunstein and Caroline Whiddon, a married couple, met in Vermont through the Me2/Orchestra, where Ronald serves as the music director and conductor and Caroline as executive director. Caroline described one critical moment early in getting to know each other:

> I ended up in the ER with him a couple times because he had moved to Vermont, and he didn't know anybody. We would eventually figure out that he was having some physical symptoms. It was lithium toxicity, and his kidneys were in trouble. I was a friend, so he eventually said, "Yeah, I've got bipolar disorder." I said, "Oh, thank God, now I know what I'm dealing with." I ordered every Kay Redfield Jamison book. I ordered *Bipolar for Dummies*. I wondered: How do I help him be successful? I said, "Let's figure this out together."

Ronald sees Caroline's help with regulating his schedule and treatment regimen as a component of a loving partnership:

> I didn't look to her as someone who would help me regulate my illness, I thought of her as someone I loved. I found out she was really, really good at managing me, which took me about five years to really accept. But since then, I've been on a roll. I've only had one depressive episode in nine years, and it wasn't that bad. Part of my job is keeping myself together. Another part is conducting. And another part is loving Caroline.

Dante and Chastity Murry, a married couple introduced earlier, work as NAMI support group facilitators in Kentucky. Dante described how setting ground rules and establishing communication strategies helps them hold each other accountable in a supportive and loving way:

We both have the same diagnosis of bipolar disorder, and we both have depression and anxiety. I also have schizoaffective disorder. When we first got together and started dating, and then when we got serious and got married, we had to set some ground rules, guidelines that we do in our support groups. We said, "We've got to sit down and say what's going to work, what's not going to work, and what our expectations are of being a married couple." And so, we did that. We wrote it down on a piece of paper. We talked about our triggers and how to work with them.

Chastity discussed how she and Dante built on these ground rules to support each other in daily life:

When Dante's having a bad day, I try to lift him up and say, "Hey, you need to get out of that bed and get going this morning." Or if I'm having a bad day, and my depression is kicking in, he gets me up and says, "Look, you've got to get your butt out of this bed, and you've got to do what you've got to do." Any time one of us feels like the other is having a bad day, and not doing something they're supposed to be doing, like their laundry or the chores in the house, then it's like, "Okay, we've got to sit down and talk about this."

Marty Parrish, a senior-level IT project manager in his late fifties who lives in Iowa, reports he has survived chronic major depression episodes since he was seventeen. He's married to Peggy Huppert, who was introduced earlier. Marty described how he struggled to maintain a mental health regimen that worked for him:

I'm hardheaded, but also determined. That helps me be successful, but it also can be a constraint when I'm trying to get well from a mental illness. You can't think your way out of it. That's the problem. I tried positive mental attitudes. In my case, it didn't work. Sometimes Peggy could tell I was slipping into depression well before I would acknowledge it.

Peggy has learned how to help Marty monitor his symptoms and respond to relapses in a proactive way. She explained:

> He'll text me in the afternoon sometimes and say, "I'm having a bad brain day. I need your help." When I get those texts, I'm not trying to get home as soon as possible. It's not an emergency. But I want to be aware. We really watch his sleep, because we know that if he goes a couple of days without getting enough sleep, that's a big red flag. And sometimes, someone has to really just kick your butt and hold you accountable, right?

Marty underscored how important it is for someone who suffers mental health challenges to have at least one person in their corner:

> Let's be honest, if she wasn't here, I wouldn't have gone through with treatment. I was trying to drop out before I even got started. You keep thinking, "This is like a broken bone. It's healed. You're good to go." Mental health is not like a broken bone. In my case, it's always there. But what I'm doing now is being more transparent with her about how I feel. I've learned to tell her if I'm not having a good day. She's going to watch too. She will, a lot of times, pick up on things before I do.

• • •

Mental health conditions add complexity to relationships. Even so, the quality of many relationships can improve in the process of learning how best to deal with those conditions together. Changing your attitude or approach, learning specific skills, attending to boundaries, and developing routines for open and honest discussions to prevent relapse are just some of the ways people have found to maintain and deepen their connection to each other.

There are multiple approaches to improving communication skills. One pathway is to employ professionals trained to help you acquire specific skills or suggest new approaches. There are practitioners in all therapeutic disciplines who have a particular interest in improving relationships. Many clinicians—including marriage and family therapists, social workers, counselors, psychologists, and psychiatrists—work with families and couples. Another approach is learning from one another in free peer support or education classes.

THIRTEEN

Navigating the Legal System

"WHAT IS THE LAW?" This all-caps question on my brother's legal pad was the central issue in one family crisis about our dad. Joe was chronicling Dad's behavior and working to understand what we could do to help get him hospitalized during an episode of severe mania and psychosis in the 1980s. Despite our loving relationship, and our encouragement to get help, Dad had fallen into a scary state. Joe noted that Dad had threatened to kill himself, had repeatedly threatened our mother, and had given my parents' life savings to a state representative to restrict the commitment laws in Michigan. I found these upsetting papers after Joe's death, and they gave me some fresh insight into the crises my family had faced. Unfortunately, this kind of urgent need to understand the law is not uncommon for families of people with a serious mental illness. Joe's question is still quite important in many circumstances. Ultimately, the law and the hospital staff saved my dad's life on many occasions.

Often when family members communicate and engage around a loved one's illness, there may not be a need to know the law. Sometimes, though, family members have the double burden of accessing information and finding care for their loved one while navigating a web of laws and regulations that, at times, seem to impede their ability to help. Since I am not a lawyer, I asked Ron Honberg, NAMI's former director of policy and legal affairs (now retired), to share the essential laws and resources for this chapter.

American society was founded on the idea that individuals have the right to liberty, and our system of law is fundamentally designed to protect the rights and privacy of individuals. Although legal protections are very important, these laws sometimes impede access to treatment for individuals whose symptoms affect their ability to make informed decisions about their own care. These protections may seem wrongheaded, and even cruel, for family members who serve as primary caregivers. Often, families give information about a loved one and are upset that they receive no information in return. Finding a balance between protecting civil rights and enabling people to help others before they come to harm or suffer needlessly is a significant challenge, one that is made worse by chronic underfunding of services.

This chapter briefly discusses some of the key legal issues that impact access and quality of care for people living with mental illness. It is not a substitute for speaking to a lawyer who understands your state's mental health law. Each story represents one family and one outcome in one state. Your local NAMI Affiliate can also be a resource to you.

Here are some key principles for families to know:

1. Most laws, procedures, and standards are defined by the individual states, though some are federal. Factors such as commitment law, visitation rights, length of stay, parental rights, and many more can vary state to state. Learning state law and consulting resources such as your local NAMI affiliate will assist you in helping a family member with a mental health condition.

2. When health care providers need information, it is important to give it to them. Give as much context to your loved one's history as you can, in writing when possible and verbally as the situation warrants. Your provider likely wants to share

information with you but may be restricted by law. Unfortunately, you may be frustrated by how little information you receive in return.

3. Dialing 988 will connect you with a trained crisis worker. Working with a trained mental health crisis responder may improve outcomes for those in distress.

Crisis and Emergency Psychiatric Assessments

In most states, emergency psychiatric assessments are a first step in determining whether a person meets criteria for involuntary inpatient commitment. When a person experiences a crisis, calls for assistance are often initiated by the individual, family members, friends, or others who know the person. Some counties have mobile crisis response teams composed of mental health professionals who will go wherever the person is. In other counties, emergency medical technicians or law enforcement officers respond to crisis calls. People across the country can now dial the new mental health crisis response number, 988, which connects you to mental health de-escalation more quickly in cases of substance use, mental health crisis, or when there is a life-threatening situation.

If responders determine that a person's symptoms are sufficiently serious, the person will typically be transported to a facility for a more comprehensive evaluation. These evaluations often occur in general emergency rooms, and frustrating delays are common. Be prepared to wait, but know that getting care for your loved one will be worth it.

Emergency psychiatric evaluations are different from civil commitment. These evaluations are typically time limited, ranging from one to ten days depending on the state. The purpose of these evaluations is essentially to determine whether the person needs civil commitment, which is typically for a longer period.

Inpatient Civil Commitment

All states have a process for civil commitment. Based on the emergency psychiatric evaluation, if it is determined that a person's symptoms are severe enough to necessitate inpatient treatment, and the person is not willing to accept this treatment voluntarily, a hearing is held to determine whether the person should be involuntarily committed to an inpatient treatment facility.

At the commitment hearing, evidence in support of the request for inpatient commitment is presented to a judge or magistrate. Because involuntary commitment is a significant infringement on a person's liberty, the person who is being considered for commitment has certain rights, including the right to be present at the hearing, to be represented by a lawyer, to provide evidence why they should not be committed, and to appeal a decision.

Nearly every state commitment statute includes danger to self or others as a criterion. Many states include additional standards, such as grave disability, commonly defined as the inability to provide for one's own basic needs, including food or shelter. The interpretation of these terms as they apply to real-world situations sometimes differs based on the beliefs of the judge or magistrate who is hearing the case. The maximum length that a person can be committed to an inpatient treatment facility also varies across states. The shortages of beds can cause delays, and shortage of appropriate community-based services can complicate the process.

Although involuntary commitment can be lifesaving, it is not a cure-all. Some people describe their experiences in inpatient psychiatric treatment facilities in negative or even traumatic terms, as discussed in chapter 6. Both individuals and families have rights. To learn more about addressing concerns for the care of a loved one in a hospital, contact your local protection and advocacy (P&A) agency or your local NAMI affiliate.

Voluntary participation in mental health treatment is always preferable to involuntary commitment. In this context, steps to help people meaningfully engage in decisions about their own care and treatment—such as shared decision-making and, where legally recognized, psychiatric advance directives (PADs)—should be utilized as widely as possible. In chapter 17, Jackie Feldman describes some proactive approaches.

Finally, it is important to recognize that involuntary commitment does not usually equate with the authority to administer psychiatric medications on an involuntary basis, and states often require a separate process for patients who may need but refuse medication. Generally, state laws set forth certain factors to consider in making these decisions, including whether the person lacks capacity to make treatment decisions, whether the administration of psychiatric medications is the least restrictive treatment available, and whether the failure to administer medications is likely to increase the length of the involuntary commitment.

Guardianships/Conservatorships

Guardianships or conservatorships, called conservatorships in the remainder of this section, are court orders giving legal authority to others to make important decisions for people with mental illness or other disabilities who have been found by a judge to lack capacity to make decisions on their own behalf. Limited conservatorships are generally specific to discrete functions, such as health care, whereas full conservatorships often apply to all aspects of the person's life who is under the conservatorship, including financial decisions.

Angela Brisbin, of Missouri, felt that several institutions missed clues that her adult son, Michael, a college student diagnosed with schizophrenia at the age of nineteen, was severely symptomatic. In Missouri, and in her specific family situation, the law gave her tools to get effective help for her son. She recalled:

Eventually we realized it was schizophrenia. We asked Michael to see a psychiatrist. He said no, he didn't think there was anything wrong with him. His illness continued to progress until Michael became extremely delusional and started hearing voices. We called an ambulance because we really wanted him to be hospitalized, and we thought that would be the route; that maybe the ambulance would take him to the hospital and involuntarily commit him.

But that was just the beginning. They hospitalized him; they started him on meds. He came home, and then we tried one medication after another, and he just kept getting worse and worse.

Angela described getting a conservatorship to have legal leverage in Michael's medication regimen:

In Missouri, unless someone is a danger to themselves or others, you cannot force hospitalization. And even once they're hospitalized, it's still difficult if they refuse the medication. To get him to take the medicine I thought he needed, I had to have guardianship. I had power of attorney, but that wasn't enough. I said, "I want to try clozapine now." And his doctor said, "Well, I just feel like it's too dangerous. You might be risking his life." And I said, "No, I think we're risking his life by him not taking clozapine."

There had been thirteen failed antipsychotics, four hospitalizations, and an overdose where he ended up in intensive care. So finally, I had to apply for guardianship of Michael for him to get clozapine. That wasn't what I wanted to do, but it was the only way I could get the local doctors here to prescribe it. Until then they had discouraged it, and Michael, who wasn't well at the time, didn't want it. Finally, I had to take legal action, and he started to get better when he got the clozapine.

When I interviewed Michael Brisbin, he recalled that it was his mother's persistence that ultimately helped him accept care. He told me:

When all of this first started, I didn't realize the value of taking medicine. I thought I wasn't sick. Mom helped me realize that I was. She has helped a lot. She researched all of this on the internet, every single night staying up hours after everyone else went to bed. So, for me, once I realized I was sick, I felt a lot more motivated to take medicine.

Angela is now studying to become a psychiatric nurse practitioner to improve access to clozapine in Missouri. Michael is on the board of directors for NAMI of Greater Kansas City and runs a NAMI young adult support group. He plans to become a social worker and work in the mental health field.

Generally, a person or organization petitioning for conservatorship must demonstrate that the individual in question lacks capacity to make informed decisions about mental health care on their own behalf. Conservatorships can be very helpful, even lifesaving, for individuals whose severe symptoms prevent them from making informed decisions. And those appointed as conservators generally have legal authority to access information about health or mental health treatment, communicate with medical or mental health providers, and serve as an active participant in the person's medical and mental health care.

For more information about guardianships, including state guardianships associations, visit the National Guardianship Association website.

The Health Privacy Conundrum

Family members frequently serve as the de facto caregivers of their adult children with mental illnesses. Yet once a person turns eighteen, medical and mental health providers often assume that they cannot communicate with family members or other caregivers unless the person specifically consents to such disclosure. In general, this is a correct assumption. However, this general principle, when applied to people with fluctuating capacity to consent due to the symptoms of their serious mental illness, can prove detrimental to recovery and care coordination.

Alice Henley, a retired educator from Connecticut, ran into this challenge with her son, John, a thirty-four-year-old musician and facilities crew member, when he was admitted to a psychiatric hospital for treatment of psychosis when he was eighteen:

> At the first hospital John was taken to, we had to fight for conservatorship to be able to have any kind of say in his care because he was eighteen at that point. They wouldn't let me in at times or give us access to him or his medical records. The conservatorship let us know what was going on, which was crucial. I remember one time, when I got there to visit him, they wouldn't let me in, and I said, "Why not?" And they said, "Well, he was acting strangely." I said, "Well, could you describe that to me?" And they said that he was walking through the hallway singing and dancing. That infuriated me because that was typical John behavior at that age. He did a lot of singing and dancing.

"I needed my mom at this point," John told me. "I needed a strong support system, and she was able to do it for me. I was out of my mind at this point. I give her credit. She's the one that pulled me through this."

Health Information Portability and Accountability Act (HIPAA)

Mental health providers often want to hear from you and, when allowed, to share information with you. The assumption that HIPAA poses an absolute barrier to communications is not only inaccurate but also detrimental to achieving good treatment outcomes and recovery. Some professionals were taught, as I was at first, to think of HIPPA in absolute terms. In actuality, the HIPAA law is far less rigid than many may think and permits communications with caregivers under certain circumstances even when the individual who is receiving care is unwilling or unable to provide consent. HIPAA permits communications with caregivers under three circumstances.

First, when the individual who is receiving mental health treatment consents to the disclosure of information. Contrary to common belief, this consent can be given by the individual verbally or in writing, though it is always advisable to get something in writing. Additionally, if the provider tells the individual about plans to communicate with a caregiver or begins to communicate with a caregiver while the individual is present and the individual does not object, that also meets the criteria for consent.

Second, a mental health provider can communicate with a caregiver when there are concerns about the person's safety or risks to others. For example, if a mental health practitioner determines that a situation is an emergency, they can share information.

Third, mental health professionals are permitted to communicate with caregivers when they determine that the person lacks capacity to make a decision on their own. This determination may be based on the discretion of the practitioner and does not require a hearing or a court order.

In view of the benefits of communications with caregivers, the process of obtaining consent from the individual receiving mental health treatment should be an ongoing process, even in cases where the individual initially withholds consent.

The Family Education Rights and Privacy Act (FERPA)

FERPA is the federal law that establishes the rights of students to protect their educational records. The law sets forth rights of parents of students under age eighteen, and these rights transfer to students once they reach the age of eighteen. FERPA also protects certain student health records. Specifically, FERPA applies to health records generated on campus, such as a campus health or counseling center. By contrast, HIPAA applies to health records generated off campus, for example at a hospital or a community mental health center. The privacy protections in FERPA are important, but they can also result in parents not being informed of health issues or crises that arise while their children are students. This can be particularly problematic when the symptoms of mental illness first

emerge, because early intervention and timely mental health treatment
are so important at this stage. Joseph Feaster Jr. of Massachusetts, who
we met earlier, had this experience:

> I remember when I took my son to college for orientation, their thing
> was, "We can't give out any information to you as the parent; we have to
> give it to the student." Well, when I subsequently got the bill, and then I
> got my son's grades, he was apparently having episodes that they never
> alerted me about.

In general, colleges and universities need authorization from students
to release health or mental health information to their parents. Parents
of children who are starting college can emphasize to their child the importance of authorizing this communication. There are two exceptions
in FERPA to this requirement: Colleges and universities may release information to parents without authorization in a) situations involving
health or safety emergencies and b) if the parent claims the student as a
dependent on their taxes. A mental health crisis necessitating emergency
transportation to a hospital or crisis center will often meet the definition
of a health or safety emergency.

Colleges and universities are in a challenging position with students
who are at a relatively high-risk developmental period in their life. One
approach that has been effective for some families is to strongly encourage their student to proactively sign permission forms in order to be informed if there is a mental health concern. This opportunity can present
itself at orientation in freshman year but can also be done later. For more
information about how FERPA and HIPAA apply to student health and
mental health information, see "Starting the Conversation: College and
Your Mental Health," a guide developed by NAMI and the JED foundation, posted on NAMI's website.

Assisted Outpatient Treatment

Formerly called outpatient commitment, assisted outpatient treatment (AOT) is court-ordered, mandatory treatment in the community. AOT is intended specifically to help individuals who repeatedly experience hospitalizations, homelessness, criminal justice involvement, or other adverse consequences due to lack of participation in treatment. Initially, AOT was primarily intended for people leaving hospitals and entering the community. However, in recent years, it has evolved in certain states as a less restrictive alternative to hospitalization for people who meet specific criteria, such as a history of dangerous behavior when untreated. Like all other mental health services, however, AOT cannot succeed if it is not adequately funded or resourced.

There is controversy around AOT laws and programs. Some critics have characterized AOT as being "forced treatment." This controversy is unfortunate, because AOT can be useful, and even lifesaving, for the small numbers of people who meet legal criteria for it. Ideally, AOT can help get services to people who repeatedly fall through the many cracks of the mental health system and experience homelessness, hospitalization, or incarceration as a result.

AOT was key to recovery for Eric Smith of San Antonio, Texas, who we met earlier. However, his parents Nancy and Brad Smith had to take drastic steps to get Eric the help he needed. Eric did not have awareness of his illness, and the Smith family felt they were out of options. A health care provider advised Nancy and Brad to get Eric care by having him arrested. Eric describes his parents' decision:

> My parents spoke with my previous psychiatrist, and they said, "Look, our son is just the worst he's been. What can we do?" And he said, "Well, the way things are set up now, the best bet for him to get the care and treatment that he needs is if he gets arrested for a low-level offense. And hopefully, before he is released from jail, he can be transferred to the state hospital if a bed opens for him there, and he could get the care that he

needs there. And then, if he's stabilized, he might be able to get some sort of outpatient care, and then live in the community."

Eric reflected:

I would consider my life having been worth living if by the time that I'm gone and my advocacy efforts have ended, no one in the United States is told by anyone in the system, "Your loved one needs mental health care for a severe mental illness. Hopefully, they will get arrested so they can get the care they need."

Although the Smiths had to take drastic and difficult measures, the judicial system was the only way they could engage Eric in care. Eric received AOT, which ended up being the best treatment plan for him. In our interview, Nancy Smith agreed:

I would say AOT saved Eric's life, because it ensured he was monitored as an outpatient, and, when he needed it, was what got him back in the hospital. We just had to call the judge and say, "Eric's meds stopped working, and he needs to be back in the hospital." It was the only way we were able to get him back in the hospital that quickly.

AOT programs should not be used as a substitute for underfunded voluntary services, but they can be very beneficial, for those individuals who, due to the severity of their symptoms, are consistently non-adherent with services and who suffer adverse consequences as a result. In our interview, Eric said:

The entire AOT treatment team is accountable to each other. The judicial/ civil legal mechanism there adds a valuable layer of accountability that does not exist without a judge, and it is a compassionate, communicative, and collaborative team effort from start to finish.

Law Enforcement Training and Crisis Intervention Teams (CIT)

For Eric Smith and his family, police intervention was the first step in getting him help through the judicial system. Many communities have relied on law enforcement to respond to people experiencing mental health crises because of a lack of mental health resources at local levels. But police responses can be unhelpful for people in crisis, and at times catastrophic. Many law-enforcement officers do not have the training or skills to respond effectively to people in crisis. Traditional law-enforcement tactics can lead to tragic outcomes, especially for people of color and those with serious mental illness. This speaks to the need for training, and for alternatives to traditional police response. Ideally, law enforcement should have very limited involvement in responding to people with mental health crises, which is why NAMI has supported the enhancement of 988 and the development of a crisis response continuum of care.

Crisis Intervention Team (CIT) programs are community-based initiatives that bring together law enforcement, mental health professionals, mental health advocates, and other partners to improve community responses to mental health crises. The origins of CIT are a core part of NAMI's story. They were first started as a result of advocacy by two NAMI leaders, Helen Adamo and Ann Dino, in Memphis. In partnership with Major Sam Cochran (now retired), Helen and Ann created the first CIT program, now well known in communities across the country.

The most well-known part of CIT is a forty-hour training for law enforcement that provides insight into mental health conditions and training on de-escalation. As part of the program, peers and families with lived experience tell their stories. People in law enforcement who have participated in CIT often cite these presentations as a particularly impactful part of the training curriculum.

Drea Landry of Delaware, an African American mother of two and grandmother of five who describes herself as "very spiritual," thrives on educating others to live their best life. In our interview, she discussed her interactions with police as a Black woman living with mental illness and her current work facilitating CIT trainings with police officers:

> Ordinarily, an adult can go missing for seventy-two hours. That's nationwide. But if you have a mental illness, they come looking for you immediately. My ex-husband, who called the police on me, told them that I had a mental illness. When they asked him if I was a danger to myself or others, he said, "I don't know what the hell her problem is." They came looking for me immediately. When they found me, the lady approached me with her hand on her gun.
>
> I said, "Listen, I had an argument with my husband. I needed to cool off so that I wouldn't break things. Please don't shoot me. Don't hurt me."
>
> That was scary. That's why I would tell the police department, when I did the NAMI presentations, "Listen to the person. I know you guys are scared, and that sometimes you never know what that person is going to be like, especially when they're heavily symptomatic. But they are speaking more truth at that moment than they are in a normal state of mind. If you listen intently to what they're saying and address it one thing at a time, it'll make things a whole lot easier than pulling your gun out."
>
> One of the things I say is, we want to get the police out of the habit of "shoot first, ask questions never," and instead, again, to just listen. Just stop long enough to listen to every single thing the person says. Before you overreact and take that extra measure, it can make a world of difference. Being a person of color, we tend to have it harder than others who are not. Therefore, we have to be more vigilant. Treat us all the same. It doesn't matter what our race, ethnicity, or creed is. We are still human beings, and we need to be listened to equally.

NAMI members throughout the country have worked with local law enforcement agencies to foster CIT and de-escalation training for law enforcement officers, and to create partnerships and procedures for coordination between law enforcement and mental health systems. These initiatives have had a positive impact on law enforcement's understanding of mental illness, increased linkages to treatment instead of incarceration, and in some instances helped prevent a tragedy.

Responses to people experiencing crises should be led by mental health agencies, not law enforcement. Some communities have implemented such crisis response systems, the most highly publicized of these being the CAHOOTS (Crisis Assistance Helping Out on the Streets) program in Eugene, Oregon. CAHOOTS teams include at least two experts in crisis intervention, including a mental health professional and a medic who is either an EMT or a nurse. Another approach to responding to crises is the "co-responder" model: partnerships between mental health and/or substance abuse professionals and law enforcement. These programs, which have been adopted in a number of communities, offer similar opportunities as other crisis response models by creating alternatives to arrests and incarceration and facilitating linkages with follow-up mental health and substance use services.

Criminal Justice Issues

The extreme overrepresentation of people with mental illness in our nation's jails and prisons is horrifying and tragic. Two million times each year, people with mental illness are booked into our nation's jails. More people living with mental health conditions are incarcerated than in hospitals on any given day. Many of those incarcerated with mental illness also have co-occurring substance use conditions. A series of court decisions have established that incarcerated individuals with serious medical conditions and illnesses have a constitutional right to treatment, though that was not the experience of many of the people I interviewed.

Eric Smith, who was arrested to try to gain access to assisted outpatient treatment (AOT), experienced firsthand how the current system of criminalizing mental illness harms everyone involved:

I'm in jail, arrested for trespassing. At times, I interacted with compassionate and empathetic police officers. Other times, I interacted with officers who threatened to harm me. I want to be very clear here that this is less the fault of the officers and more of an indictment against the way society handles putting people with a mental illness into the criminal justice system. If you task a police officer with handling people going through a severe mental illness crisis, they're being tasked to do things outside of their expertise. Don't expect that to look the way it would with a psychiatrist and a social worker.

Police are taught to maintain power and authority over people who are incarcerated. Since the goal is maintaining power and authority instead of providing the type of treatment and care that is needed for people with severe mental illness, we can see how the criminal justice system is not designed or equipped to meet the needs of severe mental illness. I was in jail for a month. No treatment for my mental illness whatsoever. My delusions, hallucinations, and paranoia were the worst they had ever been up to that point. It was an experience that I wouldn't wish upon anyone.

NAMI promotes models that facilitate diversion from criminal justice settings. The sequential intercept model promotes jail diversion at many points in the judicial process and promotes help, not handcuffs. More information is available on the SAMHSA website.

Mental Health Specialty Courts

Mental Health Courts are specialized courts established with the goal of diverting people with mental illness and co-occurring substance use disorders into treatment instead of incarceration. There are estimated to be more than 450 adult mental health courts in existence nationally, as well as additional mental health courts for juvenile offenders. Some jurisdictions also have addiction-focused courts.

Although mental health courts differ in structure, philosophy, and who they serve, most courts include judges, prosecutors, and defense attorneys who specifically focus on cases involving people with mental illness and co-occurring disorders. Rather than following the traditional model of adjudicating criminal cases and issuing verdicts and sentences, these courts aim to find consensus on an outcome that involves treatment for the defendant rather than punishment. The judge provides ongoing supervision until the person completes the program. These courts also employ coordinators, staff, and sometimes peer support specialists to help individuals find needed services within the mental health system.

Research on mental health courts suggest that they are effective in reducing recidivism, or rearrests. But their effectiveness in improving mental health outcomes depends upon availability and community support.

Mental Health and Substance Use Treatment in Correctional Facilities

Correctional facilities are not designed to provide mental health care, and, in most of them, inmates lack access to adequate—or any—care. Too often, correctional staff are under-trained and under-resourced, and they may respond harshly to people exhibiting mental health symptoms. Diversion of people with mental illness into community-based or inpatient mental health treatment programs should be the goal whenever possible.

Kimberly Comer, who we met in chapter 6, described her experiences living with undertreated mental illness in the criminal justice system:

> When I was in the county jail, I wasn't properly medicated; I wasn't seeing my therapist; there was no support system; I wasn't sleeping, and I wasn't eating. It's not where you go for wellness. Over the next eleven months, I was arrested thirteen times. Every time they'd arrest me, they'd take me off my meds cold turkey. Well, in order for my medications to be therapeutic, I must be on them a minimum of four to six weeks.

While incarcerated in a maximum-security prison, Kimberly experienced episodes of psychosis. Instead of receiving treatment, she was placed into solitary confinement, where she continued to receive no treatment.

NAMI opposes and has long fought the use of solitary confinement and equivalent forms of administrative segregation for people with mental health conditions. Solitary confinement for people with serious mental illness causes extreme suffering, disrupts treatment (if any treatment is happening), causes or worsens symptoms such as depression, anxiety, and hallucinations, and has a long-term negative impact on cognitive and adaptive functioning.

The Bottom Line for Families of Incarcerated Loved Ones

If you are concerned about the well-being of a loved one who is incarcerated, ask your family member to sign a consent form so that you can contact someone who is responsible for medical treatment in the correctional facility. Whenever possible, try to provide written information to medical staff about your loved one's mental health history, including medications that have worked in the past. If you are aware that your loved one is being mistreated, there are organizations that advocate for the rights of prisoners. The American Civil Liberties Union (ACLU) and your state's federally funded protection and advocacy (P&A) organization may also be a source of assistance.

Inside prison settings, some NAMI affiliates have set up Connections groups. Another model is WRAP, which was introduced in chapter 3. Lynn Miller, a fifty-five-year-old criminal justice advocate born and raised in Philadelphia, worked to introduce WRAP to prisons throughout Pennsylvania as the state prison system's sole mental health advocate and peer. She described a turbulent and traumatic childhood that influenced her advocacy journey, and she told me what she discovered in the state's prisons when she began her job:

I did this whirlwind tour of Pennsylvania's twenty-six prisons, every seg-regation unit, and the superintendent said, "What was your takeaway?" I said: "There's so much trauma in here. It's not just the inmates, but also the staff." He said, "So, what would you do?" and I said I would imple-ment a trauma-informed program, which we did start. The peer program in Pennsylvania's prisons had been someone else's vision, and then there I was. Now we have them in all twenty-six prisons.

And I said my other takeaway was that I should be in prison. I easily could have been. The incarcerated people were just like me. The staff thought less of them, the community thought less of them, the world thinks less of them. Yet I will go to my grave saying some of the best peo-ple I know and some of the only people I would trust with my life are sitting behind bars.

Lynn has done the best she can within the prison system, where more people reside with mental health conditions than in hospitals. It is a sad moral commentary and a call for action that this is the current state of affairs in the United States.

. . .

The legal system is almost as complex and inaccessible as the mental health system, and one of the complexities they have in common is that laws, policies, practices, and resources differ from state to state and in some instances county to county. More information can be found in the Resources section.

FOURTEEN

The Hardest Family Questions

I n my years at NAMI, I have been asked many questions by families who want the best for their family members. Sometimes I know of a research study, service, or resource I can refer them to, or I can introduce them to another NAMI family that has been through similar challenges and may have wisdom to share. Often, though, the questions are unique to each person or family, and don't have set answers. For example, some people just do not respond to the standard treatments. Others do not accept treatment, often due to the brain-based nature of their condition. These questions then evolve into deeper questions about acceptance, the ability to have relationships under difficult conditions, the role of spiritual life, and the search for meaning. Each family must answer these questions for themselves. But they do not need to do so alone.

In this chapter, a few of the many people who have faced these hardest questions share their journeys to answer them—the issues they faced, the choices they made, the wrong turns, and the unexpected revelations. They share their stories in the hopes you might learn something from them, both in terms of their direct efforts to help their family members, and the approaches they have taken to make meaning when there are no concrete solutions. These stories are, inevitably, personal, and they represent only a few of the many paths people have taken. It's important to keep in mind that these questions don't lend themselves to instant answers or quick fixes. Finding the right solutions for you, or coming to terms with the absence of them, is a journey that may take time. Connecting with others to share your experiences on that journey may be an integral part of getting there.

My adult child lacks awareness of their own illness and is refusing help. What can I do?

One of the most difficult—and common—situations families have faced is when their loved one lacks awareness that there is any reason for concern. The person denies that anything is wrong and may feel insulted or offended by the suggestion. They cannot see the problem and thus see no need to address it.

It can be easy to mistake this for willful denial, and to worry that unless we break through that denial, our loved one will likely only get worse. And it is true that a lack of awareness can correlate with forgoing treatment, refusing medication, and, often, worse outcomes. But our desperate attempts to enlighten the person we love often don't just fail; they create discord. The result is more frustration, a sense of helplessness, and even anger.

It's important to know that someone's lack of awareness of their own mental illness may in fact be a symptom of that illness. In the medical field, this symptom is called anosognosia. Anosognosia is a brain-based condition that is a feature of other brain-based conditions. It can be an aspect of Alzheimer's disease or other forms of dementia; it can also be a consequence of some strokes. When I was on a neurology rotation as a medical intern, I was surprised to meet patients who, after a stroke, forgot to wash or dress one side of their body. As their symptoms improved, they could then "see" that side of their body. In the mental health world, this phenomenon occurs primarily in psychosis-spectrum illnesses like schizophrenia, schizoaffective disorder, and, at times, bipolar disorder and severe depression. Awareness can sometimes be developed through relationship support and treatment, but often the vexing problem persists.

When someone is affected by a brain-based condition, it can be difficult to recognize or assess the extent to which their emotions and thoughts are affected by an illness process. My dad periodically experienced this state during his episodes, so I know intimately the challenge, pain, and helplessness it can generate for family members. The same microwave he truly thought was communicating to him during an episode of psychosis was just an appliance he used to heat up his coffee a few months later. We were lucky that his awareness would return once his episode ended, after months in the state hospital. He knew something had happened that prompted hospitalization, and he would take the prescribed lithium and antipsychotic medication, but he didn't want to discuss his illness or treatment. He would rather take me to a Detroit Tigers game and engage in playful stories. It was also easier for me to take all the good in him and deny his painful episodes.

That kind of denial on our part was a separate issue from that of anosognosia, which is inherent to the brain and not a conscious or unconscious choice. Dad happened to have both sides of this coin: episodic lack of awareness *and* self-protective denial after an episode. Anosognosia is the brain; denial is the mind. In fact, both of us had denial, but that can be worked on, as we saw in chapter 12. The brain dimension of anosognosia, however, is an ongoing challenge that science has yet to understand.

In Part IV, I ask two experts—Xavier Amador, author of *I Am Not Sick, I Don't Need Help*, and Kate Hardy, a leader in cognitive behavioral therapy for psychosis (CBTp)—to share their approaches to care in this critical area. Because anosognosia is brain-based, not everyone who lacks awareness of their illness can gain it—even with the best relationship support and treatment. I believe one way to better understand what your family member is going through is to listen to someone who has lost awareness, regained it, and can talk about it.

Carlos A. Larrauri of Florida, a musician, nurse practitioner, and former NAMI board member who is also in graduate school, can describe the experiences of both knowing and not knowing. His close-knit Cuban American family was a strong force in helping him access early treatment and get the psychotherapy and medications that were helpful to him. Carlos described to me his experience with anosognosia, comparing it to a fog:

There were moments early on where I had self-awareness. That's the thing. The fog kind of rolls in. It doesn't just settle all at once. At college I knew I should be doing my homework, but I was struggling to do it. I knew I should go to sleep, and I wasn't sleepy. I'm feeling more anxious. "Psychotic break" is a misnomer. People think it just happens one day—just a sudden, clean break; you've had a traumatic experience. But it's much more of an insidious process. There are periods of insight that occur. The fog waxes and wanes. My mom would say, "There were periods where I saw the real Carlos come back for a few days or hours. Then the psychosis would settle, and he would be inappropriate and not make sense."

Carlos went on to explain:

There's this lack of awareness, but it's punctuated with moments of insight that are absolutely terrifying. When you are fully aware that you're losing your mind and everything that comes with it—your sense of identity, your sense of relation to the world around you, everything you love, the people, places—and you're starting to get a sense of loss of all of that, it's a terrifying experience.

For me, with medication came self-awareness, about two or three months later. It almost felt like a lightbulb went off. I had enough insight to realize, "Well, I need to take my meds, then, because now that I'm taking them, I have a home, I have food, I have shelter, I have my basic needs," and I started to realize that I can't meet any of those needs on my own.

Carlos then used his awareness to leverage his many talents, becoming a national leader in advocacy, clinical care, and teaching in the mental health field.

The experience of anosognosia can also be poignantly logical. Like every family confronted with this challenge, Judy Harris, a retired lawyer, and her husband, Norman Ornstein, a political scientist and emeritus scholar at the American Enterprise Institute in Washington, DC, struggled to understand their late son Matthew's anosognosia. Judy recalled:

> Over time, we came to understand that our son had absolutely no insight into his illness. He was adamant that he was not sick. He believed to the core of his being that he had done something to anger God and that, as a result, God had taken his soul and was testing his faith. The only way forward was to earn back God's love. Seeing a doctor and/or taking medicine would only anger God further and destroy any possibility of having his former happy, almost idyllic, life restored.

The logical nature of anosognosia is challenging. The delusion, defined as a fixed false belief, isn't reality based, but the conclusions still followed logically. Their son's actions were completely rational if you believed what he believed.

After his death in an accident, Judy and Norm found solace in helping others. They founded the Matthew Harris Ornstein Memorial Foundation, which supports Xavier Amador in providing low-cost trainings to first responders, medical professionals, and others in communicating better with people with severe mental illness; funds a summer debate institute and tournament, honoring Matthew's enthusiasm and achievements as a champion debater; and underwrote production of the documentary film *The Definition of Insanity*, which highlights the work of Judge Steve Leifman in Miami-Dade County to decriminalize the treatment of people living with mental illness and help people with anosognosia get help and stay out of criminal justice settings.

How to cope with the loss and uncertainty that can accompany anosognosia is another common and difficult question families are forced to face. Anita Herron, introduced earlier, was confronted with this challenge directly when she realized her husband was in a different stage than her in terms of processing their son's lack of awareness:

> My husband has been at acceptance for a long time. He's a praying man; and he reads his Bible and prays that he will survive this, until maybe one day our son will have the realization. I'm not as religious. For me, there's a lot of guilt, even though you know you've done what you can. I finally came to terms with that probably a month ago. We were paying a lawyer for our son's court cases, and our son never went to court. I finally said, "We've done all we could." But there's still always going to be that guilt. I used to get so angry when someone would say, "Well, Anita, you've done all you could for him." I'd say, "Stop telling me that. There's got to be something else I could have done." So even though in your mind you know you've done what you can, you still question.

How do I cope when I don't know where my adult child is?

Some people may lose contact with a loved one experiencing severe mental illness altogether. This is an extremely challenging situation, one that can arouse intense emotions and fracture other relationships in the family as well.

Matt and Carolyn Edwards, a couple from Utah, tried for a year with little success to rebuild their relationship with their son, who had cut ties with them during his struggle with mental illness. After taking a NAMI Family-to-Family class, they gained new insight into what had been an agonizing and frustrating situation:

> It was already a nightmare for us. Our son had moved out and said he's never going to see us again. And then, in the class, someone living with mental illness shared a letter about their experience that I really felt expressed what my son must have been feeling, but not saying. It said, "Hey, why don't you understand me? Here's some of the things I experience." I

thought, man, why didn't I have that letter before? Because I honestly believe I could have avoided the catastrophe. So, I put that on me. Because, yeah, he did lots of bad things, but had I understood the "why" behind it, and the feeling behind it, I would have been much more compassionate. I would have let certain things roll off my back, been able to approach him. And with our letter to him, we sent it while he was away from us. And we said, I think we're understanding. And that's the first time he reached back out.

Developing empathy helped Matt and Carolyn reconnect with their son. But though they were reconnected with him for a while, he has since stopped reaching out, and they are no longer in contact. They believe a relapse of his symptoms is behind his disappearance. When I talked to them, they did not know his whereabouts or whether he was safe. One of the most difficult aspects of loving someone with a mental illness is the nonlinear and sometimes cyclical nature of that illness. Matt went on to share:

All my life my biggest fear was: What if one of my kids got kidnapped and I just didn't know? That, to me, would be the worst nightmare. And I feel like people with mental health conditions and their families can find themselves in that kind of nightmare. We've had people come into family groups and say, "I don't know where my child is." "We think they're in California now." "We hear from them every few months." And so, you have this child disappearance issue, even though they're adults. And how do you deal with that? Well, we're dealing with that.

Because of our experience at NAMI, we can still hang on to the hope that our son will come home. Because I understand so much more about his condition and how people who have them deal with them, I'm assuming this is one of these bad times for him. I'm assuming if he survives, he will come back, and we will meet him here again, and we will move on.

Developing their sense of empathy helped the Edwards family make sense of their son's experience. Their Latter-day Saints church, which Matt said is like a big family, has since asked them to teach NAMI Family-to-Family classes, helping themselves and others find a way to cope.

Am I a bad parent? Was this my fault?

The psychiatric profession once infamously blamed mothers for their children's schizophrenia. And despite how much more we know today about the complex neurobiological basis of mental health conditions, some of the people I interviewed still felt blamed at times for their loved one's mental health condition, including by mental health professionals, clergy, and neighbors. Self-blame is a more insidious challenge. Regardless of your child's diagnosis, it is human to wonder about your role in your child's experience and to cope with guilt and self-blame.

Karen Ranus, a Latina and native-Texan mental health advocate, described her process of working through shame and guilt after she almost lost her teenage daughter to suicide. "I made the list mentally of all the things I'd either done or failed to do that led us to wind up in that place," she told me, adding that she didn't see it as a health issue, but rather as "a failure of parenting." Karen told me about her first NAMI Family-to-Family class and what that meant to her:

I was so nervous. I walked in and here's all these people sitting in this room, and nobody had horns on their head. I say that because I was walking around with the weight of feeling like I had really failed her, like I was a terrible parent. But it was just all normal people. And a lot of it was the sense of, "I'm not alone." It's so much easier to feel compassion and empathy for other people, right? What I realized is, I was not extending that to myself, but I'm listening to other people tell their story, and I'm just like, "Oh my gosh, you poor thing. That's awful." I walked into that room with this big bag of shame, guilt, blame. And I just left that bag there. I feel like after that first class, it was just like, "Okay, this is hard, but this is not our fault."

Cathy Guild, who we met earlier, faced this question—Am I a bad parent? Is this my fault?—when she lost custody of her children in the wake of trauma and addiction. For her, the answer involved both having the courage to face the real impact of her mental health issues on her ability to parent and having the courage to seek recovery for herself. She remembered:

Someone called DSS—the Department of Social Services—on me. DSS came and saw that I was basically living in a drug den. They were going to take my children away. I cried because I felt like a failure of a mother at the time. And then I thought about it, and I wasn't being much of a mother anyway. I'd always said I wanted to be the kind of mother that my mother wasn't. I was failing miserably at that. I was not there for them. So, when DSS said that they were going to take her, I had to agree with them, and I let them.

I went to therapy, and I got through this thing. And then they said to me, "We're going to see about you getting your children back." I was floored. I couldn't believe I could have my children back in my life. They had a system. I'd call. They'd call back. So now I'm talking to my child again and I'm telling her I'm going to get better and she's going to come back into my life. She's happy. She hadn't spoken to me in three years. Now I got some recovery under my belt, I'm connecting to my firstborn. Now it's time to get my whole family together.

Cathy needed treatment to be the parent she wanted to be. Cathleen Payne, who we met earlier, also had to come to terms with the impact of her mental health symptoms on her children and find ways to help her family heal. Words said or actions done while experiencing an episode of mental illness can cause real and lasting harm to relationships. This harm can go unaddressed for the sake of moving forward. But Cathleen and Jim decided early on that for their family, mental health and healing required openly addressing the symptoms and harm. They wanted their kids to understand their mother's experience with borderline personality disorder, and to establish an open line of communication so the kids could express their feelings about negative experiences—to know that their mom's symptoms were about her and not them. Cathleen told me:

It's been a journey, some steps forward and some steps back. There were a lot of years where I was crying or yelling. I got to the point where I, almost always, would come to the kids after it happened and say, "This had nothing to do with you. This is about me. I just cry when I'm upset. My yelling had nothing to do with you."

I don't know how I learned to do that. I think it was my husband Jim's influence, encouraging me to apologize to the kids each time they could hear me yelling. So, I did talk to them a little bit about how my brain doesn't work the way everybody else's brain does.

She offered some helpful advice:

The thing I tried to model for our sons was that, if you didn't learn something growing up, you just get help and try to teach yourself. I even told my kids a long time ago, "If you ever need me to come into a therapy session and hear how you felt about me yelling or how you felt about me crying or how you felt when I didn't get out of bed and take care of you, I'm always willing to come in. Or you can tell me or write me a letter anytime. I want to hear it if there's something on your heart."

How far do I go to get my loved one care?

In a broken care system rife with shortages of beds, housing, professionals, and restrictive laws, sometimes families (and professionals) do things they wouldn't usually do to help a loved one. Dawn Brown, a mother of six who lives in Virginia, faced this dilemma. When her son, who had struggled with episodes of psychosis from an early age, experienced a particularly severe wave of symptoms, a psychiatrist advised her to take drastic steps to get her son the inpatient care and housing he needed. Dawn described their experience:

> I went to see the psychiatrist treating my son, and I'm like, "The meds aren't working. He's actively psychotic. He's talking to dead people under the stairs. He's running from aliens. He's plugging the phone into his mattress." The psychiatrist said, "Well, bring him into the office. We'll call a mobile crisis team, and we'll do an assessment here." The mobile crisis team interviewed him in the lobby, and they're like, "We can't take him. He doesn't reach the criteria yet. Put away the knives, lock the doors when you go home. Call us when he gets worse."
>
> His psychiatrist said to me, "Do you still give your son his meds?" I said, "Yeah. I have him take his meds twice a day. He doesn't refuse them." He said, "Don't offer him his meds anymore and he'll meet the criteria within a week." So, I stopped.

Within a week, her son met their criteria. But Dawn had still more to do to make sure he got the help he needed:

> They called around and found a temporary bed in a local hospital. He was finally transferred when a bed became open. Within two weeks they tried to discharge him to me. I had two little kids at home from my second marriage. I was like, "He's not coming home with me. He is still actively psychotic. I can't do it. If he'd come to the hospital with a heart attack, you wouldn't be putting him out this fast when he still had symptoms. No. You do your job."
>
> That's what the psychiatrist told me to do. He said, "They'll try to push him back home without giving him any kind of support services in the community. He's going to have a level of need that you can't provide for, so when they tell you to take him home, tell them no." And I did. It was

the hardest thing I ever did because he would cry when I came to visit him. Eventually, they started him on Clozaril. Clozaril was the light switch in his brain that brought him back. After that, he was a completely different person.

Now Dawn supervises the NAMI HelpLine, a national resource with more than one hundred volunteers across the country that receives over seventy thousand calls, emails, and webchats a year. Families are often left to navigate the broken mental health care system by themselves, and struggle to find effective treatment. As a mother with years of lived experience answering her own set of hard family questions about her son's mental illness, Dawn is better able to help others facing seemingly impossible situations and challenges.

Should I have biological children given the severity of my mental health condition?

There is much we still don't know about genetics and the specific heritability of mental health conditions. We do know they can "run in families," but the odds that a child will inherit a vulnerability to a particular mental health condition are not scientifically clear for any aspiring parent. The risk of a child developing a mental health condition is usually greater if a parent has one, but still not high statistically. For example, a parent with schizophrenia has about a ten percent chance of having a child with schizophrenia—a tenfold increase over the risk for the general public, but still relatively unlikely.

The answer to this question, then, is ultimately very personal. Some look at the risk and choose to proceed; others elect not to have biological children. Some find other ways to build a family through adoption, stepparenting, or, for those who can cover the costs, the use of donor eggs or sperm.

Genetic counselors may help inform the decision based on family history, but uncertainty is still the reality. There is some research on the best way to approach having a baby when the prospective mother or father lives with a specific mental health condition. Marlene Freeman discusses the extensive research on pregnancy if you have bipolar disorder in chapter 17.

Laura Fritz, who we met earlier, made the decision to have children after a good deal of discussion with her husband. Laura told me:

> It was definitely a thought-out decision, because there's always that chance, "Am I going to pass this down to my kids?" There's kind of a fear in that. But I feel like my kids are going to have every resource available to them, all the support in the world. They're going to be able to see me, who has gone through it firsthand and come out on the other side. They're going to have all of that at their disposal if they do happen to have this. I just want to make sure that they're equipped to handle it and that they have my support and my husband's support. So, I decided that it was worth it to have kids.

For questions with no right answers and unknown risks and benefits, creativity can be an asset. There are many ways to parent or be in a parental role. Nikki Rashes, who came to understand she had bipolar disorder after her mother, Sally, laid out the extensive family history of mood and related disorders, elected not to have biological children and to become a stepmom. She explained:

> I had decided earlier on that I did not want to have children of my own because of a fear of passing on the illness, and the idea that it would be so hard to watch someone else struggle through it, especially knowing I had given it to them. So, I didn't want kids of my own, but the man I married had three teenage children. The youngest was sixteen.

Nikki discovered just how much value she could bring to her role when her stepson started to struggle with mental health issues:

About a year after his dad and I got married, my stepson went through bouts of depression and wound up hospitalized for a bit of time. So, "Okay, I didn't think I wanted this," but at the same time, I found I spoke their language. My husband would hear something, be offended by it, get angry about it. And I'd be like, "Whoa, no, what he's saying is this. He's speaking depression, give it a minute." I could communicate with them in a way their father couldn't, and I really feel like I was put in this family for a reason.

How do I plan for my adult child's well-being after I am gone?

A heartbreaking problem I sometimes saw in community mental health was when a person in their forties or fifties arrived in our clinic brand-new to the mental health system, scared and overwhelmed, in need of housing and so much more. Their story was often the same: their last surviving parent (usually their mother) had died, and they did not know where to turn. When faced with this crisis, I always wished we could have met well before this moment of grief and chaos, with more time to plan and explore options together.

Proactive families who deal with this issue can help someone begin to find professional and peer relationships, get integrated into a clubhouse, or get on a list for housing. The loss of a parent, while profound, does not have to mean the loss of everything—such as support, love, meals, and housing. It takes some vision to plan ahead for emotional and often logistical change, but there can be some relief knowing there is a plan in place in the event of a parent's passing.

While interviewing people for this book, I came upon someone who did this work proactively to reduce difficulty later on for her son: Alice Henley, who we met earlier. Her son John was identified as having paranoid schizophrenia in his first year of college. As the years went on, she realized the importance of planning for her son:

We worked very closely with a lawyer group to set up trust and financial structures and have conversations about how things will be when we're gone. They really have done a phenomenal job in helping. And I'm comfortable with it. It is a little weird when they're talking to you and they say, "So if you die, this is what's going to happen." You kind of must take yourself out of it for a little bit, to not think about the emotion of it and just make it be the objective: How are things going to work for John and his sister? It does feel good to know that that's in place.

Each family is different, and planning will vary based on many circumstances, including the person's wishes, socio-economic realities, relationships in the family, and availability of supports. A proactive plan might look at the role of siblings, community, peer connections, and professionals, and address issues of housing, finances, qualification for Medicaid, SNAP (food), Social Security or disability benefits, and other concerns particular to your loved one's situation. These conversations aren't easy, but they do matter. The Resources section includes information that may provide some direction and help with these many issues, such as establishing special needs trusts. Planning is about resolving logistical issues, but it can also raise emotional ones. One thing I have seen, though, is that people feel relieved once they have attended to this predictable and difficult challenge.

What can I do if I don't see a path of relief from intense symptoms for my family member?

Treatments may be getting better, and science may be advancing, but another hard truth is that not everyone responds to treatment. Every research study includes people who are deemed "nonresponders" to the latest medicine, therapy, or service idea. Families who love someone who is a so-called nonresponder to multiple treatments live with a very difficult reality. After you've tried everything, it is only natural to feel helpless.

Marc DeGregorio, a retired postal worker living in Connecticut, faced this seemingly impossible challenge. Marc told me his oldest daughter has severe schizophrenia and lives in a nursing home. Though she is taking clozapine, which for many people lessens the intensity of their symptoms, her experience is still very intense and disabling. Marc has found that he is able to make meaning of his daughter's outcome through helping others. He explained:

People in the NAMI world talk about recovery a lot. I don't know what that really means sometimes. I think recovery is in the eye of the beholder. My daughter never fully recovered; she's had lulls. When I teach Family-to-Family classes, I think people need to hear my story because they need to know that could end up being their story too. Some of them think you're going to come here and wave some magic wand. I tell them that taking the course for eight weeks is not going to heal your loved one, but it can help you get better at dealing with it. Same thing for me: I don't teach the course to make her better; I do it to make myself better for her.

Marc reflected on how his feelings have evolved, and on the difficulties he's seen other men experience in accepting their children's illness:

Empathy is a big piece of how I improve my feelings about my daughter. I went from constant angst about it to compassion for her position. Her voices don't take Saturday and Sunday off. If you get into that world, you start to feel like, well, how would *you* do it? How would *you* handle every day?

Fathers have a tough time with it. They get angry at their sons, who they want to be athletes and whatever, and their dreams get dashed. If that kid got in a car accident and ended up in a wheelchair, that father would be full of empathy. But if his son has a mental illness, it becomes an anger issue. That must be displaced with compassion.

Ultimately, Marc's work with NAMI has helped him make both his and his daughter's lives meaningful, even if he can't make her better. Marc shared this insight:

Maybe the healing you get from doing these things is your own. You heal yourself so you can handle your life, rather than heal the person to make them better. It helps you heal your ability to traverse this world. Sharing with other people has been a healing experience for me. It's gotten me out of myself. It's brought me other people to listen to. If I can help, and be an ear to someone, it makes me feel worthwhile. It makes me feel like it hasn't all been for nothing. It kind of gives meaning to her losses and doesn't make her an invisible statistic, a marginalized nobody. It makes her real to people. I think I owe her that. It's not easy, but I feel very fulfilled by it. That's why I keep doing it.

· · ·

While these are some of the most common "hardest questions" families face in living with and loving someone with a mental health condition, they are not the only ones. If you are facing a hard question, NAMI's Family Support Groups and Family-to-Family classes are good places to sound out your questions and be heard. You may find answers that are concrete or connections that may help you make some sense of what you are facing. Almost every person I have met has said that, with these questions, it has made an enormous difference to not be alone on the journey to answer them.

FIFTEEN

Making Meaning of Loss by Suicide

This chapter includes content that may be distressing to
some people. If you begin to experience discomfort or anxiety as
you read, please just set this chapter aside for now. You may find
the content more helpful to you at another point in time.

"Please forgive me. My illness won today. Please look after each other, the animals, and the global poor for me. All my love, Tommy."

—TOMMY RASKIN,
in his suicide note, as reported by his parents,
Congressman Jamie Raskin and Sarah Bloom Raskin

. . .

Like cancer and heart disease, mental health conditions can sometimes claim people's lives, no matter how well they are cared for and how much they are loved. It is a very hard truth. In this chapter, I'll focus on how people face and make meaning of the uniquely painful trauma of losing a loved one to suicide. Not all deaths by suicide are caused by mental illness, but suicide is often associated with mental health conditions. It can be a consequence of untreated or undertreated mental illness, or it can happen when a person does not respond or stops responding to the treatments available and cannot see another way out of their pain.

The experience of losing someone you love to suicide is devastating. No matter how many people assure you that you are not responsible for your loved one's decision, a loss to suicide inevitably prompts questions about how you could have acted or behaved to prevent it. I felt guilty and wondered if I was cut out for the work I do when I lost a patient to suicide. As a teen, I used to lose sleep thinking about what I could do to prevent my father from going through with his threats to kill himself. The reason my own lived experience is not part of this chapter is simply luck.

This chapter can only scratch the surface of the impact of loss by suicide and shares the experiences of only a small number of survivors. Making meaning of such a loss is a complex and intensely personal journey. But for each of the people I interviewed for this chapter, sharing with others to let them know they are not alone has been a key part of the process. These people will introduce themselves, talk about what happened and what they have learned, without much additional commentary from me. We will hear from survivors who are mothers, fathers, a sibling, and an adult child when the suicide occurred, and what they have done to make meaning of their loss. When you are ready, there are many support groups and resources for people who face this uniquely difficult situation. The American Foundation for Suicide Prevention and Save.org have compiled a rich database of support groups for survivors, both in-person and online, in the United States and Canada, and searchable by zip code.

Sometimes There Are No Signs to Miss

Pooja Mehta is a twenty-six-year-old mental health and suicide prevention advocate. Her work, which also involves policy advocacy on Capitol Hill and beyond, is inspired by lived experience. She described the wrenching experience of losing her brother, who died by suicide unexpectedly:

On February 17, 2020, I took a mental health first aid class, and I got a refresher on the signs and symptoms of suicide—suicidal ideation and how to intervene. And then six weeks later, I woke up to a world where my brother was dead from suicide.

Before my brother died, I very much associated suicide and mental illness almost one to one. I knew that not everyone with a mental illness dies by suicide, but I did have this idea in my head that everyone who dies by suicide has either diagnosed or undiagnosed mental illness, and that suicide is preventable and "predictable" if you know what to look for. My brother didn't show any of those signs; not a single one. He never had any mental health issues. He never struggled with anything like that. I know there are a lot of people who would say that I'm in denial about that, but really, I'm not. In my family, we talk about this extremely openly. I asked my brother point blank at least once every two weeks: How are you actually doing? And sometimes he'd be doing fine and sometimes he'd be struggling, and we would talk about it. The last engagement he had with another person was talking to a classmate about how to divide homework problems, and I found him twenty minutes later. If you're struggling with suicidal ideation, you're not talking about homework problems. We don't understand it.

I know there's this idea that suicide is sometimes preventable, that there are signs to look out for, and this idea empowers people; it gives them a sense of hope and a sense of "I can save my loved one." But maybe not. And I'm sorry. At this point we do not know enough about why people die by suicide to always be able to identify it. Some suicide is preventable. Some people do follow those signs. Those signs and symptoms are established for a reason. And some people can be saved. We should do everything we can to make that happen. But we need to recognize that there is a lot more we need to learn before we can really start implying that all suicide is preventable.

I really struggled with that as a suicide loss survivor. Because if suicide is preventable, then the question, for the survivor community, for this club that no one wants to be a part of is, "Well, why didn't *you* prevent it?"

One thing that my therapist helped me realize is that it's not that I missed the signs; it's that the signs were not there. I relive that day over and over. Even if I had done this, even if I hadn't done that, even if I had gone up earlier or later or whatever, there was nothing I could have done, there was nothing that he let me do.

I think we treat suicide the way we treated heart attacks centuries ago. Back then, someone would be walking the street, drop dead, and no one had any idea why. Over time, we started calling it a heart attack, and then learned why it happens, and how to prevent it. Now we're at a point where we can identify someone at risk and help people live a lifestyle that will put them at less risk. But there's still a good number of folks out there where a heart attack comes just out of the blue.

My brother ordered a computer monitor the day he died, and it arrived the day of his funeral. People who are contemplating suicide don't do that. And every once in a while, I still find myself asking that question: What could I have done? And I have to stop myself and remind myself that, no, you had nothing to do with what he did; you did absolutely everything you were able to do.

Suicide Is a Medical Problem, and Nobody Is to Blame

Joseph Feaster Jr., who we met earlier, had a son, Joseph D. Feaster III, who died by suicide in August 2010. Joseph shared with me:

I feel no sense of blame at all. My son died of a medical condition. That's what my son died of. And I use the new terminology, "death by suicide." I have no problem saying it. There's nothing for me to hide or be ashamed of. There's nothing that I did or failed to do, and that's how I view it. So, when I talk to others who have lost loved ones by suicide, I say so emphatically and passionately, "No, you're not going to sit here and have this blame game. Not with me. Find someone else who can do the counseling.

If you want to talk about it from the standpoint of how you cope, then I'm more than happy to do it."

I try to educate folks. Sometimes I can speak about Joseph and not cry. Other times I speak about Joseph and do cry. I've decided that this is my ministry. Because I'm so vocal on it, I get many calls from people who are going through it, particularly caregivers. I am a resource. I chat with, cry with, do whatever I need to do in order to assist caregivers. I recognized that I'm in God's plan and it is what it is, so what can I do to help others through the process? Mainly I'm really trying to be an advocate.

Finding Community in the Process of Grief

Shirley Holloway is a longtime educational leader from Alaska. She has served on the NAMI board for six years, two as president, coming to the organization after losing her daughter Kathleen to suicide. Shirley recalled:

When we got off the plane at 5:30 in the morning in Anchorage, my two sons were standing there. I knew immediately that something had gone wrong. My oldest son had already done an identification and many of the other difficult tasks that fall to the next of kin. We went home and I think we were numb for about twenty-four hours, but then we started talking about a celebration of life and decided, "We'll do it here at home." We started the planning and I said, "I don't want people to buy flowers. I really would like people to donate to some organization that works with people who've lived through these horrendous experiences."

I reached out to a friend who ran the Alaska Mental Health Trust and I said, "Do you have any ideas?" He gave me a list and on that list was NAMI Anchorage. I called them and said, "I would like to put you in the obituary for people to donate," to which they said, "Oh, that would be wonderful." Then, all of a sudden, I said, "Do you ever visit with families who've lost someone by suicide?" And the executive director—whom I later learned was a peer and someone with lived experience—said, "No, that's not one of our activities, but I would be happy to come to your home and talk to you and your family."

The day before the actual celebration, she came with her board chairperson, a woman who was also a peer with lived experience. They sat down in our living room in a big circle with all of us, our kids, Kathleen's kids, my husband and I, and a couple of close family friends, and they told us about their own history of suicidal ideation. They were incredibly reassuring and so kind, and the big message was, "This is not your fault; this is not your doing."

We have something in Anchorage we call a Remembrance Tree. Every year we gather around a tree for people who've lost someone to suicide. We have a guest speaker and pass out little ribbons, and we write the name of our loved one on the ribbon and then we tie it on the tree.

My youngest son has given the speech to the Remembrance Tree audience for a couple years. He talked to the group about how angry he was, how angry he was at his sister, because of the way she treated me. He felt that she was disrespectful and unkind to me, that she took out a lot of her anger on me. I was amazed by how well he was able to verbalize this to the audience. And then, of course, he talked about all of the wonderful parts of her as well.

Since Kathleen passed, we've set aside an evening each year where we hold a little ceremony for the whole family. We gather and we'll all cry again and live through it again.

On Coping with Grief Through Teaching and Meaningful Creative Projects

Karyl Chastain Beal is a retired teacher and active volunteer living near Nashville. She's also the mother of Arlyn, who was presumptively diagnosed with bipolar disorder posthumously, after she died by suicide. Karyl shared:

When Arlyn died, I knew immediately that one day I'd be teaching people about how to cope after a suicide death even though I knew nothing about it at the time. I'm a teacher, and teachers naturally pass on what they've learned to others who are ready to learn. I also knew that I desperately needed to connect with other bereaved parents who might understand what I'd gone through and how I felt. So, I took steps to start a local support group for parents whose children died from any cause of death at any age. Our group met monthly.

A couple years later, I started another support group, this one online, specifically for parents who had lost their children to suicide. Support and connection were available twenty-four hours a day, seven days a week. The parents who joined were from all over the United States and other countries. We all needed the same thing: support and connection with others who reluctantly walked the same road. As I connected with other bereaved parents, I learned from them, but I also taught the others in the group while I grieved.

Karyl found new purpose not just in teaching, but in bringing together other suicide survivors to express themselves creatively, through quilting and writing:

The email group grew in numbers as more people learned about the connection. Some members expressed interest in us creating a quilt in memory of our children after we'd heard about a memorial quilt featuring squares with the faces of those who died by suicide on it. Seeing the faces of our loved ones on display was powerful, especially in a world where suicide is sometimes viewed as sinful or the result of selfishness, weakness, or cowardice. After that, every year, we made another memorial quilt.

After my husband and I moved to Tennessee, the Tennessee Suicide Prevention Network (TSPN) found me. They were putting together their first state suicide memorial quilt. I sent in a quilt square for Arlyn. TSPN asked me to take over the quilt project and coordinate the next one.

Every year TSPN displays those quilts at suicide education, awareness, and prevention events all over the state. The quilts have become a dynamic teaching aid to help those who see them understand that our loved ones aren't statistics. Their lives mattered.

Faith and Advocacy

Kristen Roper of Massachusetts is a fifty-two-year-old mother of three boys, all of whom were adopted from Russia. She is a former teacher and runs a nonprofit in memory of her son Matthew, who was lost to suicide in 2020 when he was seventeen. She emphasized in our conversation that she is most grateful to God who sustains her in all things. She said:

Matthew was a force to be reckoned with, and in no way, shape, or form did he want this to be how his life ended. I don't understand what happened in that one moment in time. But I know it's not what he wanted. He had texted his friend a couple of days before and said, "I'm getting out of the hospital again. I can't wait to get my life back." That was his final message to his best friend. It's not what Matthew wanted, and I'll never know what happened. But I know Matthew was a fighter. And sometimes the illness wins.

I had heard about the Samaritans 5K walk last summer. And I thought, "You know what? It would be really nice to do something, because between losing Matthew and the pandemic, it was a really difficult time." So, I called some close friends and family and thought I could raise maybe $500. It grew and grew. One of my cousins said, "If we're going to do it together, wouldn't it be fun to have T-shirts?" We turned our T-shirt design into a logo and ended up with the largest team: 135 members, from Alaska to Germany, all over Massachusetts, New England, Idaho, everywhere. My wish to raise $500 turned into more than $16,000. Honestly, it's a testament to my Matthew—his beauty, his power, his amazingness; no one wants to let him go. And I think it was because of who he was that everyone wanted to be part of it. They want to be part of Matthew;s Crew.

On the Samaritans Walk, we saw other people gathered with Matthew;s Crew signs and T-shirts. And then other people that we bumped into along the way were asking, "What is this Matthew;s Crew? We keep seeing people like you everywhere."

It was very, very powerful, and I felt very inspired. And we realized we can't just stop with a walk. I think it's divine that this is something I'm being called to do. That Matthew's story can't end on the day he died; his story needs to continue.

Our mission is threefold. The first part is working to change attitudes and perception through conversation. Nothing's going to change until we shift how society views this. The second part is to raise funds for mental health initiatives and suicide prevention programs. And the third part is to engage the health care system. I feel incredibly strongly that Matthew was failed over and over, from the pediatrician on up.

Kristen again highlighted how important her faith was to her:

My faith is super important. I don't know how I would still be here today, still be doing this without it. I don't know how people get through life without their own faith in whichever way they practice. For me, it's everything. And I would say that to my children: "My most important job is not to raise you to just be good men, but to raise you so that your soul makes it to heaven, because that's where eternity is. My faith, and our faith, is the most important thing I can give you."

Advocating for a Better Approach to Suicide Prevention in Colleges

Phil and Donna Satow of New York founded The JED Foundation in 2000 after the loss of their son, Jed. Donna told me their story:

"If love could have saved him, this wouldn't have happened." Those are the powerful words that Andrew Solomon wrote to me when my son Jed died by suicide in 1998. When you have been through this kind of trauma, there are certain things that stick with you. Learning that my love could not have saved my son was a profound thought and a motivation. It made me think that maybe I could find a path out of this terrible hurt.

Jed was my third, and youngest, child. He was very engaging, smart, and gifted. He had an incredible sense of humor and was very insightful. He wasn't perfect. He had issues, like everyone does. He was impulsive and struggled with a learning disability. But we—the people who knew and loved Jed—never saw his impulsivity as lethal.

Parents can often minimize these things, considering it a phase that their child will manage and emerge from relatively unscathed. But there is an intense psychological autopsy that happens when you lose someone to suicide. As we went through this process, we realized there had been many warning signs. Sometimes, however, the red flags are subtle. Especially if you don't know to look for them.

As time passed, I found myself on a relentless quest to do two things: I wanted to figure out why this happened to Jed. That's a question I am still chasing. I also wanted to understand more broadly how to prevent suicide in young adults.

This kind of trauma changes your trajectory. Initially, you're so bereft that you don't know exactly where to go. But if you can bring yourself to start moving forward, your pain can fuel a passion that begins to heal you. Phil and I were inspired to figure out what happened, and to do something to help other families avoid the tragedy our family experienced.

We started by meeting with the president of the large university that Jed was attending. He looked at us and said, "I have 35,000 kids. What would you have me do?" This question started us thinking that perhaps there was something we could do. We brought together a dozen bright minds in child and adolescent psychiatry, public health, psychology, and education to share ideas. Our goal was to reach as many schools and students as possible, using a model framework to identify and support these young adults comprehensively and prevent suicide.

We thought that if we could influence colleges—and now high schools—to reach their students early, and get them talking to friends and professionals, help them think of solutions to problems, and give them the tools to make it real, we would build a strong safety net. We wanted to give young people a sense of belonging and a feeling of hope and empowerment in who they are and want to be, so they could thrive.

That was our vision. We adapted a model that had been extremely successful in lowering suicide rates in the Air Force. We tweaked their model to create a comprehensive approach to mental health promotion, and to substance use and suicide prevention awareness [in colleges and universities], that would bring whole campuses together to work toward the same goal. Now, we have expanded that approach to reach high schools as well.

There are currently four hundred JED Campuses nationwide and more than fifty high schools in our recently launched JED High School program. Our comprehensive approach reaches nearly 5 million students across the country.

I am so deeply gratified by all JED's accomplishments. Yet it won't bring my Jed back. I know so much more now. I understand what happened with Jed intellectually, but emotionally I'm not sure. That gaping, painful hole persists. But the fact that my grandchildren know the JED Foundation, that they feel proud that their uncle inspired this work, and that something meaningful has come from his loss, is a solace—and a huge incentive that keeps Phil and me going.

To learn more about the JED Foundation, visit their website.

Finding Other People

Lisa Fabian is a fifty-nine-year-old single woman who lost her father, who had lived with bipolar disorder, to suicide. She shared:

When my father was quite depressed, I knew it. He would become very quiet and kind of restless, walking around, and sometimes going to the basement to cry. I was just a kid, and to hear your dad cry was heartbreaking. He would try to say things to not scare me, but it was stilted. It would be, "I love you girls and your mother so much." Or, "I'm sorry." "I'm sorry, I'm sad. I'm just feeling sad." I did not understand what it meant.

My dad did pretty well on lithium. He was compliant and was thrilled that it was helping him. He didn't struggle much with side effects. But there were what I call breakthrough episodes every few years. When he turned about fifty, he began to rapid cycle and it never got under control.

I was twenty-seven when he died. My sister found him. My own making peace with this is that he just wore out. At my wedding the year before, he was using every ounce of strength to be there, my mom was propping him up. He was quite depressed at that time, but still stood up and made a sweet little toast. I value that too.

When my father died, my mom didn't want to talk about it. We didn't have a funeral. I did call quite a few of my friends who I discussed this with, or people who knew my dad. I was doing that to connect, but I still felt alone. I got one card from somebody who I just knew as an acquaintance. She knew people I knew, and somehow heard and sent me a note. She had lost her father, a few years before, the same way. Though we never spoke until just a few years ago, I saved that card. That card meant as much to me as anything else that happened. Because I felt like there was somebody out there who got the depth of pain I was in.

I contacted a psychiatrist and started going to therapy in Chicago. I was struggling with this, because I had really just been getting to the point where I could love him, care about him, provide support, but not feel that it was my job to keep him safe, and I, shortly thereafter, got the call that he had died.

In the survivors of suicide support group that I went to many years later, we came up with this metaphor about being on an island; that we were on an island by ourselves, we felt by ourselves with this loss. But as we talked, we were learning that there were other people on the island,

and we were on the island together. When somebody decided to leave the group, for instance, this one guy who was just raw and sweet said, "Just remember that we're all here on the island for you."

It is sometimes quite difficult to have these conversations with people in the grief support groups. I have distance from the death, but that doesn't mean I don't feel what they're feeling, maybe more than is all that healthy. For most of the people in there, the death of their loved one is really fresh. Is it going to be discouraging to them that somebody thirty-three years into their journey is still seeking something? I felt kind of like the wise old aunt.

But for me, there came a point where thinking about my dad brought more happy memories than pain. It took a long time. It doesn't mean the pain isn't still there. But I'm so grateful to have had him for a father, to have learned from him, and that's dominant. And I tell the people I talk to, it will come; that will come. People don't totally get past it, ever. And they need to understand that, in a way, that's reassuring. Because you don't want to lose the connection.

Many support groups are available for survivors of suicide loss. You are not alone.

SIXTEEN

Family Advocacy

Helping to care for someone living with a mental illness can be a very big job.

The idea of having the time or energy to become an advocate for other families, and for systemic change, may seem far-fetched. But you may find yourself doing just that in the process of advocating for your own family members. You might also discover a new sense of purpose in engaging the "big issues," like opening the conversation about mental health in public settings, and fighting for better research, funding, and services.

In this chapter, family members talk about what they have done to help each other, to promote openness, and to advocate for improved care for people who've gone through experiences like those of their loved ones. Each person's passion to make change is rooted in their own personal experience. They also forged new connections and found healing by joining the peer community of families. But just as their engagement in advocacy changed their own lives, it also changed the larger world. Most of the major progress in mental health legislation and mental health system change is a result of the collective force of advocacy. There is still much advocacy work to be done, and your passion and personal experience can make a difference.

There are many avenues through which to advocate for mental health. In this chapter, we'll hear from people who were primarily engaged in advocacy through NAMI: by helping to pass along what they learned by teaching courses; by taking advantage of the Smarts for Advocacy training to learn skills to advocate in other forums; or by getting involved through one of our 650 state and local affiliates to advocate for particular policies. For example, one policy that advocates have rallied around is funding culturally informed mobile crisis services people may need when they call 988, the new mental health emergency number.

Advocating for One Family at a Time

One simple and important form of advocacy involves letting other families know that they're not alone, helping them learn more about mental illness, and encouraging them not to place blame on themselves.

In the mid-1980s, medical professionals directly blamed Gary Mihelish and his wife Sandra for their son Kurt's schizophrenia diagnosis. Gary, a retired dentist from Montana, didn't believe that could be true. He recalled:

> After Kurt's first hospitalization, they brought Sandra and me up to have a consultation with a psychiatrist and a psychologist. When we stepped out of the room, they didn't close the door completely, and we heard the psychologist say to the psychiatrist, "There's something terribly wrong with that family."
>
> And I looked at Sandra and I walked back into the room, and I told them, "This is baloney." I said, "I know we don't know everything, and I don't know what's wrong with my son," but I said, "I don't think his family is the problem here."

When Joyce Burland, the creator of NAMI Family-to-Family, came to Montana and taught the course, it changed everything for Gary and Sandra. Today, professionals are taught not to blame families, but this difficult history of blame is critical to understanding the formation of NAMI and the creation of Family-to-Family.

"The Family-to-Family program saved our marriage, no doubt," Gary said. "And it saved Kurt's life, too, because we began to understand." For Gary and Sandra, Family-to-Family provided a framework for navigating the complicated and confusing world of mental health care and helped strengthen their coping and communication techniques. They resolved to teach the course so that other families would gain the understanding that conditions like schizophrenia and bipolar disorder were not their fault, and to develop strategies to move forward. They have now taught the Family-to-Family program thirty-five times. Gary and Sandra have impacted many hundreds of lives for the better.

As there is still so much shame and secrecy about mental health conditions in society, one simple and effective advocacy tool is to share your experiences with other families. Many people who have made the decision to "go public" with their story find a warm reception and note that taking this initiative encourages other people with lived experience to share their stories, too. Telling their truth not only creates space for others to do so; it also creates community.

Kumi Macdonald shared in chapter 10 about how in the Japanese culture in which she was raised, the usual response to her expressing concerns about her mental health was to "suck it up." Kumi decided to change that pattern—first in her family, and then in her community. Here is how she advocates for parents to be more open to getting help for their children in Hawaii:

A lot of times, moms think their child's emotional or behavioral issue will go away, and I'll tell them, "It may not go away. It might, but it might not. And do you want to take that chance?" I say, "Let's get it at stage one, before it's a stage four, like cancer. Let's get it early; don't wait until you must go to chemo." That wakes them up. The second thing I say is: "Don't be ashamed." It's very, very embarrassing for an Asian person—I think even if you're not Asian—to admit that you need help. I always tell them, "It's not embarrassing; you don't realize how many people are going through it."

They see here's Kumi, she has a good family, a good life, and she went through it; okay, maybe it's not so embarrassing. That helps, to join with them. I noticed that when I started sharing my story, people came out of the woodwork. People I knew for thirty years said, "My family too!" And I said, "Why didn't you tell me this for thirty years?"

Karen Ranus, introduced earlier, knew nothing about mental illness until her teenage daughter was hospitalized. She found a NAMI support group, and that encouraged her to share her story in other places, like her local Catholic church:

I feel like people are hungry for you to open the door. Every time I tell the story, I just open the door and say, "Hey," and I've rarely seen a person who hasn't wanted to walk through. It's very interesting because all of us on the exterior can look like we've got it all together, and therefore, how can a family who functions at that level have something like this happen? It happens because this is a health issue, and genetics play a big part. To me, understanding that was powerful.

I felt the most powerful way I could share who NAMI was, what they did, and what they were capable of doing, was to share my own story. I still remember, I had been asked to write a piece for a Catholic newspaper, and it was one of the first times that somebody asked me to write something. Somebody through church had heard the story. I remember writing this piece, and I had my daughter read it. I said, "Are you sure? Because this isn't just my story. It's really your story. You really do have to be okay with this." And she's like, "Totally am." I still remember to this day, she said, "Mom, if we saved just one life by you sharing that story, it's totally worth it."

Advocating at the System Level

Mental health services have been systematically underfunded, ignored, or allowed to be second class to medical benefits in health insurance policies for decades. Advocacy, through laws and policy, has been a critical component of changing this frustrating reality.

There are many examples of successful advocacy efforts that have begun to turn the page on a long history of devaluation and underfunding of mental health services. This advocacy happens at federal, state, and county levels, and first-person experience frequently changes both minds and laws. The 2021 passage of the 988 crisis call legislation, a result of many advocates demanding better access to crisis care, is the most recent example. The federal Mental Health Parity and Addiction Equity Act of 2008 was the result of a multiyear advocacy effort to end discrimination in insurance coverage and payment for mental health services.

Few believe that we have achieved true parity, and advocacy and lawsuits today continue to help define what parity means in practice. Another important arena for mental health advocacy is the criminal justice system. The tragic consequences of police mishandling of mental health crises regularly make headlines.

Denise Paley is a fifty-one-year-old white woman who works as a regional sales manager and lives in Connecticut. She is the proud mother of two boys, one of whom lives with mental illness. Denise faced an extremely difficult situation when her son had a mental health crisis and went missing. Law enforcement in her town did not have the training to respond adequately. Denise explained:

> It was so abundantly clear to people who knew my son that he was having a mental health episode, except for law enforcement. We had said to the officers, "We think he's having a break. We think he's not in his right state of mind." That's the language we were using. And they literally said, "He's not having a psychotic break that we can determine. He's not a danger to himself because he made no overt statements that he was going to harm himself. You just need to let him cool off."
>
> It's such a shame. So, part of it is devastating for me. Part of it just really made me more aware and feel I need to do something about it.

Determined to change things for other families in crisis, Denise became a legislative advocate for improved police training:

> I need to speak out, and I need to help encourage people to get the education. You can't intervene if you just don't know how. And I'm sure they really thought they were doing the right thing.
>
> So, my state senator put forward two bills to address what happened with my son. One of them was for the Crisis Intervention Team Training, and it got picked up, and it's being rolled into a bigger bill. And I testified about the fact that the other town where he was finally arrested does have Crisis Intervention Training. And if they didn't, he could be dead now.

Denise continues to advocate for improved police training, along with thousands of others.

NAMI Roots in Research Advocacy

Like service advocacy, neuroscience advocacy is in NAMI's DNA. It started when original members wanted to better understand the science behind their adult children's conditions and rebut misguided, nonscientific theories that blamed parents. The relationship between NAMI and the National Institute of Mental Health is longstanding. I asked the late Eleanor Owen, one hundred years old when we spoke, who attended the first NAMI convention in 1979, to share her recollections of the first get-together:

> We were on the stage, mostly parents across the country who had come together. I asked the audience, "Is there anyone who has a loved one with schizophrenia who has been impacted by the closure of state hospitals?" A field of hands went up. After the panel, a leader from NIMH came backstage and said to me, "We had no idea."

Leaders from NIMH now attend every NAMI convention to communicate the latest developments in science to the people who need to know the most.

NAMI's influence on NIMH continued through the 1980s and '90s as NAMI itself continued to develop. Demanding more science-based answers, NAMI successfully fought to double the research budget of NIMH in the 1990s. After E. Fuller Torrey, the first NAMI psychiatrist, appeared on *The Phil Donahue Show* to advocate for more research funding to understand serious mental illnesses, the fledgling NAMI national office, then consisting of one room, was flooded with mail. This outpouring of need and frustration led to a massive and successful NAMI petition campaign to drive increased congressional funding for NIMH brain research on serious mental health conditions.

"This was a vivid illustration of NAMI's growing grassroots clout," Ron Honberg, a staff member at the time, told me. "Being able to generate 400,000 signatures, truck these signatures up to Capitol Hill for a press conference, and getting a celebrity like Patty Duke [an actress living with bipolar disorder] to talk about why research on mental illness was so important, showed the influence of the NAMI family movement."

Laurie Flynn of Virginia, who had become NAMI's executive director only a few months before, recalled that, despite the truckful of signatures, it took a lot more work to put NAMI at the center of the research advocacy map:

I'm on the job a couple months and we've opened all that mail that came from the *Donahue* show. I wanted to make an appointment with Shervert Frazier, who was the new director of the NIMH. After a bunch of calls, I got an appointment. I go out to the NIMH, and I have this brief, pleasant, but utterly non-substantial conversation. I thought, "This is not working."

We sent out a letter to the affiliates that we had—less than one hundred chapters at the time. "These people are going to help us; they just don't know it yet. Two things you need to do. Connect with your local university and watch for whenever Dr. Frazier or anyone from NIMH is showing up to give a presentation. And ask this question, 'When is NIMH going to do something about psychosis and schizophrenia?'

It only took a few of those encounters and I got a meeting with him. I got right in, and he was much more interested.

NAMI believes in science. That was a meeting ground. They saw we were willing to work hard, willing to sign up for clinical trials; we were going to Congress and demanding more money. They didn't have a constituency that was active like that before NAMI. They wanted us because we were a great constituency to promote science. At the same time, our advocacy for more research money came with strings attached: "You're going to have to focus some more money on the folks we are taking care of."

Studies are ongoing to create better medications with fewer side effects—a core need for many living with illnesses on the psychosis spectrum, such as schizophrenia. NAMI and NIMH have a collaborative relationship to get the best science to the people who most need it. Still, the quest to understand the biology underlying mental health conditions, and how best to approach it scientifically, has been elusive and frustrating.

Thanks to persistent advocacy and dedicated leadership from many parties, there is now a five-year, NIH Foundation–led, $100-million public/private research partnership called the Accelerated Medicines Partnership (AMP Schizophrenia) dedicated to promoting the collaborative development of new medicines for treating schizophrenia. AMP Schizophrenia is the first initiative of its kind. The Foundation for the NIH, NIMH, interested pharmaceutical companies, NAMI, and other nonprofit groups have joined this important endeavor. The goal of AMP Schizophrenia is to find new biological targets to inform potential new medication discovery. We need better treatments, and this may be one way to get there.

Carlos A. Larrauri, introduced earlier, co-chairs the steering committee for AMP Schizophrenia. His own lived experience gives him a unique
and valuable perspective in this leadership role. He is helping to lead the
largest coordinated effort to find new treatments for a condition he lives
with every day. Carlos told me:

It's been the highlight of my professional career thus far. It's like being a
kid who grew up wondering about the moon and the stars and then being
asked to work for NASA. My first scientific paper that I wrote in seventh
grade was on schizophrenia. I chose schizophrenia because I read *A Beautiful Mind*, and I was moved by it. I sent it to my family friend Joe
Gonzalez-Heydrich—who I call Saint Joe—who's a psychiatrist, and he
said, "This is great. You got the enlarged ventricles. You're going to get an
A+." Fast forward two decades later, I have schizophrenia, and here I am
working on AMP with Saint Joe, who is part of the Schizophrenia Biomarkers Consortium. Co-leading AMP is a way of making sense of the
experience, coming full circle in my life.

Altruism drives participation in and advocacy for better research. So
does honoring a loved one. To honor their son Peter's life, George and
Jutta Kohn founded the Peter Corbin Kohn Endowment, which supports NAMI's annual research award recognizing America's leading researchers in advancing neuroscience and mental health treatment. Jutta
wants people to remember and acknowledge her son's life and death,
even when they don't know what to say. She told me:

Right after Peter died, people wouldn't even mention it. When someone has mental illness, they tiptoe around the discussion. Just acknowledge it in some way. You must talk about the loss because it makes the
life of the person who died meaningful. If you don't mention it, it's like
the person never existed. It's the worst insult. That's part of the reason
why we set up the endowment, because he *does* exist. He had a life.

With the endowment we wanted to show that his life deserves to be respected.

When Peter died, we had to write his obituary. We decided to mention NAMI for charitable donations in Peter's name, but people didn't know Peter was sick. The doctor made us very aware that once you put NAMI in the obituary, people would know Peter had a mental illness.

Jutta told me that after they named NAMI in the obituary, they noticed that others followed in the ensuing years.

My conversation with the Kohns reminded me of when my family faced the same question. When my own father died, we too had to decide which charity to select to honor his life. Joe, Sue, and I advocated for NAMI, but, of course, the decision was our mother's. Mom and Dad had been together for sixty-three years. She hesitated but vowed to think it over. I knew that meant no and decided to let it go. The family had lived in silence for decades, and I saw nothing to indicate that Mom had any appetite to change that.

Later that day, in the surprise of my lifetime, she said, "NAMI it is." I was never prouder to be her son. Mom had overcome eight decades of social attitudes and barriers at long last. On one level, an obituary that included Dad's vulnerability seems a tiny gesture, but it was so meaningful in the context of the silence in our family about Dad's mental illness. My mom's acknowledgment still moves me even now, fifteen years later.

When we got to the funeral home, the director said to us, "I had never heard of NAMI, but just this morning I had a family of a sixteen-year-old boy ask to mention the same charity." My heart sank for them. Our family, who had lost our eighty-seven-year-old patriarch, and the heartbroken family of this young man who had lived seventy fewer years than Dad did, shared the same pain. I suspect we also shared the same hope— for a world where people with mental health conditions are acknowledged, valued, and respected.

We are not yet there, and there is so much to be done. Anyone who has walked a few miles in these shoes knows this to be true. We can walk much farther together.

As physician and educator Philip A. Lederer said to me in our interview, "The question is, what do you really want to fight for? You don't want to fight alone. No, you can't fight alone."

PART IV

Best Practices

SEVENTEEN

Experts Answer the Most Frequently Asked Questions

A s NAMI's chief medical officer, I have been asked thousands of questions over the years. For this book, I asked some of the leading thinkers in the United States to help answer the most critical questions in short, nontechnical terms.

Accessing care

Q: How do I find a good therapist?

A: As both a therapist and an employer of many therapists, I believe therapy is an incredibly powerful force for change. That change is rooted in finding the best possible match between client and therapist.

To start, always be sure that any therapist you consider is licensed in your state. This ensures that their education and practice are up to the important professional standards of their discipline. To check a license, go to the official website for your state (ny.gov is New York's, for example), search for a "Check a Professional License" page, then enter the discipline (psychology, social work, etc.) and the therapist's name and location; this should be enough to verify that their license is in good standing.

Some therapists begin with a phone call while others will ask to meet before taking you on as a client. They will likely talk about their style of therapy, and they should begin with an assessment to make sure they are a good match for the kind of work you are intending to do and the improvements you'd like to see. The therapist may ask you questions about how your emotional concerns affect your daily life, or about previous diagnoses other providers may have assigned to your struggles. They should also consider the impact of your racial, cultural, gender, sexual, and all other relevant identities on your life. Then you would decide together on the kind of work you might do to bring about change by crafting a plan for your treatment.

A good therapist also brings a professional level of kindness and compassion to this process. This means they should help you to feel human in your struggle and respect what you are going through—everyone deserves that. While they will likely ask you to work hard in observing your life and its patterns, they should do that in an environment where you feel confident that they "get you," and want for you what you want for yourself.

Lastly, the therapist should be committed to change. They should make you feel like they've signed up to help bring improvements to your life, not just "check in" every week without directing any real energy toward your goals. A good therapist will suggest alternatives to treatment if you aren't seeing any improvement, and a good therapist would be receptive if you brought up concerns about the work you are doing together or their methods of practice.

Let's face it: Therapists, and the ways in which they work, are diverse. Some are very formal and will give you worksheets and homework; others might ask if you want to walk outside while you talk; some might even swear during sessions. All these factors could work for you if the therapist is professional, if you are comfortable with them, and if you are seeing desired change.

But what if you don't like the match? Discuss this with your therapist and consider making a change and/or checking out other therapists. You may need to call your insurance provider and let them know you need to do that, and you may need some persistence to navigate their rules, and to enlist their help in finding a good match in or out of their network. In the end, it may be very much worth the effort.

JEN ERBE LEGGETT, MSW, LICSW, is CEO of the Leggett Group, a Boston-based therapy group practice that advocates for increased access to therapy as treatment for the general public.

. . .

Q: How do I approach getting help if the therapist doesn't look like me and may not understand my racial and/or cultural experience?

A: This is an important but complex question for people of color. For example, as a Black psychiatrist, I have observed that, for many Black people, the experiences with the mental health system often come during other stressful times, which may feed into a general mistrust of the system. The stigma of mental illness, combined with the historical mistrust of the health care system, can lead to real mistrust. Furthermore, seeking mental health treatment continues to be a deeply embedded taboo for some in the Black community, resulting in reluctance to ask for help or even acknowledge the need for help, often with lethal outcomes. Unfortunately, there are too few therapists from the most marginalized groups in any behavioral health profession to match with people seeking services from those specific groups. The wait to see those that are available can be long, leaving those in need without immediate help.

Let's first acknowledge that you should feel good about the decision you have made to seek help. Remember, it's okay to say you're not okay. Therapy should be a safe space for you to express concerns and discuss any issues causing distress, including racism, sexism, or other forms of culturally marginalizing behaviors.

Then be prepared to do an FTD or *Fit, Trust, Discuss* check with yourself and the therapist.

- **Fit** matters, but it can come in many different forms. Ask questions if you wonder how the therapist will handle issues of race, gender, or sexual orientation if you raise them. Ask yourself whether it is more important to have a shared identity or an ally in your journey to healing.

- **Trust** takes time! Don't expect to make permanent decisions at your first visit. Every relationship requires taking a chance with trust. Be sure to trust your instincts—the response to examples of everyday racism, whether in the initial evaluation session or later in the therapeutic relationship, can tell you a lot about how a therapist outside your own race might handle uncomfortable conversations that arise during the course of treatment.

- **Discuss** what's on your mind, not just what you think you *should* talk about! Be as open as possible and explain what you expect as best you can in the initial session. Start a discussion about your real self—the "you" that is normally kept in the background in interracial relationships (especially in professional settings). Hopefully the therapist will demonstrate an openness to listening to you and learning about your life experiences and their impact without judgment, assumptions, or disbelief.

It can be a challenge to find a therapist who shares your racial, ethnic, or cultural identity due to limited availability issues, but if you can find someone who helps you on the path to being your best self and provides a safe, therapeutic space to address your needs, it will be well worth the effort.

ALTHA J. STEWART, MD, is director of the division of public and community psychiatry at the University of Tennessee Health Science Center.

. . .

Q: Would I benefit from new technology such as mental health apps? How do I choose from the many apps that are available?

A: Video visits for mental health are an effective and common way to obtain mental health help—especially since the Covid-19 pandemic. But beyond these telehealth visits, there is a raft of new technologies being adapted for use as mental health tools—like wearable sensors, smartphone apps, and virtual reality. A search for "depression" or "anxiety" in an app store will reveal thousands of products ready for sale and immediate download. But how do you know which ones to pick and which to avoid? This can be hard because data about an app's effectiveness is not often accessible and clear, and most of these products exaggerate their claims and minimize risks. To help you make the most informed choice, we have created a four-step process for evaluating an app or other health technology based on years of research, partnerships, and experience using apps in mental health care.

Step 1: Privacy and Security. The first thing to look for is how the app or technology keeps your mental health data safe and private. In 2021, *Consumer Reports* found that some of the most popular mental health apps still have serious privacy flaws that allow data to be freely shared. While looking over a privacy policy is never fun, it is worth spending the time doing so, or asking a friend to help, if you are considering using an app that asks for information you would not want to publicly share. Through the American Psychiatric Association's App Advisor project (visit psychiatry.org and search for App Advisor) there are videos to help you know what red flags to look for, and through the Mobile Health and Index Navigation Database (MIND; mindapps.org) you can sort over five hundred mental health apps by privacy (and other) features.

Step 2: Evidence. The second factor to consider is the quality and quantity of evidence about the app's effectiveness. Research suggests most app descriptions do not present all the facts about how well an app works. While many may make medical claims, most new apps are only defined as "wellness devices," and thus are not bound to follow the marketing rules that apply to medications or therapies. For apps that make extraordinary claims, you should demand extraordinary evidence. While most apps cannot boast that today, we do know that apps that connect you to peer support or to another person are more likely to be effective and helpful. Again, you can sort through the evidence and more features at mindapps.org.

Step 3: Ease of Use. The next step is to consider how engaging the app is to use. While apps may be easy to download, research suggests that the average mental health app is never opened more than a few times before it is abandoned. Each person has different engagement styles, so thinking about what factors make the apps you already use and like appealing is helpful in identifying the engagement factors to seek in a mental health app. For some, this will be a chatbot, and for others it might be a video or lots of data and graphs. There is likely no one perfect match, but finding an app that can keep you engaged is the key to sustained use and meaningful change. Mindapps.org can also help you search engagement features.

Step 4: Sharing Capabilities. Mental health is a part of your overall health, and you don't want to isolate it from the rest of your health care. Thus, finding apps that make it easy to export and share your data with those you trust, like your treatment team, may be advantageous. Increasingly, apps can share data with your medical record; those apps that let you control where and to whom your data goes will promote better integration of your mental and physical health. Of course, some people may prefer not to share personal health data except on an as-needed, explicitly designated basis—or not to share it at all—so you will again want to evaluate this aspect of the app through the lens of Step 1.

Technology in mental health is both new and evolving. These steps should help you find what might be helpful and safe for you.

JOHN TOROUS, MD, MBI, is director of the digital psychiatry division in the department of psychiatry at Beth Israel Deaconess Medical Center, a Harvard Medical School–affiliated teaching hospital. He serves as editor in chief for *JMIR Mental Health,* is the web editor for *JAMA Psychiatry,* and currently leads the American Psychiatric Association's Health IT Committee.

• • •

Q: When seeking addiction treatment, besides location and whether the facility accepts my health insurance, what qualities should I be looking for?

A: I know firsthand the stress and uncertainty that can come with assessing addiction treatment options. My son Brian cycled through eight different treatment programs. Not one of them offered care that was rooted in evidence or science. Throughout these struggles, my family felt isolated, alone, and judged—and so did Brian. Tragically, Brian died at just twenty-five years old.

After Brian's death, I struggled with two questions. What could I have done differently as a father? And what could be done to spare other families the tragedy my family had suffered?

What I discovered destroyed me all over again: Proven research sitting there, buried in medical journals, that could have helped my son and millions of others. What was missing was an organization to get this information on effective addiction treatment implemented.

I founded Shatterproof to do just this. Our organization is working to revolutionize the addiction treatment system so that the millions of American families struggling with this illness can easily find effective, science-based care. First, we established a standard of care for addiction treatment: the National Principles of Care. These eight principles promote the use of key clinical best practices that improve outcomes for those with substance use disorder. They have been adopted by twenty-three large health insurers representing almost 200 million people.

Next, we created ATLAS, the Addiction Treatment Locator, Assessment, and Standards Platform. ATLAS empowers those impacted by addiction to cut through confusion, deception, and misinformation when searching for treatment, and allows them to navigate to high-quality care while also accelerating the delivery of these clinical best practices. TreatmentATLAS.org is a trusted website for individuals with substance use disorders and their loved ones, empowering them to do three things: receive a science-based recommendation on the appropriate level of addiction treatment that meets their needs (e.g., outpatient, residential), receive a science-based recommendation on additional services needed (e.g., medications for opioid use disorder, mental health services), and locate a facility that provides these recommendations using evidence-based protocols.

After taking our quick, confidential Addiction Treatment Needs Assessment, you'll receive the first two recommendations most appropriate for you or your loved one. You can start browsing treatment providers to locate one providing the recommended level of care and additional services using evidenced-based protocols. ATLAS allows you to search and filter treatment options by location, substance focus, insurance type, and more. ATLAS also clearly indicates whether treatment programs align with the Principles of Care.

ATLAS launched in six pilot states in 2020: Delaware, Louisiana, Massachusetts, New York, North Carolina, and West Virginia. In 2021, we announced ATLAS would be expanding to five additional states: Florida, New Jersey, Oklahoma, Pennsylvania, and California, and has since expanded even further to Connecticut, Indiana, and Wisconsin. We are continuing conversations with additional states across the nation to expand the impact of this valuable platform.

My son didn't see a world where he could be seen as normal—as a young man who got sick, got treatment, and then got better, finding a path toward a full and fulfilling life. Together, we are changing this for families across the country. Shatterproof is here to support families navigating this process at all stages. Visit shatterproof.org for more resources. You'll find the National Principles of Care on the homepage of TreatmentATLAS.org.

GARY MENDELL is founder and CEO of Shatterproof.

Helpful Tools

Q: I've heard that the Wellness Recovery Action Plan (WRAP) is a particularly effective, structured "self-help" program for people recovering from mental health conditions. What is it and how does it work?

A: When I began trying to find a way to stop my extreme mood swings from destroying my life back in the late 1980s, I was told that *recovery* is not a word that should be used with regard to mental health issues; that it was not possible to recover and maintaining this "false hope" was a form of denial. Nevertheless, I persisted and was determined to find a way. Since I was not getting the help I needed from care providers, I instead sought answers from other people who had experienced mental health issues. I asked how they coped with their condition, how they had gotten better, and how they were staying well. Over one hundred people volunteered for my first study.

I learned from them that recovery required five essentials. You must:

1. have hope
2. take personal responsibility for your health and wellness
3. educate yourself

4. advocate for yourself
5. have a strong system of support

I tried the strategies other people were using to get better—and I got better and better. Then I started sharing what I'd learned in workshops and at conferences and even wrote a book. In 1997, I was working with a group of people who were looking for a way to structure their "wellness tools" so they would be effective. They came up with a unique self-help system: the Wellness Recovery Action Plan.

Once I developed a WRAP for myself, that was a new beginning for me. Before WRAP, I had gotten well enough to work and take care of myself, but not well enough that I was truly enjoying my life. WRAP got me there, and it is my guide to daily living. It is my answer when I am having a hard time.

To develop a WRAP, you start by developing a list of wellness tools—simple, safe, and usually free things you can do to help yourself get well and stay well—and a description of yourself when you feel the way you want to feel, so you can refer to it when you are having a hard time. For example, you might find that going on a walk helps with sadness, or listening to familiar music reduces anxiety, or that calling a friend can help with loneliness.

Then, from your list of wellness tools, you select a "short list" of the tools you know you need to use every day to feel your best. This is your daily maintenance plan. Next, you make a list of stressors or triggers—things that, if they happened, would be upsetting, and the wellness tools you would use if these stressors or triggers came up. Then, write down your early warning signs, a list of signs that things are not quite right with you, such as sleep disruption or loss of interest in normal daily activities, and the tools you will use when you notice these signs.

"When Things Are Breaking Down" is a critical section of your Action Plan. Here you identify the signs that things have gotten much worse and then develop a very structured plan of the wellness tools you will use at this critical juncture to prevent a crisis. Your WRAP also includes an intensive crisis plan to fill out and share with your supporters so they will know what to do for you if you can no longer care for yourself; there you list the signs that indicate that others need to take over, designate who you want to take over, and describe what you want them to do. There is also a post-crisis plan for navigating that often difficult time after a crisis and before you are ready to once again use the daily maintenance plan.

WRAP has stood the test of time and has been well studied in rigorous research trials. It is what I, and people all over the world, use to get well, stay well, and do what they want to with their lives. I review and update my WRAP from time to time when my circumstances have changed or when I feel that it is not working for me as well as it should. This is my plan. I am the expert on it, and I use it daily. It has saved my life.

The only one person who can develop your WRAP is you, the person who will be using it. You can reach out to others for ideas and support with your WRAP, but you are the "bottom line."

In 1997, **MARY ELLEN COPELAND, PHD,** worked with a group of people who experience mental issues and together they developed WRAP. Dr. Copeland is the author of *Wellness Recovery Action Plan* and other books that describe the WRAP process.

• • •

Q: Do I (or does my family member) need a crisis plan or a psychiatric advance directive?

A: Benjamin Franklin once said, "An ounce of prevention is worth a pound of cure." This remains sound advice. When facing any situation, it is better to be aware of what is coming so that we can shape our reactions and minimize any negative impact or consequence. Folks living with mental illness, and the family, friends, professionals, and systems of care that support them, should see crisis situations as opportunities to learn what's necessary to prevent harmful consequences—or future crises.

We can learn from our past experiences, build in different supports, and explain our preferences, in order to change our responses and the responses of our environment, and work to ensure a positive resolution to a crisis situation. One way of doing this is to create a crisis plan.

A crisis plan is a *written* plan meant to identify mounting symptoms and behaviors that indicate that an evolving situation might lead to a mental health crisis, and to identify the triggers that can incite, or exacerbate, crisis situations. It also delineates what approaches have worked or not worked in the past and offers your perspective on what supports will best help in resolving the crisis. It should be created when you or your loved one is clinically stable; be informed by recollections of recent events; and be reviewed and updated after each crisis to reflect new "discoveries" of what proved helpful and what did not. I always recommend keeping the plan on one sheet of paper that you or your loved one can carry in a wallet or purse. It's also helpful to distribute crisis plans to supporters: other trusted family members, friends, designated emergency rooms, and personnel (who can transmit information to admitting units), current care providers, clergy, primary care physicians, mobile crisis teams, and local law enforcement. This way, everyone is informed, and there is consistency in interventions and treatment response. Supporters of people who are vulnerable to crisis would benefit by building skills to de-escalate situations and improve interactions with those who live with mental illness.

A crisis plan should include the following information:

Demographic information: Name, age, date of birth, address, phone number, diagnoses (medical and psychiatric), pharmacy information, insurance provider information, and contact information.

Supports: Names and phone numbers of trusted folks (family, friends, teachers, co-workers, faith leaders, treatment providers) that you consent to have emergency care providers contact regarding clinical information and for treatment planning. The plan can also indicate facility preferences should admission be necessary.

Triggers and blockers: What symptoms should be monitored? What has caused symptom flare-ups in the past? Daily life stressors like social isolation, irregular sleep, poor nutrition, or stopping meds? Or are there job-related, financial, or housing issues? Are there relationship conflicts or losses or substance use? If you or your loved one begin to sustain known stressors, then it's important to be prepared to use available assets to mitigate or prevent harmful consequences.

Medication: Include a list of all medications you currently take, reason for use, and dosage; medication allergies should also be noted.

Treatment choice: What medication/treatments have worked? What has not worked, or should be avoided? What do you or your supporters feel are your strengths? Your vulnerabilities? Do you find listing some short-term goals to be helpful or hurtful? For example, wanting to be a stable, calm, loving parent can provide an emotional anchor for someone in crisis, or it can trigger unrelenting feelings of remorse. It varies from person to person, so this must be adjusted accordingly. Examples of crisis planning worksheets can be found at mhanational.org/crisis-planning-caregivers.

Psychiatric Advanced Directives
Some states allow for legally binding documents called psychiatric advanced directives. These legal documents, completed in times of wellness, make it possible for people with mental illness to determine what kind of care they would like to receive in a crisis should they not be able to make decisions. Psychiatric advanced directives can be a lifesaving tool. They help ensure that your or your loved one's voice is heard, and also facilitate dialogue with providers. They are similar to crisis plans but may contain more directives (what the patient will accept or disallow), are legally binding, and are state specific. If you're interested in creating a psychiatric advanced directive, you can find more information at www.nrc-pad.org.

JACKIE MAUS FELDMAN, MD, DLFAPA, is professor emerita, department of psychiatry and behavioral neurology at the University of Alabama at Birmingham and associate medical director of NAMI.

. . .

Q: How do I use my own lived experience to become a peer specialist?

A: Only a very small fraction of people who live and recover with a mental health condition become peer specialists—those living a life of recovery who also work professionally to help others as part of a treatment team. When I first entered the field, I thought many more individuals would take up the challenge. But I've come to realize that to do this work, one should have a sensitivity to inequality, discrimination, traumatization, and marginalization that drives their passion to make peer support their life's calling. For me, that sensitivity is a hard-earned product of lived experience. Being able to help others is in part about going through some things yourself.

I never knew I had a mental illness until I was told I had one. Most of my life leading up to that moment, the people who knew me best described me as a "wild child." But that wild child had been deeply affected not just by a mental health condition but also by traumatic experiences of racist violence, including: 1) encountering a dead body hanging in a tree on my way to fish as a child in Mississippi, 2) being assaulted with a beer bottle full of urine at age thirteen by three white men riding in a pickup truck while I was coming home from school, and 3) being pelted by a mob throwing rocks while protesting segregation in high school.

I also had lived experience of accomplishment, pride, and success. After college, I escaped the oppression of the South by joining the Navy, where I earned individual citations, early promotions, the Navy Achievement Medal, and graduated from the prestigious Naval Postgraduate School. I benefited mightily from concepts that were the bedrock of

Navy service, like duty, honor, integrity, and esprit de corps. But my buoyant, fulfilling Naval career soon gave way to difficulty finding and maintaining employment commensurate with my education and experiences. I bounced from job to job and town to town, and I had more than one failed personal relationship.

My journey to becoming a peer specialist started when the drug court referred me to a treatment facility to be a designated subject-matter expert on treating co-occurring disorders. One of my responsibilities was to digest as much of the contemporary research literature on my condition as I could. That research gave me my first insight into my own condition and sparked my interest in knowing and understanding contemporary thought leadership on behavioral health. My next stop was as operations officer of NAMI Tennessee. It was there that I learned about advocacy, with an emphasis not just on how to advocate but what to advocate for. And just as important, I discovered the strength derived from being part of an organized network of individuals living with a common purpose and singular identity. Recovery for me was about being mentored, educated, and respected by individuals I came to consider guardians of the principles of recovery, who continue to have a profound effect on my life.

Becoming a peer specialist means taking full account of your lived experience—what it has been, what it is now, and what you aspire for it to be in the future. When we're able to use that experience to benefit and serve others, it becomes a force multiplier. The authentic lived experience of a peer specialist, along with treatment and therapeutics, can truly benefit people seeking recovery. I consider myself very fortunate to have found a vocation in which I can make use of everything I've lived and learned to lift up others and, in doing so, bring out the best in myself.

Requirements for becoming a peer specialist vary from state to state. Doors to Wellbeing, a program of the Copeland Center, has a complete list of training and certification requirements and appropriate contact information for each state (Doorstowellbeing.org). Recently the Substance Abuse and Mental Health Services Administration (SAMHSA)

collaborated with federal, state, tribal, territorial, and local partners—
including peer specialists—to develop the National Model Standards for
Peer Support Certification, inclusive of substance use, mental health, and
family peer certifications. These National Model Standards closely align
with the needs of the behavioral health peer workforce, and subsequently,
the overarching goal of the national mental health strategy (https://store
.samhsa.gov/sites/default/files/pep23-10-01-001.pdf).

CLARENCE JORDAN, MBA, CPS, is director of clinical programs,
Carelon Behavioral Health (Elevance), responsible for Carelon's national development and implementation of the use of peer specialist
in treatment, wellness, and recovery. He received the SAMHSA 2010
Voice Award and the 2014 Peer Specialist of the Year Award, and was
selected as a member of the SAMHSA Technical Expert Panel for the
National Model Standards for Peer Support Certification.

. . .

Q: Can a job be a mental health intervention?

A: Yes. This question shifts the focus from what is important to professionals and industry to what is important to everyday people who live
with a mental illness. Operating on a deficit model, in a health care system structured around insurance funding, professionals provide medications and therapies that suppress symptoms but typically do not improve
social function. Yet people living with mental disorders prefer a model
that emphasizes their strengths, choices, resilience, and goals.

The ideology of "recovery" refers to the potential for a meaningful, functional life, not a complete absence of symptoms. People can live with
symptoms if their life has meaning and satisfaction. As one of my mentors,
Pat Deegan, described her own recovery journey, her doctor said she was a
treatment success when she was heavily medicated, unable to focus her
thinking, and smoking cigarettes in front of a television all day. However,

Pat wanted a full life. She learned to live with fewer medications and some symptoms, returned to college and graduate school, and became a successful psychologist, wife, and mother. Along her journey, she has helped tens of thousands of people start their own journeys of recovery. Many with a mental illness have more modest but equally meaningful functional goals.

As the mental health field slowly embraces recovery, we are also beginning to address social determinants. Employment is a central social determinant of health because it influences other social factors: income, housing, social support, friendships, and community integration. When people have earnings from a job, they have opportunities to pursue other goals. In addition, employment helps people with mental health conditions to increase self-efficacy, self-esteem, and symptom control, and enhances their ability to structure their days. Employment is an effective treatment because it helps people to function and to manage their illnesses. In this sense, a job is arguably the most effective and cost-effective mental health intervention that we currently have.

A fundamental development in employment services for people with a disability has occurred over the past twenty-five years. Following years of ineffective interventions, we now have an evidence-based, cost-effective approach called Individual Placement and Support (IPS supported employment) that helps most people with disabilities to become successfully employed. The only requirement is that a person must want a job. Supports are put in place to make that happen in competitive work roles, and individuals are taught how their benefits can be coordinated with a work income. The IPS specialist helps with the employer as needed and helps the individual on important questions, such as the disclosure of disability to the employer to help get and keep the jobs that they want. IPS specialists continue supporting the client after obtaining employment for as long as they want.

A strong evidence base shows that IPS enables people with mental health conditions to obtain jobs that align with their interests and skills, and to maintain competitive integrated employment for years. The evidence is particularly strong for people with a serious mental illness.

The tragic reality, however, is that while 60 percent of adults with serious mental illness express a desire to work, only 2 percent have access to IPS services. The reason is simple: Even though IPS is cost-effective, the available funding mechanisms are complex and inadequate. Professionals, hospitals, and the pharmaceutical industry spend millions of dollars on lobbying, and the government funds the treatments they prefer rather than the services that people living with mental illness want and need.

IPS is currently available in nearly every state, the District of Columbia, and thirty other countries. You can find out where IPS services are offered in your state and advocate for IPS services by calling the governor's office, the Department of Mental Health, and the Department of Vocational Rehabilitation.

ROBERT DRAKE, MD, PHD, is a professor of clinical psychiatry at Columbia University and consultant to the Substance Abuse and Mental Health Services Administration and Westat.

• • •

Q: How can I improve my cognitive functioning to do better at work?

A: Cognitive functioning refers to mental abilities (or thinking skills), such as attention and concentration, memory, organization and planning, problem-solving, and thinking speed. People with better cognitive functioning are more likely to be employed, perform better on their jobs, and earn more money, both in the general population and among those with serious mental illness. Unfortunately, mental illness symptoms can negatively impact people's cognitive functioning depending on both the severity and the diagnosis. However, effective vocational rehabilitation programs, such as supported employment, can help people with serious mental illness get and keep competitive jobs.

The good news is that there are ways to improve cognitive functioning, and a new psychiatric rehabilitation approach called cognitive remediation has proven effective at improving cognitive functioning in people with serious mental illness. Cognitive remediation is a program that may employ several different methods to enhance cognitive functioning, including computer cognitive practice exercises; strategy coaching by a trained facilitator to improve performance on those exercises; and learning self-management strategies for improving cognitive performance in everyday situations—such as removing distractions to improve attention or repeating back information to improve memory. Cognitive remediation programs vary in the specific cognitive enhancement methods they use, with some programs using one method, others using two different methods, and still others using all three methods. The programs also differ in whether they are broadly focused on improving cognitive abilities and overall functioning or are specifically focused on enhancing cognition in order to improve work outcomes.

The Thinking Skills for Work (TSW) program is a cognitive remediation program we designed specifically for people who want to start working or improve their work performance. The TSW program is generally provided to people who are enrolled in a vocational rehabilitation program. In addition to improving cognitive abilities, such as memory and problem-solving, the TSW program teaches cognitive skills for improving confidence and developing a positive "can-do" attitude when faced with cognitively challenging situations. Increasing self-efficacy and motivation to do one's best can enhance the effort, and the persistence an individual invests in tackling difficult work-related tasks will maximize their success in achieving their employment goals. All three cognitive enhancement methods described above—computer cognitive training, strategy coaching, and teaching cognitive self-management strategies—are included in the TSW program. A series of ten educational handouts on topics such as recognizing your strengths, challenging negative thinking, improving attention and concentration, and overcoming memory problems are used to facilitate teaching different cognitive self-management strategies.

Controlled research on the TSW program has shown that individuals who receive TSW in addition to vocational rehabilitation improve more in both cognitive functioning and competitive work outcomes than people who receive vocational services alone. The TSW program has also been found to be effective in helping people who have not previously benefited from vocational rehabilitation get and keep jobs. Furthermore, people do not have to experience cognitive challenges in order to profit from the TSW program. *Everyone* can benefit from improving their thinking skills for work, regardless of their level of cognitive functioning.

You can learn more about TSW in our book, *Cognitive Remediation for Successful Employment and Psychiatric Recovery: The Thinking Skills for Work Program.*

SUSAN MCGURK, PHD, and **KIM MUESER, PHD**, are both professors in the departments of occupational therapy and psychological and brain sciences and faculty members of the Center for Psychiatric Rehabilitation at Boston University.

. . .

Q: As a person with a mental health condition, what are my rights in housing and in the workplace?

A: *Rights to Housing:* The federal Fair Housing Act prohibits discrimination in housing against people with disabilities, including people with mental illness. These antidiscrimination protections apply to both the sale and rental of housing. They also apply to evictions or attempts to evict people from housing based on their disabilities.

In addition to individual protections, the Fair Housing Act also applies to broad-based laws or policies that have the effect of restricting housing for people with disabilities in communities. For example, the US Supreme Court has determined that zoning laws that exclude group homes or other congregate housing for people with disabilities from specific neighborhoods violate the Fair Housing Act.

The protections of the Fair Housing Act are not absolute. For example, although a landlord cannot evict someone because they have a mental illness, they may be able to do so if that person violates the terms of their lease. The key is that the same rules must apply to everyone, whether or not they have a mental illness or another disability.

The Fair Housing Act also requires landlords to make reasonable accommodations in rules, policies, and practices to enable a person with a mental illness or another disability to succeed in obtaining or maintaining housing. This can include permitting another person to support and assist the individual with mental illness meet the terms of their lease.

Rights to Employment: Federal law also provides certain protections for people with mental illness or other disabilities against discrimination in employment. Title I of the Americans with Disabilities Act (ADA) makes it unlawful for private companies with fifteen or more employees to discriminate against people on the basis of disability, including mental illness. This applies to all aspects of employment, including hiring, firing, leave, and promotions.

A separate section of the ADA also prohibits employment discrimination by state and local governments; and another federal law, the Rehabilitation Act, prohibits discrimination by the federal government and by federal contractors.

The ADA specifies that people with disabilities must be qualified to perform the essential functions of the job. However, as with the Fair Housing Act, the ADA encourages employers to provide reasonable accommodations that will enable people with disabilities, including mental illness, to successfully carry out their job responsibilities. The determination of whether an accommodation is reasonable occurs on a case-by-case basis. Examples of reasonable accommodations may include adjustments in work hours, relocation of workspaces to areas free of unnecessary distractions, and the granting of leave for medical appointments or treatment.

To find out more about the Fair Housing Act, including how to file a complaint, visit the US Department of Housing and Urban Development website at https://www.hud.gov/program_offices/fair_housing _equal_opp.

To find out more about the employment provisions of the ADA, including how to file a complaint, visit the Equal Employment Opportunity Commission website at eeoc.gov/disability-discrimination.

In addition to federal laws, many states have laws that provide protections to people with mental illness or other disabilities from discrimination in housing or the workplace. The National Disability Rights Network website can direct you to protection and advocacy organizations and client assistance programs that understand the relevant laws in your state: ndrn.org/about/ndrn-member-agencies.

RON HONBERG, JD, is the former national director of policy and legal affairs for NAMI.

. . .

Q: I lost my job during the Covid-19 pandemic, and when the eviction moratorium ends, I'm going to be out on the street. Even though I've been taking my medication, I'm either super anxious or super depressed, and my OCD has flared up to where it's unbearable. Am I experiencing a mental health condition, or is life just really stressful and depressing?

A: More often than not, society regards mental health as an individual issue—a "character flaw" or private condition that we don't like to talk about, and that we are each responsible for solving ourselves. Relatively few people think about how wider social and structural issues might be putting us at higher risk of having mental health conditions in the first place.

But if you don't know where your next paycheck is coming from or are wondering how to put food on the table for your family or can't imagine securing affordable quality childcare when you do find work, then all that can worsen your mental health. Similarly, if you are incarcerated or victimized by the criminal justice system or struggling with housing and homelessness, your mental health might also get worse. And, of course, when you need to talk to a mental health provider but the care is inaccessible or unaffordable, or they don't "get" what is or isn't acceptable in your culture, this can also be a detriment. Whether the negative impact is temporary or leads to chronic and more severe issues, it is clear that social and health system forces—and the stress and trauma they inflict—can exacerbate mental health conditions for people who are vulnerable due to genetics, individual behaviors, or other risk factors. Nowhere has this been more apparent than with Covid-19, which has clearly worsened our collective mental health, especially that of children.

As a whole, we have begun to recognize the role of society, policy, and the environment on physical health conditions—say, the impact of tobacco use or toxic air pollution on lung disease; the role of food systems and highly processed, high sugar foods on diabetes; and the consequences of lead paint exposure in early childhood development. However, we have largely failed to acknowledge that mental health conditions, like depression, anxiety, and substance use disorders—and even more severe conditions, like schizophrenia and bipolar disorder—have clear connections to issues like poverty, housing, education, and employment.

If, as a country, we can begin to accept that social forces, bigger than any one individual, can impact mental health, then we can begin to devise collective solutions. Those solutions require changes in public policy and the people who we elect to make those policies. Thus, we must, as a people, make mental health and the so-called social determinants of mental health a political issue and hold our leaders accountable for advancing those protective policies. Such policies would help make mental health care more accessible, affordable, and of higher quality; expand the availability of affordable housing and effective long-term drug addiction treatment; increase living wages to make daily life easier for more people;

improve education systems; and reduce the negative impact of our criminal justice system, among other things.

We live in a divided and polarized time, but mental health might be one of the last truly bipartisan issues left. It affects almost all demographic and social groups relatively equally, even if the outcomes are dramatically different based on the color of your skin, your income, or where you live. Our fragmented and dysfunctional mental health care system hurts us all. We have already heard encouraging rhetoric and seen encouraging attempts at bipartisan legislation emerging around mental health, which should give us hope that on this issue, at least, politicians may still be able to reach across the aisle to make change.

It is essential that we educate ourselves on how policy choices in health care, housing, and other related areas can impact mental health in negative and positive ways; and we must use our energies to organize our communities and advocate for officials who support the positive ones. So learn what you can, call your elected officials, participate in "get out the vote" campaigns, and most important, *vote* for better mental health for all.

ASHWIN VASAN, MD, PHD, is the 44th commissioner of the New York City Department of Health and Mental Hygiene. Dr. Vasan is the former president and CEO of Fountain House, a national nonprofit fighting to improve health, increase opportunity, and reduce social and economic isolation for people with serious mental illness.

Self-Care and Ways to Reduce Medical Risk

Q: How can I quit smoking without making my psychiatric symptoms worse?

A: The good news is that people who are able to quit smoking on average report significantly *improved* psychiatric symptoms. After six months, people who quit smoking have significantly lower levels of depression, anxiety, mixed anxiety and depression, and perceived stress than those who continue smoking. And the effect is large—about as large as the effect of an effective antidepressant medication.

People who smoke report that smoking a cigarette (or cigar or vape) reduces their negative emotions—in particular, their anxiety. This is true. If this is the case for you, it makes sense that you would worry that quitting smoking will worsen any symptoms that smoking seems to improve. What many people don't realize is that the anxiety, depression, and stress that smoking a cigarette relieves are in large part caused by nicotine withdrawal. People begin to experience nicotine withdrawal between cigarettes, and nicotine withdrawal for most people is most severe first thing in the morning, after having no cigarettes throughout the night while sleeping. People who quit smoking have lower levels of anxiety, depressive, and stress symptoms about two weeks after quitting because they are no longer experiencing withdrawal symptoms between each cigarette—especially first thing in the morning.

The issue here is that there is overlap between nicotine withdrawal symptoms and psychiatric symptoms. The excellent news is that the effective medications to help people quit smoking increase quit success rates for people with serious mental illness by three- to fivefold (300 to 500 percent), and they do this by preventing nicotine withdrawal symptoms. Thus, neither quitting smoking nor using medications—such as varenicline, dual nicotine replacement therapy (patch plus gum, lozenge, inhaler, or nasal spray), or bupropion—worsens psychiatric symptoms. And using a medication to minimize nicotine withdrawal symptoms during an attempt to quit can greatly reduce the nicotine withdrawal symptoms of anxiety, depressed mood, and feelings of stress that feel like worsening of symptoms associated with a mental health condition. New guidelines recommend that every smoker try a medication to help them to quit, even those who feel they may not be ready to try to quit. This is because taking one of these effective medications reduces the feelings of nicotine withdrawal between cigarettes and increases people's confidence that they can and may be ready now to try to quit.

A. EDEN EVINS, MD, MPH, is Cox Family Professor of Psychiatry, Harvard Medical School; founding director, Mass General Hospital Center for Addiction Medicine; and director for faculty development at Mass General Hospital's department of psychiatry.

· · ·

Q: My antipsychotics are helping me, but I worry about the risk of weight gain and diabetes. What can I do to reduce my risk of medical problems while taking this medicine?

A: Many types of antipsychotic medications can increase appetite, lead to weight gain, and contribute to diabetes risk. This side effect is not your fault but is something to understand and plan for. Further, not all antipsychotic medications have the same metabolic effects. If you have questions about the specific medications you are taking, speak with your psychiatrist or prescriber. You can also consult your primary care doctor and ask both these doctors to speak with each other—and you—about your heart health. This coordination can ensure that it's clear who is doing this critical monitoring. For antipsychotic medicines that can cause these symptoms, it also important for you to know that you should have your weight, cholesterol, and hemoglobin A1c (a measure of diabetes risk) checked annually as part of regular preventive care depending on your age and other risk factors.

Regardless of what medication or medications you are taking for psychiatric symptoms, there are steps you can take to be heart healthy and move toward a healthy weight. And if you are considered overweight by your doctor, losing even a few pounds can have a clinically significant positive impact on your health.

Making changes to diet and exercise is challenging for many people. It can be more challenging if a medication affects your metabolism, or your sense of hunger, like some antipsychotics. It's important to remember that you don't have to change everything all at once. Creating new habits can take time, and it's okay to start slow and have success with one healthy habit first. It's okay to stop and start with healthy behaviors, too.

Our body manages the calories in nutritious foods differently than with calories that come from highly processed foods containing lots of fat, salt, or sugar. There are several high-impact health behaviors you can adopt to lose weight or maintain a healthy weight without needing to count calories. Some of them may already be familiar:

1. Avoid beverages with high sugar content.
2. Avoid junk food, including overly salty, sweet, and greasy foods.
3. Eat smart portions. This can be eating less than you would usually eat.
4. Eat more vegetables. Vegetables are low in calories and high in fiber.
5. Exercise for twenty minutes each day, focusing on moderate intensity aerobic exercise, like going for a brisk walk. Two ten-minute periods of activity may be easier to start with for those who are not currently active. In addition to helping you lose weight or maintain a healthy weight, exercise leads to increased energy and better sleep, improved mood, and improved blood sugar and blood pressure.
6. Self-monitoring, or tracking your eating, exercise, and weight, is also recommended. Tracking can increase self-awareness and help you identify areas for improvement, create realistic goals, and see progress being made. There are many new apps and technologies that can help with tracking, but just keeping a daily logbook using pen and paper can work just as well.

Even small changes to eating and exercise behaviors can lead to weight loss and help build confidence to make bigger changes. The goal is to create sustainable healthy habits.

NAMI has a resource called Hearts and Minds (found on the NAMI website) that outlines more details of these side effect risks and practical proactive approaches you can take to promote your health.

In addition to adopting these healthy lifestyle changes, there are prescription medications that are sometimes used to help people lose weight. Your doctor may prescribe such a medication if you have a high BMI ($\geq$ 30 kg/m2), or if you have a BMI $\geq$ 27 and a weight-related medical condition. These weight-loss medications can lead to significant weight loss and are often taken long-term to avoid weight regain. More research is needed on the impact of these anti-obesity drugs among persons living with serious mental illness, including using in combination with healthy behavior lifestyle change. If you are interested in these medications or have questions, please speak with your physician about whether they would be advisable for you.

GAIL L. DAUMIT, MD, MHS, FACP, is the Samsung Professor of Medicine at Johns Hopkins University School of Medicine.

Questions about Family

Q: How can I best help my daughter deal with a traumatic event that happened at her afterschool program?

A: Let me respond to your question from a perspective that might surprise you: neuroscience. Over the past several decades, in part thanks to increasingly sophisticated brain-imaging machines, we have learned more about what makes our brain-body system work best, and how to help deepen our own and our children's natural capacity for resilience. And, fortunately, there are some very easy and practical ways that this information can be used. So, let's apply some of it to your daughter's situation.

First, the fact that your daughter told you about what happened to her is a sign that she sees you as a protector. A sense of safety is one of the most essential factors in shaping our way of being in the world.

Neuroscience has shown that in the midsection of our brains, each of us has two little structures called amygdalae that act as our brain-body's smoke detector. They are always scanning for potential threat. When they are "alert," we feel fearful and anxious and unable to focus on anything other than getting out of danger. Your daughter's sense of safety has been compromised. So, step one is for you to find as many ways as you can to help your daughter feel safe. At home, this could mean maintaining her favorite rituals, offering her choices about when or how to do things, and pointing out when she takes care of her needs (brushing her hair, making her bed, etc.). Things like this help remind her that she has the power and the ability to manage her environment at home.

Another ingredient that is important to the brain and how we function is the quality of our attachments. When we have relationships that matter to us, we feel safe. When we feel safe, we can build better relationships. They go hand in hand. Talk with your daughter and highlight the positive relationships in her life. Who have been her favorite teachers and why? What kinds of friends does she like best, and what kind of a friend is she? When I work with people who are suffering, I usually try to shift their attention away from what is making them upset and to focus on their resources. Resources are people, activities, and things that bring us a sense of joy, calm, or security. The questions I have suggested above are what I call resource questions. The longer you can keep your daughter talking about her resources, the safer she will begin to feel. Her amygdala can then stop being so hypervigilant.

You'll be able to tell whether your daughter is experiencing a deeper sense of calmness by paying attention to her breathing—is it deeper rather than shallower?—and the tension in her body—does she seem a bit less tight, more relaxed? If she's breathing deeply and holding her body without tension, then the part of the brain-body system that calms us and decreases activation is operating.

Here's the good news: You have a lot more control over how your brain works than you realize. This amazing power is called neuroplasticity. We change our brain through what we pay attention to. Learning to shift attention from negative or scary things to resources, and practicing doing so whenever the negative things rear their heads (as they will), begins to enlist neuroplasticity. The neural pathways for the positives get stronger and the ones for negatives start to get pruned away. If you can help your daughter shift her attention to positives when that scary experience comes to mind, she will build a deeper zone of resilience; and when hard things happen, she'll be better able to deal with them.

Make a safety plan with your daughter for how to handle the after-school problem. Ask her what would need to happen for her to feel safe going back to the program. Initially, she'll probably say "nothing will," but that just means her amygdala/smoke detector is still on high alert. Not to minimize what happened—it is natural that she would feel fear. But coming up with a plan can start to create new possibilities: Who does she trust in the program? Can the two of you talk to that person, or is it okay with her if you call that person? Can she stay close to the adults, so she knows the mean kids won't bother her? Can she ask friends in the program to do something fun with her so she's not alone? It is probably a good idea for her or the two of you to talk with her main teacher to help build a sense of safety back during the main part of the school day. The more things you do to build safety and relationship, the more you will be building a brain that can bounce back from difficulties.

Finally, each evening before bed, sit together and review the resources of the day. You can even suggest that she keep a little notebook and write them down so she doesn't forget. This will help with sleep. And as she tells you who or what is on her list, be sure to ask at least two or three "curiosity questions" to draw her out about each item. Keeping her brain-body system attentive to those resources for a bit longer is an easy and important way to deepen her resilience. You may even share some of your own resource experiences. It's a lovely way to end the day.

LAURIE LEITCH, PHD, is cofounder and director of Threshold Global Works.

. . .

Q: How do I know if my teen's behavior is just part of normal teenage development, or if it is potentially symptomatic of a mental health condition and warrants an assessment?

A: There is no doubt about it: Being the parent of a teenager is hard. Teens are experiencing multiple changes and challenges during this period of development, from increasing academic demands and more complex peer relationships to discovering their identity and attempting to gain more independence from their family. Many parents tell me that they are often scratching their heads trying to figure out why it is that the child who used to follow them around the house, talking nonstop and frequently seeking out their affection and attention, is now easily irked by their mere presence and avoids any attempts to engage in a conversation about their feelings.

Parents should know that it is typical for teens to experience some mood-related fluctuations, and that it may be hard for them to put into words exactly how they are feeling—which is why your teen may prefer not to engage in a lengthy discussion with you about their emotional state. Also, teens are still learning how best to deal with stressful situations and still trying to identify effective coping strategies that they can use to navigate difficult emotional states. Some adults may know that when they feel anxious or overwhelmed, they can engage in certain activities, such as exercising or setting boundaries with others, to help regulate their emotions; teens are still learning what strategies are most effective for them.

However, behaviors that may seem to be typical for teens—such as spending more time in their rooms and appearing more withdrawn from family, as well as being more oppositional—could also be signs of a bigger problem. As a child psychiatrist, I remind parents that while their teens will experience a wide range of emotions, if they notice that the intensity of their teen's emotional state, and/or their behavior, interferes with their ability to function and accomplish daily activities, then that is a sign that they need help. Signs of difficulty in functioning can be seen in multiple aspects of life: A teen who is missing multiple days of school, is falling behind in multiple classes, and has a drop in their grades may be struggling academically due to some mood-related difficulties. Also, if a couple weeks go by and you notice that your teen is no longer interested in hanging out with friends or participating in extracurricular activities they once enjoyed or has lost interest in their physical appearance in terms of grooming or showering, then an appropriate next step would be to schedule an appointment with their pediatrician.

Parents can have difficulty recognizing that their child may be struggling with a mental health condition, or they may feel unsure about how to approach having a conversation about their concerns since mental health was never discussed within their own families when they were teens. As parents, it is important to know that mental health is part of overall health, and that providing the tools and support for teens to effectively manage their moods will have a positive impact on their overall development. Although it may be hard to overcome the fear of going outside cultural or family norms to get your child mental health support, finding help is crucial if your child's ability to function is impaired.

CHRISTINE CRAWFORD, MD, MPH, is associate medical director of NAMI and assistant professor of psychiatry at Boston University School of Medicine.

. . .

Q: My child has started to struggle in school, takes longer than she should on homework, gets lost in her thoughts during class so she can't pay attention, and talks negatively about herself. I'm concerned she might have ADHD. What exactly is ADHD, and how worried should I be if she does have it?

A: Having attention-deficit hyperactivity disorder (ADHD) is like having a Ferrari engine for a brain, but with bicycle brakes. The challenge is to strengthen the brakes so the Ferrari can win races instead of spinning out on curves. With the right help, people of all ages who have ADHD can become champions. But without the right help, they will likely face many roadblocks.

If your child gets the right diagnosis and proper interventions, their life will improve. The only question is, improve by how much? With the right help, the answer is: a lot!

The tip-off that your child might have ADHD is unexplained underachievement. No matter their age, if they are not doing as well as their native talent predicts they ought to be doing, consider the diagnosis of ADHD—before you ascribe the problem to lack of effort. Millions of people with undiagnosed ADHD are lectured year after year about trying harder. But telling a person with ADHD to try harder is about as helpful as telling a person who's nearsighted to squint harder.

Furthermore, when the diagnosis is missed, when instead a "moral diagnosis" is applied—lazy, willful, undisciplined—then the truly pernicious disabilities of shame, fear, and the belief that they are "stupid" will set in.

The underachievement that so characterizes undiagnosed ADHD derives from the negative symptoms of the condition: distractibility, impulsivity, and restlessness or hyperactivity. Keep in mind, though, that each of those negative symptoms has a flip side that is powerfully positive. The flip side of distractibility is curiosity; the flip side of impulsivity is creativity; and the flip side of hyperactivity is energy, which at my age of seventy-one, I'm very glad to have. I have ADHD myself, and I wouldn't trade it for the world.

A quick clarification: While the diagnosis is called ADHD, we often shorten it to just ADD. What's the difference? Strictly speaking, there is no ADD, only ADHD. But there are two subtypes of ADHD: "primarily inattentive" and "combined type" (the combination being inattention plus hyperactivity and impulsivity). It is important to know that a person can have ADHD without the *H*—without any sign of hyper-activity or disruptive behavior; this is the type that's common in girls and women. The main reason that ADHD is notoriously missed in females of all ages is that they show no signs of disruptive behavior. But they have tremendous difficulty staying focused and so they under-achieve. They have ADHD, and thus, they deserve treatment every bit as much as disruptive males.

Untreated, ADHD of both subtypes can lead to a lifetime of frustration, disappointment, addiction, depression, unemployment, isolation, even early death. This is a high-stakes game, but one with potentially excellent outcomes. As devastating as undiagnosed ADHD can be, people who have ADHD often soar to the top, including Nobel Prize winners, self-made millionaires and billionaires, world-class artists, inventors, athletes, surgeons, and scientists. You name the field, and you can find a person with ADHD at the top of it.

As for getting a diagnosis, you'll need to consult with a professional who has extensive experience with ADHD. Contrary to popular belief, there is no foolproof test for ADHD. The diagnosis resides in your history. Once you know your child has it, treatment begins with education. Learn as much as you can about the condition. The goal is to maximize the positives of ADHD and minimize the negatives. Thankfully, we have many tools to make this happen.

Most treatment plans include coaching or tutoring to help improve organizational skills; an exercise program, since exercise is great for your brain; counseling to help defuse the struggles that so often crop up in couples or families with ADHD; attention to sleep, nutrition, and screen time; and the development of positive human contact in place of shame and isolation.

Medication—stimulant medication as well as others—can also be dramatically helpful. The two main stimulants we use to treat ADHD are amphetamine, common brand name Adderall (first used in 1937 to treat what we now call ADHD), and methylphenidate, common brand name Ritalin (first used in 1955). The stimulants have the best track record in terms of efficacy. Non-stimulants that have proven useful include bupropion (Wellbutrin), atomoxetine (Strattera), guanfacine (Intuniv), and, off-label, amantadine (Symmetrel). One medication or another works about 80 percent of the time. By *works*, I mean it targets symptom improvement with no side effects other than appetite suppression without unwanted weight loss.

Properly supervised, medication for ADHD is both safe and effective. But unsupervised, these medications, especially the stimulants, can be dangerous. They can be abused, bought and sold on the street, and potentially lead to severe medical complications. However, all the dangers can be avoided if you have a good doctor working with you and your child.

Like millions of people who have this condition, I've achieved my dreams in life, and I'm small potatoes compared to many others. Don't fear this condition. Instead, embrace it. Learn all you can about it and turn ADHD into your special power. Take seriously the major problems it can cause, but then get the right help to turn it into your close friend and ally.

EDWARD M. HALLOWELL, MD, is founder of the Hallowell ADHD Centers and author of twenty-two books, including *Driven to Distraction* (1992) and *ADHD 2.0: New Science and Essential Strategies for Coping with Distraction—from Childhood through Adulthood* (2022).

Communication Strategies

Q: What if my loved one doesn't do what needs to be done to get better? How should I talk to them about it?

A: Concerned family members are among the most motivated people I've encountered. They want to do the right things to help their loved one, and, like doctors, to "first, do no harm."

Ironically, though, a helper's first instincts about what to do may be unhelpful. In developing the conversation style called motivational interviewing, we termed this the "righting reflex"—the natural desire to make change happen and set things right. It's done with the best of intentions. We see what's wrong, we know what should be done about it, and think we will help by sharing this information with the person we are concerned about. Unfortunately, most of us don't respond well to being told what to do.

When it comes to making a change in our lives, the central issue is often ambivalence. When someone is doing something harmful or potentially so, it's very likely that part of them already knows it's not a good idea. For example, what cigarette smoker these days is unaware of the real health risks, harm, and costs of smoking? At the same time, most people who are considering (or being told they should) change feel reluctant to do so. They see both pros and cons of change; they want it and don't want it simultaneously. For example, they don't like the chronic cough they've developed, but they still enjoy that first cigarette with their morning coffee or rendezvousing outside with fellow smokers on a break at work. It's as if there is a committee in their head debating whether to quit. Some members favor making a change; others oppose it and may be fearful, unwilling, or defiant.

Now consider what happens when someone who is ambivalent talks to a helper with the righting reflex. The helper argues that it's important for the person to change, explains what could happen if they don't, and urges them to do it. When an ambivalent person hears an argument for one side of their dilemma, the normal response is to defend the opposite side. In other words, you wind up acting out the person's own internal ambivalence, where you're speaking the pro-change lines and eliciting their arguments against change. That might be therapeutic, except that we tend to believe what we hear ourselves say more than what others tell us. Thus, the effect of arguing *for* change is often to cause people literally to talk themselves *out* of the change. It has the opposite effect from what you intended, and nothing changes except perhaps your own level of frustration.

Motivational interviewing is a skillful way of inviting people to voice their own motivations for change. It involves asking questions to which the natural answers are reasons for change. You're not installing motivation, but rather evoking what is already there. Some example questions are:

- What would you say are some good reasons to stop smoking?
- How important do you think it is to take your medication, and why?
- If you did decide to get help, what qualities would you look for in a therapist, given what you know about yourself?

Ask with curiosity, then listen attentively to the person's answers. If you encounter resistance, don't push back or argue against it. Ideally, it's the person rather than you who is voicing the arguments for change. This is not easy to do at first, especially when you feel a sense of urgency about your loved one's health. But it works.

One practical response to a loved one's ambivalence is a double-sided reflection that acknowledges both parts of the person's ambivalence. Start with the reluctance, insert an *and*, then state a pro-change reason that the person has expressed. The order matters: reluctance first. For example:

- You don't like some of the side effects of your medicine, and at the same time you know it helps you a lot.
- Part of you wants to manage on your own without help, and another part hopes that a therapist would have some good ideas.

If you find yourself arguing for change while your loved one argues against it, don't continue. That will only cause your loved one to dig in. Wait for another opportunity to start over, asking questions that will invite your loved one to answer with their own reasons for change.

WILLIAM R. MILLER, PHD, is emeritus distinguished professor of psychology and psychiatry at the University of New Mexico.

• • •

Q: I'm worried about someone. How should I approach a person in my life who might be experiencing suicidal thoughts?

A: We care about the people in our lives. Whether they are our children, parents, a spouse, siblings, friends, or coworkers, we can care for them by being attentive to each other's mental health. We all have mental health, just like we all have physical health. Some of us have greater vulnerabilities to particular health issues, including mental health conditions; some of us also become at risk for suicide. When someone you love is struggling, and especially if they become at risk for suicide, there are things you can do to open up space for increased connection and support.

The key is to trust your gut when you sense someone you love is struggling and take the step to begin a dialogue. Are they not behaving like themselves? Are they giving any hints about possibly feeling hopeless, trapped, overwhelmed, or as if they are a burden to others? If that's the case, the most important thing you can do is let them know you care; that you want to understand more about what they're experiencing. And if there are any hints of deteriorating mental health, ask them directly (in private) in a matter-of-fact way, free of shame or judgment: "Are you thinking of ending your life?" You could start by expressing care and concern: "I care about you, and I've noticed you haven't been yourself lately. You seem more . . . [fill in the blank and feel free to use the words they've used to describe how they've been feeling: frustrated, worried, sad] than you've been in a while, and I'm wondering how you're doing." Let them know it's normal to struggle with life's challenges, and that you're there for them, whatever it is they're experiencing.

If the person hesitates or says they don't want to bother you with their problems, reaffirm in your own words that you want to be there for them. Once they open up about what they're going through, avoid the temptation to problem-solve: Your role is to actively listen. Repeat what they're saying so you are sure you are understanding their perceptions correctly and so they know they're being heard. Reassure them that it's okay to talk about their experiences and their feelings. Ask for more detail, and remind them that just because they're struggling now, doesn't mean they'll always feel this way.

If you get the sense the person may be more comfortable talking with someone else, you might ask, "Is talking to me about this helping you right now? Or is there someone else you'd feel more comfortable with, who we can bring in to help support you?"

If the person divulges that they're thinking about killing themselves, stay calm, listen to them, and ask follow-up questions, such as "How often are you having these thoughts?" and "What do you need to do to feel safe?" You can thank them for trusting you to share about these experiences. Remember that most people who are having suicidal thoughts aren't about to act on them. And not only has research shown that allowing them to share their experience with suicidal thoughts doesn't increase risk, but you might open up the possibility for the person to take a step toward professional help or to develop or use their safety plan—a tool that helps people develop strategies that work best to keep them safe during moments of crisis—just by actively listening and caring.

Let them know that connecting (or reconnecting) with a mental health professional can truly make a big difference in their situation. You might say, "I really think talking to a professional can help you gain some perspective and help you with some new strategies." Then, offer to help them connect with a mental health professional. You might sit with them while they call their insurance or go online to find a mental health professional or substance use program. Or you can offer to do these things for them. If they're not ready to take these steps, leave them with contact information for resources, such as the National Suicide Prevention Lifeline (dial 988), the Crisis Text Line (text TALK to 741741), or, for LGBTQ youth, the Trevor Project can be found at thetrevorproject.org or 866-488-7386. If they seem to be in immediate danger, meaning if they are in the act of or moving immediately toward self-harm, call 988 for guidance.

If the person is in treatment, you could consider alerting their provider—ideally with the person's consent or participation. Even though health professionals don't always have permission to communicate about a person's treatment or clinical status, they can always receive information, and sophisticated clinicians will find ways to communicate appropriately in order to engage designated family members or friends optimally and appropriately.

However the conversation goes, following up later is a simple way to let the person know you genuinely care about them, and that nothing is going to change that.

By noticing how the people in our lives are doing, opening up these kinds of dialogues, and staying connected, we can make our communities safer and work to ensure that we care for our mental health in the same way we would our physical health, in an ongoing and proactive basis.

CHRISTINE YU MOUTIER, MD, is chief medical officer of the American Foundation for Suicide Prevention.

• • •

Q: How do you talk to someone who says, "I'm not sick!"?

A: People with schizophrenia and related disorders, like bipolar disorder, can frequently appear to be in denial. As it turns out, denial is rarely the problem. Instead, they have another symptom of their mental health condition called anosognosia. Having this symptom is the top predictor of who will refuse medication; and of who will stop taking medication if they are on it. As such, this symptom of unawareness is a huge problem for professionals and families alike.

So how do we help someone who has anosognosia? How do we help someone who is absolutely certain that nothing is wrong with them and thinks that everybody who is trying to help them is dead wrong? Like the science on anosognosia, the research on how to help is enlightening.

My colleagues and I conducted research on a program I developed called LEAP (Listen, Empathize, Agree, Partner). Using LEAP, you'll first learn to stop doing much of what you've been doing. That's what I had to learn to do when talking to my brother, who had schizophrenia and anosognosia, and who refused all help, including medications. I realized that I had been doing the same thing over and over again—telling him he was ill and needed help—and expecting a different result. According to Einstein's definition of insanity, I was insane!

I don't say this to belittle myself. After all, I was doing what any loving brother would try to do for a loved one with a mental illness. I was trying to prove to him that he was ill and needed to see a psychiatrist. But with every attempt I made, he pushed back, moving further and further away from accepting any kind of help. I finally learned that telling him he was sick and needed drugs was *guaranteed* to be counterproductive. So I stopped. That is the cornerstone of the LEAP approach. Instead, I focused my efforts on listening to him, being empathic, and building a relationship in which he felt truly respected and not judged. I even apologized for all the times I told him he was ill and needed treatment. I promised him I would never do that again, and I kept that promise. The result of my focus on the relationship—instead of on pushing him to develop insight—was that he ultimately accepted a long-acting injectable antipsychotic medication, which he took for the rest of his life, for eighteen years. He did not die from his illness; he died when he was hit by a car while walking on a pedestrian sidewalk.

The tragedy of my brother's untimely death is offset, in my mind and heart, by the eighteen years during which our relationship was healed and he was in treatment. During that time, he worked volunteer jobs and had friends and a girlfriend. He was in recovery.

So how does LEAP work? It works by using seven communication tools designed to create the nonjudgmental and respectful relationship my brother and I enjoyed. Using LEAP, you will:

Listen	Reflect without judgment, reactions, or contradictions
Empathize	Express empathy for feelings coming from delusions, anosognosia, and desires
Agree	Find areas of agreement—abandon your goal of getting the person to agree that they are sick
Partner	Move forward to achieve common goals that you *can* partner on
Delay	Delay giving hurtful and contrary opinions— redirect and ask permission
Opinion	With humility, give your opinion while respecting the person's perspective
Apologize	Apologize for acts and interactions that feel disrespectful, frustrating, or disappointing

What I learned, and the research confirms, is that we don't win on the strength of our argument; on our rational explanations of why the person we care about needs help. We win on the strength of our relationship.

There is hope for people with anosognosia—it just lies with us and how we talk to them.

XAVIER AMADOR, PHD, is CEO and board chair emeritus of the Henry Amador Center on Anosognosia and author of *I Am Not Sick, I Don't Need Help!*

EIGHTEEN

State-of-the-Art Care and Research for Specific Conditions

This chapter is designed to have leading researchers and clinicians answer important questions related to specific mental health conditions, such as bipolar disorder, addiction, psychosis, and others.

Depression Spectrum

Q: What is cognitive behavior therapy (CBT)? And what happens during a CBT session?

A: Cognitive behavior therapy (CBT) is an evidence-based form of talk therapy that has been extensively researched and found to be very effective in treating a wide range of mental health conditions (e.g., depression, anxiety, post-traumatic stress disorder [PTSD], substance use, schizophrenia); medical problems with psychological components (e.g., chronic pain, hypertension, chronic fatigue syndrome, IBS); and quality-of-life issues (e.g., anger, insomnia, procrastination, public speaking anxiety, and relationship difficulties). Research shows that for many conditions, CBT is as effective as—or even more effective than—medication and is generally better than medication in preventing relapse. CBT and medication are also often used together.

CBT is based on the theory that the way individuals *view* a situation is more closely connected to their behavioral and emotional (and sometimes physiological) reactions than the situation itself. For example, let's say the situation is that you sent your friends a text but didn't hear back. If you're depressed, you might think, "They don't like me anymore." You would then feel sad, and you might avoid reaching out to them again. But if you think, "What if something bad has happened to them?" you'll probably feel anxious, your heart might start beating faster, and you might try calling them right away. So, it's not the situation itself that *directly* affects how you feel and what you do. It's what you're *thinking* about the situation that leads to your reaction. People's reactions always make sense once we know what they're thinking.

When individuals are distressed, some of their thinking is inaccurate and/or unhelpful. One important part of CBT is helping people learn to *identify* their distressing thoughts and *evaluate* how realistic or helpful their thoughts are. When individuals think more realistically, they feel better and can act more effectively. Another important part is helping individuals solve their current problems and learn needed skills, such as effective communication or scheduling their time. When clients' difficulties are very longstanding, and when a focus on the present is insufficient, therapists might also suggest the possibility of exploring the meaning of childhood experiences. CBT therapists are not limited to using cognitive and behavioral techniques, though; we might use techniques from any evidence-based treatment.

Early in treatment, we help clients identify their aspirations and values and then set specific goals they want to achieve. At each session, we do a mood check so we can make sure that clients are making progress. We ask for an update from the previous session and check to see if anything important is happening in the coming week. Then we might review the action plan, the self-help assignments we collaboratively created in the previous session.

Next, we work with clients to set an agenda for the session. We ask what problems clients want help in solving—or what goals they want to reach. We help clients set priorities among these problems, and then start working on the goal or problem clients feel is most important to them. We collect more information, look out for inaccurate or unhelpful thoughts or beliefs, and work together to form a strategy, which might involve problem-solving, evaluating clients' thoughts, and/or teaching them skills. Then we ask clients what they want to remember and do about the problem or goal in the coming week, and we make sure this action plan is recorded.

The relationship between the therapist and client is highly collaborative. Therapists endeavor to use essential counselling skills such as conveying warmth, empathy, and a sense of shared humanity. We help clients feel safe with us. We're transparent, educating clients about their diagnosis, sharing our treatment plan, and providing rationales for the techniques we want to use. We seek feedback during and at the end of sessions. When clients give us negative feedback, we positively reinforce them for doing so and then collaboratively figure out a strategy to address the problem.

We tell clients that the way they're going to get better is by making small changes in their thinking and behavior every day. We teach them skills that they practice in and out of session throughout treatment. In essence, we teach clients how to be their own therapist. Many will need just six to twelve sessions; others will benefit from a longer course of treatment and/or periodic "booster" sessions when new challenges arise.

When we treat individuals who have been diagnosed with a serious mental health condition (on either an inpatient or outpatient basis), we have found that a variation of CBT, Recovery Oriented Cognitive Therapy (CT-R), is more effective. In this approach, we focus on eliciting and strengthening individuals' positive thoughts and beliefs. An important feature of this approach is to jointly engage with individuals in doing activities in line with their values, aspirations, and interests, in which they gain a sense of pleasure, connection, and/or competence. Then we help them identify the positive meanings they received from participating in the activity. While engaged in normal, everyday activities, their positive and negative symptoms reduce. Over time, we find that they are able to operate more and more in an adaptive mode.

DR. JUDITH S. BECK is president of Beck Institute and clinical professor of psychology in psychiatry at the University of Pennsylvania.

• • •

Q: What is neurostimulation and where is the research going? Could it help me or my family member?

A: Neurostimulation refers to a family of interventions that use devices to stimulate the brain. The ones that are clinically available for the treatment of mental illness include electroconvulsive therapy (ECT), transcranial magnetic stimulation (TMS), vagus nerve stimulation (VNS), and deep brain stimulation (DBS). There are other devices that are still at the experimental stage, including transcranial direct current stimulation (tDCS), magnetic seizure therapy (MST), focused ultrasound (FUS), and transcranial laser. What these devices have in common is that they use various forms of energy (electricity, magnetic fields, light, or sound) to change activity in the brain. These techniques offer the hope of providing effective treatment when medications fail, because they can target the circuits in the brain thought to cause depression and other disorders. Each device has its own unique risks and benefits, so let's explore them one at a time, with a focus on the ones that are currently available for treatment today.

ECT involves the use of electricity applied to the scalp to induce a seizure. The procedure is done under anesthesia, so you are asleep for the entire process. The seizure typically lasts about a minute, and the procedure is repeated three times a week for four to six weeks. Among the

FDA-approved devices, ECT is the most effective and rapidly acting in the treatment of severe depression, in both unipolar major depressive disorder and bipolar disorder. There is also evidence that ECT can be a helpful intervention for people with schizophrenia, particularly those who also have depression. ECT can work even when other treatments fail, and it is highly effective in preventing suicide. It is something to consider in cases of severe depression, including psychotic depression, catatonia, and with individuals having thoughts of suicide. A known side effect of ECT is memory loss. Steps can be taken to reduce the risk of memory loss, such as using Right Unilateral electrode placement (this refers to where the electrodes are placed on the head) and ultrabrief pulse ECT (which refers to how long, in milliseconds, each electrical pulse lasts). It is important to talk to your doctor about which type of ECT is recommended, what measures will be taken to reduce memory loss, and what treatment you will need after ECT to prevent relapse.

TMS involves the use of magnetic fields to induce small electrical currents in targeted circuits in the brain. The procedure does not require anesthesia, so you are awake for the entire process. You will feel a tapping sensation on your scalp, and hear a clicking noise during the stimulation, so you'll need to wear earplugs to protect your hearing. TMS is typically done five times a week for four to six weeks. TMS is FDA approved for the treatment of adults with depression who have failed to respond to prior treatment, for treatment of obsessive compulsive disorder (when coupled with exposure therapy), and for smoking cessation. TMS can work when medications fail, but it is important to know that TMS is generally less effective and works more slowly than ECT. TMS is something to consider when medications are not working, and when there is not a pressing need for the rapid response desirable in treating severe depression and acute suicide risk; in those cases, ECT may be the better choice. The side effects of TMS include headache, scalp discomfort, and, in rare cases, seizure. Your doctor should screen you for seizure risk factors. It is important to ask your doctor what strategies will be used after the course of TMS is completed to prevent relapse.

VNS involves the surgical implantation of a pacemaker-like device in the chest. The device is attached to thin wires, implanted under the skin, that deliver tiny electrical pulses to a nerve in the neck called the vagus nerve. These electrical pulses trigger changes in brain activity. VNS is FDA approved for treatment of resistant depression when at least four previous treatments have failed. It takes much longer for VNS to work than for ECT—typically months instead of weeks—so ECT remains the treatment of choice for severe depression when rapid response is needed. However, VNS could be considered if ECT fails to be effective or if there is difficulty sustaining remission after ECT. The side effects of VNS include hoarse voice, neck or tooth discomfort, and dry cough. The surgery itself entails risks of bleeding and infection. It is important to ask your doctor about how rapidly to expect the VNS to work, about the risk of interaction between VNS and diathermy (which refers to the application of energy to the body to produce deep heating of muscles and joints), and about precautions that need to be taken after VNS surgery when undergoing Magnetic Resonance Imaging (MRI).

Like VNS, DBS involves the surgical implantation of a pacemaker-like device in the chest. In the case of DBS, however, the device is attached to thin wires, implanted under the skin, that deliver tiny electrical pulses directly to the brain. The wires pass through a small hole that is made in the skull. DBS has a Humanitarian Device Exemption (a medical device that is approved for marketing and use without requiring evidence of effectiveness) for the treatment of treatment-resistant obsessive-compulsive disorder (OCD). DBS carries all the risks of brain surgery, which include bleeding, infection, stroke, seizure, and other serious complications. Research studies are underway to evaluate the effects of DBS in treating other conditions such as depression, post-traumatic stress disorder, and schizophrenia.

In short, neurostimulation devices offer hope for effective treatment when other approaches fail. This field is rapidly evolving, and it is exciting to see the number of newly FDA-approved treatments for mental illness expand as the research matures.

SARAH HOLLINGSWORTH ("HOLLY") LISANBY, MD, directs the Noninvasive Neuromodulation Unit, a pioneering translational research program in the National Institute of Mental Health's Division of Intramural Research Programs (IRP) specializing in the use of brain stimulation tools to measure and modulate neuroplasticity to improve mental health.

. . .

Q: I've tried almost every medication and therapy, as well as a combination of treatments for my depression, but nothing seems to work. What are my options?

A: Endless trial-and-error of depression treatments is a deeply frustrating and discouraging experience that many people face. Some end up with treatment-resistant depression (TRD), which generally refers to the failure to respond to adequate treatment trials and could include antidepressants or evidence-based psychotherapies. Diagnosis of depression is difficult: Doctors are using subjective measures on a heterogeneous population to target an illness of which there are many variations. While patients with TRD may feel as though a successful treatment will never be found, I instead argue that many of them are misdiagnosed or inadequately treated.

Key elements of a sufficient treatment trial include both adequate dosage and duration of treatment (note that *dosage* here may refer to either medication dose or frequency of therapy visits). Generally, a patient (and/or their family) collaborates with a doctor regarding treatment alternatives, including psychotherapy, psychopharmacology, exercise, and brain stimulation, then chooses and begins a course of treatment. The length of time to begin seeing improvements is different for every individual, but generally those being treated with antidepressants may notice improvements within two to four weeks, and those in therapy may notice improvements in one to two months.

There is currently no readily available brain or blood test to help identify which treatment is best for a patient, although there are some tests
that may suggest which antidepressants *not* to use based on genetic testing. Much of my research involves identifying biosignatures and biomarkers that could potentially distinguish which treatments might be
most promising for a particular person. A biosignature is a unique description of you and your illness. For example, with a sore throat, your
doctor will check for fever, body aches, white blood cell count, and other
symptoms. That information, combined with test results, helps to identify the specific germ that is making you ill.

Knowing the specific cause of illness guides your doctor to the most
efficient treatment. With depression, just as with any other illness, it is
necessary to identify which tests provide the best answers for a particular
patient. There are many socio-demographic, lifestyle, clinical, psychological, and biological variables in play. Biomarkers are biological indicators
that can point us toward a definitive diagnosis or treatment plan. With a
biosignature, you would be able to undergo the treatment plan that has
the best chance of succeeding first, instead of trying several different
options until one works.

The most promising biosignatures for personalized depression research
are brain tests, blood tests, and the gut microbiome. In my lab, an elec-
troencephalogram (EEG) measures the electrical activity of the brain via
electrodes placed on the scalp. This is a quick, affordable, and portable
way to identify subtypes of depression. My team has used EEG to distinguish between two different subtypes of depression and post-traumatic
stress disorder (PTSD) and to develop an algorithm that identifies the
best treatment plan. Another brain test we know of that can signify depression is a functional magnetic resonance image (fMRI) that provides
a map of the brain and its activity. Blood tests identify inflammatory
markers in the blood. Inflammation is the body's normal response to
infection or injury, and we have proteins in our blood that increase or
decrease this inflammation. Since increased pro-inflammatory markers
have been found in patients with high rates of suicidal ideation,

blood-based biomarkers may help us identify those at risk. Lastly, the gut microbiome consists of natural bacteria in the digestive tract and is an additional promising biomarker of depression. This research is still in its early stages, and thus not yet typical in standard clinical practice, but as more evidence becomes available, particularly tests that can be done at point of care, more providers will be able to provide these opportunities to their patients.

Recent research has also highlighted ketamine and transcranial magnetic stimulation (TMS) as promising new antidepressants. Ketamine, a medicine commonly used in anesthesia, has been shown to reduce suicidal thoughts in adults *within hours*. TMS, in which a machine is used to deliver magnetic stimulation to a specific area of the brain, is already an FDA-approved treatment.

Precision medicine for depression is on the horizon. With more research and perseverance, we can get it to all people who need it.

MADHUKAR H. TRIVEDI, MD, is professor of psychiatry, chief of the Division of Mood Disorders, and founding director of the Center for Depression Research and Clinical Care at University of Texas Southwestern Medical Center. He is president of the American Society of Clinical Psychopharmacology.

Obsessive Compulsive Disorder

Q: What is the psychotherapy of choice for obsessive compulsive disorder (OCD), and where should I look for treatment resources?

A: Finding the right treatment for OCD can be challenging. Most people living with OCD in the United States have never received treatment. Those who have been treated likely waited almost two decades after their symptoms began before they received care. Many factors can get in the way of getting treatment for OCD, including misdiagnosis, limited provider availability, shame about symptoms or receiving mental health care, costs of care, and not knowing where to get treatment. Individuals with OCD from communities of color likely face even greater hurdles to getting care. However, because OCD usually does not improve on its own, it is essential to get treatment early.

The psychotherapy of choice for OCD is cognitive behavioral therapy (CBT)—particularly a specific type of CBT called ERP—meaning exposure with response (or, sometimes, ritual) prevention. ERP usually involves three to six months of weekly fifty- to sixty-minute sessions. The therapist guides the patient to gradually face anxiety-provoking situations that trigger obsessions (exposure) and to stay in those situations without using compulsions or other safety behaviors they might typically rely on to lower anxiety (response or ritual prevention). ERP is based on the premise that, although compulsive behaviors may reduce distress in the moment, they increase distress and the need to perform those compulsions in the long run, fueling a vicious cycle. In ERP, facing anxiety without using compulsions allows you to instead let anxiety reduce naturally on its own; test unhelpful beliefs that compulsions have been fueling (for example, "I have to do X to stay safe/keep something terrible from happening"); and learn that you're able to tolerate obsessions without doing time-consuming compulsions.

In addition to ERP, cognitive therapy, or a combination of cognitive therapy and ERP, are also effective treatments for OCD that fall under the broader CBT approach. Cognitive therapy involves identifying unhelpful beliefs common to OCD, such as "I can't tolerate being anxious" or "If I am not extremely careful, it will be my fault if something terrible happens," and learning to evaluate those beliefs in a more accurate, balanced way.

To find a provider who treats OCD using CBT treatments, like ERP and cognitive therapy, you can use online search tools from reputable professional organizations. The International OCD Foundation (IOCDF .org), Association for Behavioral and Cognitive Therapies (ABCT.org), and Anxiety and Depression Association of America (ADAA.org) allow you to search for specialist CBT (and specifically ERP) for OCD providers. That said, it can be difficult or expensive to find face-to-face CBT for

OCD. A newer alternative is online or smartphone-delivered CBT. When looking for these treatments, be aware that some publicly available apps are of poor quality or have low standards for privacy and security. Frameworks like the American Psychiatric Association's app advisor and the M-Health Index and Navigation Database (mindapps.org) give guidance for choosing apps based on quality and security, and can be helpful in navigating and reviewing available mental health apps.

HILARY WEINGARDEN, PHD, is an assistant professor at Harvard Medical School and a psychologist at the Center for OCD and Related Disorders (CORD) at Massachusetts General Hospital.

SABINE WILHELM, PHD, is a professor at Harvard Medical School and director of the Center for OCD and Related Disorders at Massachusetts General Hospital.

Borderline Personality Disorder

Q: Why is dialectical behavior therapy (DBT) recommended for people who struggle with emotion regulation?

A: The simple answer: It works. There is more research evidence supporting the use of DBT for emotion regulation than any other treatment approach. Emotion dysregulation refers to an individual's poor ability to manage emotional responses or to keep them within an acceptable range of typical emotional reactions. It is an uncomfortable state characterized by intense nervous system upset, distorted thinking, and heightened sensitivity. More simply, emotion dysregulation is like living with all your emotional nerve endings painfully exposed. Although it is typically a childhood problem that resolves itself as the child learns emotion regulation skills and strategies, it may continue into adulthood.

DBT was crafted for those who live with this intense emotion regulation problem—the kind that makes you feel life is intolerable, the kind that makes you say, "I can't stand it!" and leads to hopelessness and impulsive, often self-destructive behavior. Ultimately this painful experience can lead to suicide. Although emotion dysregulation is present in almost all problems of human suffering and is a shared characteristic of substance abuse and many behavioral health categories (so this includes ADHD and other processing disorders), individuals who are diagnosed with borderline personality disorder have the highest rate of suicide across all psychiatric diagnoses.

Marsha Linehan is a social psychologist who spent years as a young adult struggling with her own mental health issues. She was hospitalized more than once and had recurrent suicidal thoughts. One of Marsha's oft-cited quotes is that during this difficult period, she "vowed to get out of hell and then go back and get the others there out." And that is what she did. She developed DBT after she noticed that standard behavior therapy was not effective for chronically suicidal clients, describing them as "emotional burn victims."

For decades, I watched Marsha craft, develop, test, refine, and retest the treatment strategies of DBT with the help of her students and research staff. When it became clear that the technology of behavior change alone was not enough to help individuals cope with traumatic invalidation, she incorporated mindfulness and acceptance, primary building blocks of distress tolerance, into the treatment model, making DBT the first of the western psychotherapies to incorporate mindfulness. DBT has never stopped evolving. Marsha frequently stated that when a treatment more effective than DBT was developed, she would happily shift her scientific focus.

Comprehensive DBT, needed by those who experience acutely severe emotional distress, has five parts: 1) individual therapy with a DBT trained clinician, 2) DBT skills that teach new ways to react and respond to distressing events, and 3) between-session coaching. Additionally, DBT is uniquely offered by 4) a team of therapists treating a community of clients and includes 5) additional therapeutic modalities where needed, e.g., medication, family work, etc. Its use is supported by over thirty-five randomized controlled trials (the research "gold standard"). Treatment generally lasts from four to six months to one year.

A fast-growing body of research supports the use of DBT Skills as a standalone treatment for people with a variety of less severe problems, and this growing research is worth following. DBT-LBC.org (Dialectical Behavior Therapy-Linehan Board of Certification), originally founded by Linehan, maintains a directory of certified individual DBT therapists and certified DBT programs. Certification by DBT-LBC is currently the only way to assure that a therapist has demonstrated they can conduct DBT with fidelity to the model. If you or someone you care about is experiencing intense and out of control emotions, or lives with recurrent thoughts of self-harm or suicide, consider DBT.

ANDRÉ IVANOFF, PHD, is professor and director of the DBT Intensive Training Program, Columbia University School of Social Work, the president of Behavioral Tech, and chair of the board of directors of the Linehan Institute.

Trauma

Q: I have been through a life-threatening psychological trauma and have been having flashbacks, nightmares, and feel cut off from my feelings. What are the best kinds of psychotherapy treatments for dealing with trauma? What kind of research is happening for trauma?

A: Experiences like flashbacks, nightmares, and emotional numbing can be symptoms of post-traumatic stress disorder (PTSD), a condition that involves reexperiencing a traumatic event, avoiding things that are reminiscent of the trauma, having increased negative thoughts and feelings, and feeling on edge after the event. PTSD occurs when a person's natural recovery response after a trauma becomes stuck. About 9 million adult Americans have PTSD during a given year, but many more struggle with symptoms that are distressing but not severe enough to be diagnostic of full PTSD.

Thankfully, PTSD is treatable. The most effective treatments are talk therapies, which help the person to be less haunted by their trauma, to come to terms with what happened, and to develop new, more helpful ways of thinking and behaving. In one form of talk therapy called prolonged exposure therapy, the person gradually revisits their trauma memory and situations they have been avoiding in order to lessen the hold the trauma has on them. Cognitive behavioral therapies, such as cognitive processing therapy help change unhelpful beliefs related to the traumatic event and encourage healthy behaviors to aid recovery. Eye movement desensitization and reprocessing (EMDR) attempts to change the way the trauma memory is stored in the brain by having the person focus on the memory while also tracking a back-and-forth stimulation, e.g., following the therapist's fingers or a light moving left to right with their eyes or listening through headphones to a tone played alternately in the left and right ears. One theory of how this therapy works is that recalling a traumatic memory while engaging in another task at the same time lowers the vividness of the memory and its emotional charge, thereby allowing the person to work through the trauma.

Unfortunately, these therapies for PTSD do not work for everyone. Dropout is a common problem, and about half of people with severe PTSD do not access treatment at all. Although less studied than traditional talk therapies, there is some evidence for somatic therapies, which are based on the notion that trauma is stored in the body and not just the brain, and that the body can be used as a tool for healing. For example, one of these therapies, somatic experiencing, involves increasing awareness of bodily responses and learning to shift uncomfortable sensations stemming from trauma to sensations of well-being, so that negative emotions from the trauma are released from the body.

Recent research has also examined whether therapy can be more effective if combined with psychedelic drugs, which are substances that powerfully change how people perceive, think, and feel. The most studied of these treatments for PTSD is MDMA-assisted therapy. MDMA, the pure form of the drug recreationally known as Ecstasy or Molly, is a stimulant that appears to dampen fear, increase empathy, and allow people to be more in touch with their emotions. In combination with therapy, MDMA is believed to help unlock the mind's natural healing process, making it less frightening for the person to revisit their trauma, feel the emotions they need to feel in order to heal, and develop new, more helpful insights about what happened. MDMA is given during therapy with specially trained therapists; it is not prescribed afterward. On average, people who complete this treatment have meaningful reductions in PTSD that are larger than those receiving the same therapy with a placebo; the treatment appears to be safe, dropout is low, and improvement lasts at least one year after treatment. But more research is needed to confirm its effectiveness and to determine how it compares to standard therapies.

The US Food and Drug Association is currently reviewing a New Drug Application for MDMA-assisted therapy for PTSD. It would be the first psychedelic-assisted therapy approved by the agency and would require the US Drug Enforcement Administration to reschedule the pharmaceutical form of MDMA under the Controlled Substances Act, where MDMA is currently Schedule I, a designation for drugs with no accepted medical use and a high potential for abuse. Research on Schedule I drugs is difficult and costly, so reclassifying pharmaceutical MDMA to a less restrictive schedule would open the door to much-needed additional research on this promising treatment.

DIMITRI PERIVOLIOTIS, PHD, is clinical psychologist at the VA San Diego Healthcare System and clinical professor at the University of California San Diego School of Medicine department of psychiatry.

Addiction

Q: My psychiatrist says that I must stop drinking before he can treat my depression. Is that true?

A: That's a great question, and one I get frequently. When I first started out in this field over thirty years ago, there was a tendency not to acknowledge co-occurring substance use disorders (SUD) among people with psychiatric illnesses. Rather, depression in somebody with alcohol use disorder (AUD) was all attributed to the alcohol: "If they just stop drinking, the depression will go away." While it is true that chronic alcohol use can mimic major depression, it is also true that major depression and AUD co-occur more frequently than either condition appears by itself in the general population. When referencing the big epidemiological studies that demonstrated this fact, I was once told that I was "just giving alcoholics an excuse to drink."

Luckily, the field has evolved, and we understand that it's not either/or (either AUD or depression), but frequently it's both/and. In those cases, the most effective treatment is integrated treatment for both disorders. So the suggestion that depression treatment should occur after the AUD treatment actually runs counter to the current recommendation, which is based on decades of clinical outcomes documented in the literature. And the treatment regimen for people with co-occurring disorders—alcohol counseling and psychotherapy, plus an antidepressant and a medication for AUD (e.g., naltrexone)—is appropriately more complex than a regimen for somebody with just one of the disorders.

This leads me to consider another question that I hear frequently: "Isn't it true that psychiatric medications are not effective in somebody who's drinking?" The simple truth is that studies suggest that psychiatric medications are both safe and effective in people with co-occurring mental illness and SUD, so there is no reason to delay starting psychiatric medications in people with co-occurring disorders.

Another consideration is taking medications for AUD. When I first started treating people with co-occurring disorders, I heard more than once that prescribing medications for people with AUD was akin to encouraging them to "chew their booze." Unfortunately, enough people internalized that phrase that I found I had to defend the practice of such prescribing. Fortunately, we have learned a lot in the past thirty years. First, SUD is a chronic illness, comparable to other chronic illnesses, e.g., diabetes, high blood pressure, and depression. Like other chronic illnesses, SUDs may be characterized by periods of improvement and exacerbation and variable adherence to the recommended treatment plan—think, for example, about how people with diabetes may struggle to observe diet and exercise recommendations. And as is the case in treating other chronic illnesses, beneficial medications are typically one component of a multi-faceted treatment regimen. Furthermore, the medications for AUD—disulfiram, naltrexone, and acamprosate—are not chemically related to alcohol and, therefore, do not have the same effects on the brain.

How about medications for opioid use disorder (OUD)? I still hear from people: "Isn't taking medication for OUD just like exchanging one addiction for another?" I would say that, if somebody tells you that recovery that includes medication is just addiction to a different drug and not a true recovery, you should feel confident to say the following: First, medications are not "drugs," with all the negative connotations that come with that term. They are medications, like penicillin and aspirin. Second, anybody who has been addictively dependent on a drug (e.g., fentanyl) knows that the addiction takes over your life and affects every aspect of living in a very negative way. The drug becomes the main—indeed, only—relationship in your life. Treating a SUD with a medication, however, facilitates a healthy recovery process, helping restore order in one's life rather than promoting disorder. A picture of somebody hooked on oxycodone juxtaposed to a picture of that same person prescribed buprenorphine would resemble the "before and after pictures" one sees in advertisements for life-changing products. Indeed, the medications may be lifesaving; a recently published study demonstrated that a year after a non-fatal opioid overdose, people treated with either buprenorphine or methadone were significantly less likely to die from any cause compared to those people who were treated with no medication. Incidentally, this mortality rate disproportionately affects people of color.

This leads me to one final question that I hear: "Doc, am I going to have to take this medication for the rest of my life?" The answer usually is "Maybe, maybe not. Let's get you free of the drug that may well kill you; then we can think together about slowly tapering the medication, if you want to do so." In my clinical practice, I have treated patients for whom the medication is for the rest of their life, and patients who, with the right combination of recovery supports, are able to slowly taper off the medication. This is similar to people with diabetes. Some of those people make such great strides with diet and exercise that they can stop taking metformin (a medication for type 2 diabetes).

In the end, people with co-occurring disorders are a heterogeneous group of people, and no one treatment approach works for everybody. What does work is an integrated treatment approach—which might include individual and group treatments either with or without medications—that addresses both the psychiatric and addiction conditions.

MARK ALBANESE, MD, is medical director, Physician Health Services, Massachusetts Medical Society, and assistant professor of psychiatry, Harvard Medical School/Cambridge Health Alliance.

Bipolar Disorder

Q: Do I have to take these meds for my bipolar disorder forever?

A: This is one of the most frequent questions posed by people with bipolar disorder. Because forever is a very long time and people can feel that taking medications forever seems like a terrible burden, I try to be as thoughtful as I can and provide them with data.

First, it is helpful to discuss the course of bipolar disorder and how medications can help people feel well and function as best as they can. People with bipolar disorder tend to have multiple episodes of mania, hypomania, depression, and mixed mania/depression along with other challenges, including anxiety and problems sleeping. Without medications, they have over a 90 percent chance of having another mood episode after they recover from an acute episode. With the appropriate medications, they have less than a 30 percent chance of having another episode. Some people have a lower chance and others have a higher chance of another episode with treatment (more on that later). For those interested in decreasing the probability of recurring disruptive and painful mood episodes, it makes sense to continue medications.

Second, all medications have unwanted side effects, including those used for bipolar disorder. Finding the right balance between the positive effects of medications (preventing episodes) and side effects requires good communication with one's prescriber as well as careful monitoring. If the medications are helping, then it makes sense to try to find the best methods to manage the side effects or to find an alternative treatment.

Third, one of the most difficult challenges is when people who have had several mood episodes, respond well to treatment, and are free of mood episodes for years then question whether they need to continue medications. As Justice Ruth Bader Ginsburg wrote in her dissent for the *Shelby County v. Holder* case, "Throwing out preclearance [for changing voting laws] when it has worked and is continuing to work to stop discriminatory changes is like throwing away your umbrella in a rainstorm because you are not getting wet." But I appreciate the dilemma: Is someone doing well because they are taking medications, or do they just no longer need the medications and would do fine without them? If someone decides that they don't want to take the medications anymore, one path is for them to gradually discontinue medication with careful monitoring and supervision, while understanding that they are taking a risk that the episodes will return. While some people may do okay, unfortunately most will not. The key is to have shared decision-making between the people who take medications and their treaters.

Finally, because a minority of people might do okay without medications, it will be important in the future to find out who needs to continue to take medications and who does not. By having people with bipolar disorder collaborate with their clinicians and organizing data about outcomes in a learning health care network, we can all work together for better outcomes.

ANDREW A. NIERENBERG, MD, holds the Thomas P. Hackett, MD, Chair in Psychiatry at Massachusetts General Hospital, and is the director of the Dauten Family Center for Bipolar Treatment Innovation, and a professor of psychiatry at Harvard Medical School.

· · ·

Q: Besides medications, what else can I do to reduce my risk of bipolar episodes?

A: There are multiple ways people living with bipolar disorder can improve their risk of recurrence. I'll focus first on two core strategies that are particularly powerful.

Nurture Good Sleep Habits

Sleep is a weathervane for psychiatric conditions. Depression and many of the mood states of bipolar disorder are often accompanied by abnormal sleep patterns: sleeping too much, too little, or experiencing frequent awakenings through the night. Seemingly trivial worries may also interfere with sleep, and poor sleep leads to more stress and a vicious cycle ensues, which may lead to poor choices and desperate behaviors.

A satisfactory sleep pattern that is consistent over time is key to health, yet many people with bipolar disorder experience ongoing chronic sleep problems. Disrupted sleep patterns are typically part of the symptoms of bipolar disorder. Good sleep often means the disorder is well managed, while bad sleep portends problems. People living with bipolar know that a sleepless night is often an urgent indicator that something is going very wrong. Intermittent sleep disruptions may be related to situational stress, an argument, or conflict resulting in reactive ruminations that spill into the night. But whatever its origins, a night without sleep is often followed by mania. Sleep medications like benzodiazepines and hypnotics may work only temporarily and are not a viable long-term strategy. What can you do to up the odds of a good night's sleep?

The first step is getting a handle on the nature of the problem. There may be underlying conditions, beyond bipolar disorder, that are interfering with sleep. Are you a snorer? Sleep apnea is a condition that is associated with excessive snoring and being overweight. Soft tissue in the neck can restrict air passages, resulting in snoring and periods of slowed or stopped breathing that keep you from deep sleep. An overnight sleep study can diagnose this condition, and a physician may recommend using a bedside device called a CPAP machine to improve air flow when asleep. Are you drinking alcohol in the evenings? How much coffee do you drink during the day? Substances such as alcohol, caffeine, or stimulant medication may contribute to sleep disturbances. An evening glass of wine, for many, will disrupt sleep patterns or diminish the quality of sleep. While alcohol is initially relaxing, it is quickly metabolized and may result in middle-of-the-night awakenings as it leaves the system. Do you sit in bed with a bright-screened tablet as you are getting ready for sleep? Light—particularly the blue light emitted by LED bulbs and phone and computer screens—interferes with your circadian rhythm (the natural, internal process that regulates sleep).

The second step is action. Ask your medical provider whether a sleep study is indicated. If you drink alcohol on a regular basis, ask yourself how important it is in your life and whether you can curtail drinking. Can you avoid using screens for several hours before bed—or at least make use of options on many devices to filter and reduce blue light? While you should exercise caution about regularly taking medications that are solely intended to encourage sleep, ask your doctor about the risks and benefits of having an "as needed" medication on hand to address intermittent sleep problems, and what the minimal dose might be for you.

Lastly, try to resolve conflicts or find a peaceful state of mind before going to bed. That's easier said than done, but it will help to learn and practice a relaxation technique or a form of meditation. Know that sleep problems are common in bipolar. There are other strategies available to address sleep issues, including a form of cognitive behavior therapy, CBT-insomnia, that can help you establish and maintain good sleep hygiene.

Establish and Maintain a Daily Routine

Having a routine is both one of the more effective—and most challenging—strategies for maintaining stability in bipolar disorder. A routine means keeping a regular schedule: getting up at the same time every morning; starting work or activities at a defined hour; eating healthy meals at regular times; and observing a regular bedtime. Disrupted routines are often a signal of trouble ahead and potential mood swings that can easily end in an episode of mania or depression, or a combination of the two. Interpersonal and social rhythm therapy (IPSRT) is an innovative form of psychotherapy that specifically helps you focus on establishing and maintaining a routine to help your body regulate.

In addition to focusing on sleep and routine, there are many other things you can do. For example, working with a psychotherapist can help you identify patterns and stresses and develop new ways of understanding and managing them. Exercise can both help with sleep and be part of a healthy routine. Support groups like NAMI or the Depression and Bipolar Support Alliance (DBSA; dbsalliance.org) can help you find community and reduce isolation.

Together We Can Learn More

We know that healthy lifestyles help everyone thrive. But the substantial differences in how people with bipolar disorder experience life means that we must truly study the disorder over time—ideally, lifetimes. That way, we can learn more about what causes, prevents, and treats episodes effectively, and what strategies a person with bipolar disorder can employ to live a fulfilling life.

If you want to join the largest long-term follow-up study of people living with bipolar disorder to help us unravel some of these challenges, contact the Heinz C. Prechter Bipolar Research Program at the University of Michigan (prechterprogram.org). This program began in 2006 and is committed to engaging those with bipolar over their lifetime to learn about bipolar disorder and the sustaining elements of the illness, and how these elements can be managed so that everyone with bipolar will live a fulfilling and meaningful life.

MELVIN MCINNIS, MD, is the Thomas B. and Nancy Upjohn Woodworth Professor of Bipolar Disorder and Depression and the director of the Heinz C. Prechter Bipolar Research Program at the University of Michigan.

. . .

Q: I want to have a baby, but I have bipolar disorder. Would I have to stop taking my medication?

A: Many women of reproductive age have psychiatric disorders that are chronic or recurrent and require medication maintenance to stay well. Unfortunately, there is a common belief—even among some health care providers—that women cannot take psychiatric medications during pregnancy, and that psychiatric medications are less important than those prescribed for "medical" disorders. The truth is that some psychiatric medications have been very well studied in terms of their effect during the perinatal period (pregnancy and postpartum), and women are often surprised and reassured by the data. It's also true that acute and serious psychiatric illnesses are detrimental to the mother's well-being, and to obstetrical and neonatal outcomes. These are important considerations both for you and your health care practitioners in making risk/benefit decisions about medication use during pregnancy.

How women with bipolar disorder should be treated during pregnancy is a topic of great importance and frequent misunderstandings. The risk of relapse to a mood episode is high if mood stabilizing medication is discontinued, and the postpartum period may be the most exquisitely risky time of life for severe mood episodes. Although treatment decisions are ideally tailored to the individual, the use of mood stabilizers during pregnancy is critical to wellness for most women with bipolar disorder, and the use of mood stabilizers postpartum can treat and prevent severe illness, including postpartum psychosis.

That said, some mood stabilizers are potentially risky to take during pregnancy. Birth defects, or major malformations, occur in about 3 percent of babies born annually in the United States, and some medications may raise that risk. Since about half of pregnancies in the United States are unplanned, it's imperative that women of reproductive age, and girls younger than reproductive age, use medications that would also be reasonably safe for use during a pregnancy. Women with bipolar disorder may begin treatment at a time when having a baby is not in their plans, but later find themselves ready for motherhood, so safety in pregnancy should be a factor in selecting medications from the very beginning.

Which mood stabilizers are safest? Lithium is associated with a small risk of cardiovascular malformations with first trimester exposure. However, the risk is low enough that many women who respond well to lithium are advised to continue it. Valproic acid (Depakote) is the mood stabilizer with the highest risk of major malformations and long-term poor neurocognitive outcomes for children. It is recommended that girls and women of reproductive age do not receive treatment with it at all. Even with use of contraception, the rate of serious birth defects is too high to accept the risk. Lamotrigine (Lamictal) is well studied during pregnancy and does not appear to be associated with any type of birth defect, nor does it have a negative impact on neurocognitive development in children. Atypical antipsychotics as a class do not appear to increase the risk of birth defects in the studies conducted to date, though we have more information for some antipsychotics than we do for others.

The risk of relapse for women with bipolar disorder is heightened in the postpartum period. Women who stopped taking mood stabilizing medication during pregnancy are usually advised to restart it immediately after delivery. Another major consideration is postpartum maternal sleep. Sound sleep is critical to mental health for all of us, but it is particularly important for people with bipolar disorder. A plan to get help with infant care and feedings at night can often make a major difference. Psychotherapy and support groups are also extremely helpful in counteracting the isolation and loneliness women can feel as they deal not only with the demands of new motherhood but with psychiatric disorders and medication decisions.

Bipolar disorder presents challenges across pregnancy and the postpartum period, but with careful planning and support, there can be healthy outcomes for both you and your baby.

MARLENE P. FREEMAN, MD, is a professor of psychiatry at Harvard Medical School and associate director of the Ammon-Pinizzotto Center for Women's Mental Health at Massachusetts General Hospital.

Psychosis Spectrum

Q: My child's thinking has started to seem unusually paranoid; they are isolating from us and others and may even be hallucinating. What is the best way to help?

A: Your child may be experiencing an episode of psychosis. Psychosis refers to a state of mind characterized by an impaired sense of reality, in which the individual has delusions (such as paranoid thoughts of being surveilled or the target of a conspiracy), hallucinations (such as hearing voices), and/or difficulties organizing their thoughts. Psychotic illnesses typically begin in the teenage years or young adulthood. In the United States, about 100,000 individuals annually experience a first episode of psychosis. Causes of psychosis can include schizophrenia, bipolar disorder, severe depression, substance misuse, and, less commonly, another medical disorder.

If you suspect or know that your child is experiencing psychosis, early intervention greatly increases the odds of a better outcome. Early diagnosis and the right treatment within the first two to three years can decrease relapses of psychosis by over 50 percent and reduce the disability associated with a psychotic illness.

Your first step is to identify the right treatment setting. Look for a local program that offers a team-based approach to treatment, also called coordinated specialty care. These programs are now available in most states. If symptoms are severe and there are safety concerns, hospitalization may be necessary, but the goal is to transition to outpatient or partial hospital care as soon as the acute symptoms are stabilized. Whether your child is first treated in the hospital or as an outpatient, the team will first carry out a comprehensive assessment—including laboratory tests as needed—to determine the appropriate diagnosis.

The team will then develop a treatment plan involving a combination of services. The team psychiatrist may prescribe and monitor low doses of antipsychotic medication to ensure the most benefit, at the lowest dose, with the least side effects. Ideally, a clinician trained in cognitive behavioral therapy for psychosis (CBTp)—a form of CBT adapted specifically to target psychotic symptoms—will meet with your son or daughter once a week for therapy sessions focused on learning to handle ongoing symptoms and developing healthy coping skills. Clinicians will also address any other mental health conditions that may accompany psychosis, such as depression or substance use. The team will also engage your child in other individual or group therapy sessions designed to help strengthen cognitive (such as memory and problem-solving) and social skills, with a goal of getting them back on track at school or work. They will also educate you and your family about the illness, provide support, and teach you effective ways to deal with crises.

After starting treatment, your child is likely to quickly feel better, though some symptoms may continue at a milder level. Your young adult may be reluctant to accept the illness or the treatment. Having a mental health condition that can manifest in psychosis is a profound life challenge that can be hard to accept, especially at a time of life when you are developing an independent adult identity. Acceptance is a process, and this is a lot to accept for all involved, including the parents. Open and honest discussions with your child, collaborative decision-making between your child and their clinicians, and this new approach to early intervention focusing on strengths and goals rather than symptoms and deficits, will all be helpful. The frequency of treatment sessions may decrease as your child stabilizes, but ongoing collaboration, monitoring, and treatment with a trusted clinician is important to minimize the risk of relapse.

MATCHERI S. KESHAVAN, MD, is Stanley Cobb Professor and academic head of psychiatry in the department of psychiatry at Beth Israel Deaconess Medical Center and Massachusetts Mental Health Center, Harvard Medical School, and the editor of *Schizophrenia Research*.

· · ·

Q: When is it time to consider clozapine for people with schizophrenia? Is it the drug of last resort?

A: Clozapine is the only medication that is approved by the FDA for treatment resistant schizophrenia (TRS). But what does TRS really mean? TRS refers to the 20 to 30 percent of people with schizophrenia who don't respond fully to other antipsychotic medications. People with

TRS continue to have bothersome hallucinations or delusions despite taking an antipsychotic medication as prescribed. Being diagnosed with TRS doesn't mean that you are getting worse or are opposed to treatment. TRS doesn't mean that the situation is hopeless. It does mean that clozapine may be a more helpful medication for you. For people with TRS, there is about a 40 to 60 percent response rate for clozapine, 10 percent for atypical (second-generation) antipsychotics, and 0 percent for typical (first-generation) antipsychotics. Clozapine tends to work better to decrease delusions and hallucinations than it does to address mood and cognitive symptoms of the illness.

Clozapine should not be thought of as a last resort treatment. *The American Psychiatric Association Practice Guideline for the Treatment of Patients with Schizophrenia* recommends that if a person doesn't respond to two different antipsychotic medications, clozapine should be the next drug considered. But clozapine is underutilized in the United States, and, many times, prescribers don't think their clients are "there yet." There are no blood tests or imaging studies that can be used to proactively determine whether someone would benefit from clozapine. But studies do show that after someone doesn't respond to that second non-clozapine antipsychotic, they are unlikely to respond to the third, the fourth, and so on. Often, the delay in starting clozapine can result in significant and prolonged suffering.

There needs to be a careful shared decision-making discussion about whether clozapine is the right medication for you or a loved one. Clozapine can have side effects, and some of them can be very serious. For example, in about 1 percent of people who take clozapine, the levels of neutrophils, the white blood cells that fight off infection, can become dangerously low. For this reason, a health care team monitors the absolute neutrophil count by a lab test weekly for the first six months someone takes the drug, then every other week for another six months, and once monthly indefinitely after a year. This routine monitoring helps prescribers stop the medication if the neutrophil count gets too low. Additionally, clozapine can cause an inflammation of the heart muscle, seizures, constipation, and weight gain. Clozapine can make people feel tired, drool, or get dizzy when they stand up. Prescribers will monitor for these side effects, and there are evidence-based strategies to help mitigate each of these problems.

To us, one of the worst phrases that we sometimes hear is, "Oh, that's just this person's baseline," when what the speaker means by "baseline" is that the person is experiencing severe, sometimes intolerable symptoms. Their attitude is, "That's just how it is, and nothing can be done." Don't accept this. We encourage you to expect and push for more, and for your care to be optimized. A decision to pursue clozapine is about not accepting the status quo. It is about believing that recovery is possible. For many people, the trade-off between the benefits and side effects is worth it, and clozapine can be game-changing for many and even life-saving for some.

ROBERT O. COTES, MD, is associate professor of psychiatry at Emory University School of Medicine.

DONNA ROLIN, PHD, APRN, PMHCNS-BC, PMHNP-BC, is clinical associate professor and the director of the psychiatric mental health nurse practitioner program at the University of Texas–Austin.

• • •

Q: Are there any treatment options for someone dealing with psychosis other than adding more medications? Can talk therapy help?

A: Cognitive behavioral therapy (CBT) is one of the most well-researched, proven-effective forms of talk therapy. More recently, CBT has been adapted into an evidence-based intervention specifically to support people experiencing symptoms of psychosis—both "positive" symptoms (as in symptoms that are added on to a person's experiences), like delusions and hallucinations, and negative symptoms (as in symptoms that reduce or take something away), like difficulty with focus, motivation, and daily functioning—and other mental health problems that may underlie or occur simultaneously with psychosis. Cognitive behavioral therapy for psychosis (CBTp) is typically offered as an individual therapy—though it may also be offered in group settings—and typically as an adjunct to medication management.

Although CBTp is grounded in general cognitive behavioral therapy, important adaptations have been made to ensure its effectiveness for people with psychosis. If you decide to try CBTp, you should seek a clinician who has been formally trained in it and who is engaged in good quality consultation or supervision. While there are new initiatives to train frontline providers in "CBTp informed skills" in order to broaden access, you are more likely to get the most benefit by working with a well-trained and experienced therapist.

A CBTp clinician initially works to develop a strong and trusting therapeutic relationship with their client. This phase (referred to as "befriending") may take more or less time, depending on how amenable the client is to participating in treatment and how adept the therapist is at establishing rapport. Family members eager to get the "real therapy started" may find this introductory phase frustrating, but studies have shown CBTp to be ineffective unless a strong therapeutic alliance has been established. Once that bond has been established, the clinician and individual jointly develop shared goals to work toward over the course of therapy.

CBTp clinicians are trained to adopt a stance of curiosity about the experiences reported by their clients. Their role is not to convince clients that delusions, hallucinations, voices, premonitions, etc., are not based in reality but rather to offer a safe place to explore both these experiences and clients' interpretations of them. CBTp takes the position that the client's interpretation of their experiences can significantly increase distress and impact functioning, more so than the event itself. For example, someone experiencing voices might interpret them as the voice of the devil, indicating that they are a bad person, resulting in them staying in their room and reading religious texts. The goal of therapy might be to help that person explore different possible interpretations—for example, the voices could be coming from somewhere or something else; they could be hallucinations; they could signify that the client is actually a good person and is being tested—or to examine different ways of responding to the experience that would help the client move toward their chosen goals. For example, if the time the client spends reading religious texts is distressing, an option might be to set limits on that time and focus their time on something else, such as enrolling in an online college course.

Together the client and clinician develop a "formulation"—a shared understanding of the paths that have led the client to where they are today and the steps that can be taken to move toward their goals. Developing this formulation will typically involve exploring early experiences and how they have impacted the clients' view of themselves, the world, or other people. Then, as both client and therapist develop a deeper understanding of the client's inner life, personal history, struggles, desires, and goals, they begin discussing possibilities for change, and how to implement them. In this way, CBTp aims to support individuals to become their own therapists. Together the client and therapist identify "homework" that encourages clients to practice skills they'll need to move in the direction they want to go outside of sessions and report back on their effectiveness. Family members can be important in supporting their loved ones to practice these skills. Finally, CBTp therapy ends with "wellness planning." Together the therapist and client focus on steps to be taken should a return, or exacerbation, of symptoms occur.

KATE HARDY, CLIN.PSYCH.D, is co-director of the INSPIRE Clinic, a person-centered program providing interdisciplinary and evidence-based care for people experiencing psychosis, at Stanford University School of Medicine.

Research to Help Get Better Tools

Q: We need better medications. What new medications are being brought to the market for treatment of mental illnesses?

A: Psychiatric disorders are among the top leading causes of disability worldwide, and there is an urgent need for new treatments. Research focused on understanding the natural history, developmental trajectory, and pathophysiology of psychiatric disorders has led to the identification of new biological approaches for drug development and for early intervention to maximize clinical benefit and reduce disease burden in individuals living with mental illnesses. In the past two years, six new drugs have been approved by the US Food and Drug Administration (FDA) as new medicines for the treatment of depression and schizophrenia:

New Rapid-Acting Medications for Depression

Major Depression and Suicidality. Spravato (esketamine nasal spray) is a next-generation rapid-acting medication for adults with treatment-resistant depression (TRD). Foundational clinical research on the use of ketamine in TRD by the National Institute of Mental Health (NIMH) and other leading investigators led the industry to invest in the development of esketamine. Ketamine analogs comprise the first new class of antidepressants to be developed in several decades. Esketamine's speed of action makes it especially valuable in treating suicidality in adults with moderate to severe major depressive disorder (MDD), and the nasal spray is approved for use in adults in conjunction with an oral antidepressant medication.

Pregnancy and Postpartum Depression. The period after childbirth carries a risk for women to develop a severe and long-lasting depression. The novel, rapid-acting antidepressant Zulresso (brexanolone) is a gamechanger for women with postpartum depression. Brexanalone is a bench-to-bedside success with basic research on derivatives of the hormone progesterone by NIMH investigators and others spurring its development. Brexanolone injection is approved to treat postpartum depression in adult women with an episode of major depression starting in the third trimester of pregnancy or within four weeks after delivery. Women are asked to suspend breastfeeding while receiving treatment until more is learned about the safety of brexanolone in nursing infants.

New Medications and Developments for Schizophrenia

Long-Acting Antipsychotics. Long-acting injectable antipsychotics have been developed for treating individuals with schizophrenia who relapse for failing to consistently take daily oral antipsychotic medications. Invega Hafyera (paliperidone palmitate extended-release injectable) is the newest of the long-acting antipsychotic medications currently available in the United States. The new extended-release technology for twice-a-year injection is anticipated to reduce relapse frequency and hospitalization rates in adults with schizophrenia.

Antipsychotics and Weight Gain. The NIMH CATIE trial (Clinical Antipsychotic Trials of Intervention Effectiveness) showed that olanzapine was more effective for the treatment of schizophrenia than other antipsychotic medications except for clozapine. Yet weight gain and risk for diabetes are substantial side effects of chronic antipsychotic medication use. Lybalvi (olanzapine and samidorphan) is a new combination treatment that offers the efficacy of olanzapine with less weight gain.

Additional Approvals and Emerging Biological Approaches

Caplyta (lumateperone) is a new mechanism antipsychotic drug that adds to the arsenal of medications available to treat adults with schizophrenia. It is also approved for the treatment of depressive episodes in adults with bipolar disorder, either alone or in conjunction with other medications (lithium or valproate). Cobenfy (xanomeline and trospium chloride) is the newest antipsychotic medication to be approved to treat schizophrenia in adults and the first novel mechanism therapy for schizophrenia in decades.

Information about the pharmacologic mechanism of action of these drugs can be found at the Neuroscience based Nomenclature website (https://nbn2r.com).

Looking to the future, several additional new mechanism of action drugs are in clinical development as potential medications for schizophrenia and major depressive disorder, with several under FDA review. In addition, the new Accelerating Medicines Partnership Schizophrenia program is conducting a comprehensive, longitudinal characterization of individuals with clinical signs of high risk for psychosis to enable a better understanding of the early stages of illness and the development and testing of new drug mechanisms for early intervention in schizophrenia (visit ampscz.org for more information).

LINDA BRADY, PHD, is director, division of neuroscience and basic behavior science at the National Institute for Mental Health.

. . .

Q: I know we need better treatments. Is participating in research a way to help us get there?

A: Essential to the development of new treatments are the many thousands of people who volunteer to participate in National Institutes of Health (NIH)–supported studies. None of these studies can move forward without the many individuals who generously give their time, effort, energy, and hope to improve our understanding of mental illnesses and identify and test new treatments. One example is a major National Institute of Mental Health (NIMH)–funded effort to understand the effects of trauma on mental illness, the Advancing Understanding of RecOvery afteR traumA (AURORA) study. AURORA scientists visited dozens of emergency rooms across the country, talking with people who had been through traumas and asking if they would be interested in participating in a study to learn more about the psychological and neurobiological effects of trauma. Thousands of people agreed to participate. As a result, these scientists are revealing with unprecedented detail the events that lead from traumatic experiences to post-traumatic stress disorder (PTSD) and other mental illnesses, as well as the specific characteristics that help resilient individuals recover.

The NIMH, one of the twenty-seven institutes and centers of the National Institutes of Health (NIH), is the primary federal agency in the United States responsible for conducting and supporting mental health research; it is the largest funder of mental health research in the world. For more than seventy years, NIMH has supported both basic and clinical science, striving for prevention, recovery, and cure. NIMH-funded studies help establish our understanding of the basic biochemistry of communication in the brain—findings that enabled the development of the most significant classes of medications we use to treat mental illnesses today. Translational studies conducted in the NIMH Intramural Research Program on the NIH campus and in NIMH-funded research in labs around the country have led directly to the development of the newest psychiatric medications, such as esketamine for treatment-resistant depression and brexanolone for postpartum depression, both approved by the US Food and Drug Administration in 2019. NIMH-supported scientists have also been at the forefront of psychotherapy research, leading to groundbreaking psychotherapies like dialectical behavior therapy (DBT), which has been shown to reduce suicidal and self-injurious behavior for individuals living with a range of mental illnesses.

Even now, scientists around the country and the world are busy asking scientific questions that will help improve care for everyone with mental illnesses in the future. They're studying how to reach and care for adolescents and young adults at risk for developing schizophrenia and what approaches health care professionals can use to reduce suicidal behavior. They're looking at how to increase mental health care availability and acceptability in minority communities and maximize the chances of recovery from PTSD. These and many other studies promise to pave the way for a more effective, equitable, and efficient mental health care system and improve the lives of the millions of individuals living with mental illnesses, their families, and those in their communities.

Consider, too, the Accelerating Medicines Partnership Schizophrenia program (AMP SCZ), a similar-sized effort to develop and test new treatments for young people at risk for developing schizophrenia. AMP SCZ is a partnership between NIMH, NAMI, and several other government, nonprofit, and pharmaceutical industry organizations. But most of all, it is a partnership with thousands of teenagers and young adults around the world who are volunteering to participate, donating their data and their clinical records to make sure we can continue to improve treatments available for people with schizophrenia.

If you or someone you love has a mental illness and is interested in participating in an NIMH-funded study, you can find out more information about how to participate on our website, www.nimh.nih.gov /health/trials. The site has information about studies conducted on the NIH campus in Bethesda, Maryland, and studies supported by NIMH being conducted at sites all around the country and the world.

NIMH research is paving the way for prevention, recovery, and cure, making a difference for individuals, families, and communities bearing the burden of mental illness. Getting involved in research can make a difference for you, your family, and generations to come.

JOSHUA A. GORDON, MD, PHD, is the director of the National Institute of Mental Health.

ACKNOWLEDGMENTS

I want to thank the large and talented village it took to create NAMI's first book.

I knew NAMI deserved a book, as I had met so many resilient and remarkable people in NAMI over the years. NAMI's CEO Dan Gillison was very encouraging the first time I pitched him the idea. Thank you, Dan, for believing. Will Lippincott, our agent from Aevitas, became a friend and a trusted guide through the journey. He escorted this rookie author through the peaks and valleys of the writing and publishing process with endless support and a likable, professional approach that helped build bridges when bridges were necessary. Will introduced me to Lisa Kaufman, who was critical to organizing and editing this work. My weekly calls with Lisa became a source of delight to me with equal parts humor, collaboration, and productivity that I will always cherish. Lisa's thinking and smart edits were substantive and critical to making this book happen. There would be no NAMI book without Lisa.

Jordan Miller worked tirelessly as my NAMI copilot and project manager, sitting (virtually) beside me through 150 hours of interviews and serving as the beloved connective tissue that created and maintained a beautiful community of the voices featured in this book. She remained dedicated to this project from proposal to final draft, and many of her thoughts, ideas, and observations from her first year working at NAMI helped to organize a massive amount of content into digestible themes and chapters.

Along the way, we were joined by Alexa Zielinski, a great writer and analytical thinker who reviewed thousands of pages of transcripts with a sharp and compassionate eye. She quickly became an integral part of the team, elevating many of the chapters in this book to greater levels of depth, demonstrating both empathy and brilliance. Jordan, Alexa, and I drilled down chapters from initial outlines to quote and story excavation, to curation of themes and editing. I looked forward to each of our meetings. Together, you two brought fun and keen eyes and ears to the adventure of writing this book.

At NAMI, many hands helped, for which I am deeply grateful. Thanks to the entire NAMI team involved in making this publication happen. Luna

Greenstein helped with editing for NAMI style, voice, and organization; she also redid a challenging chapter right down to the studs. Teri Brister, Dawn Brown (HelpLine), Hannah Wesolowski, Shannon Scully, Christine Crawford, Fredric Miggins, Barb Solish, and Jessica Edwards reviewed content and gave helpful feedback. Dawn Brown (Cross-Cultural Innovation), Kenya Phillips, and Sean Stickle offered important additions. Danielle Hall, Lindsey Brown, Matt Raymond, Richele Keas, and Glenn O'Neal helped with communicating about our newborn project. Sue Medford, a NAMI treasure and friend to all, shared her wisdom forged as the stalwart executive assistant to NAMI's CEOs for decades. Retired NAMI legends Bob Carolla, Mike Fitzpatrick, and Ken Norton gave me thoughtful input, and Ron Honberg coauthored the law chapter. In the break of a lifetime, many years ago, Rona Purdy flew to Boston to recruit me to NAMI. I am grateful to you every day, Rona. The NAMI founders were well ahead of their time and created a movement. I was humbled to write NAMI's first book, and I never forgot that I was standing on the shoulders of these giants.

Arooshe Giroti, Elizabeth Rockett, Lili Rodgers, and Bulldogs Andres Martin, Laelia Benoit, Kai Shulman, Georgia Spurrier, and Ashley Clayton helped with research.

At Zando, Molly Stern, Quynh Do, Andrew Rein, Nathalie Ramirez, Chloe Texier-Rose, Sarah Schneider, Maya Raiford Cohen, and their team were inspiring, focused, and collaborative to help get this project completed. Thank you for believing in this vision and for being my perfect publishing team.

Many leading experts across the nation answered my request to summarize decades of their work in a short Q&A for the public in this book. You graciously gave your time and shared your wisdom for the greater good. Thank you for giving to the public, to NAMI, and for all the work you do.

Many of my friends, most who do this work every day, looked at drafts along the way and gave helpful feedback, including Mike Kahn, Nat Kuhn, Seth Rafal, Jack Lloyd, Deirdre Calvert, Jemima Theork, Amy McHugh, Robert Accordino, Jay Mamon, Susan Abbott, Steve LaMaster, Mary O'Byrne, Steve Rosenfeld, Jackie Feldman, Joe Shrand, and Tony Sossong. Marsden McGuire helped with VA resources. Matcheri Keshavan, my academic leader, kindly supported this endeavor and also reviewed a key chapter. Marty Derda, my lifelong friend, served as unofficial therapist throughout the writing and editing process. Ann Katz, my actual therapist, helped me understand my family so that I could talk about them with ease.

I was very fortunate that my family stepped up for me. My fabulous daughters—Megan, Katie, and Clare—were all helpful reviewers who lovingly supported my vision and me as I processed the writing experience. You bring me joy every single day. My stepkids, Brooks and Owen, listened patiently and with a smile as I bounced early ideas off them and were generous with their perspective. My nephews, Jason and Rob, and nieces, Lauren and Angie, gave me helpful feedback and encouragement. My cousin Jim kept the happy memories and our shared playful stories of my father alive in my mind's eye. This helped me excavate the harder times about my father.

My beloved Kelly Douglas was all in right from the first idea. She read and helped me reframe early drafts and fully supported me to realize a dream. Her way of being also inspired me. Many years ago now, when I first took Kelly to see the closed and decrepit Northville State Hospital, where so many hard memories lived for me, she joined with me and has never left my side. We were parked in the now overgrown parking lot. I was sharing my difficult memories and was upset and teary. A security guard pulled up and asked us what we were doing there. I was too upset to talk and without missing a beat, Kelly looked straight at him and said, "We had family here and just need a minute." *We.* She did not want me to feel alone. She witnessed my difficult experience and joined with me. This book and the feeling that I was not alone began right there in that parking lot more than a decade ago. Thank you, Kel. You are perfect for me.

My biggest thank-you goes to each of the remarkable people who courageously shared their story for this book. You are changing the world and will help many. I was inspired, humbled, and moved by every single conversation. Your candor, strength, humor, pain, and individual perspective taught and enriched me. I deeply hope I captured some of your lessons well in this book, and I know the outtakes could be a fabulous book of its own.

Each of you is a hero of mine in our shared mission to live the truth that you are not alone.

Brenda Adams
Haley Amering
Danny Anastasi
Wendy Ascione-Juska
Sukhmani Kaur Bal
Diane Banks
Chrissy Barnard
Cynthia Berkowitz
Janet Berkowitz
Sascha Biesi

Ronald Braunstein
Angela Brisbin
Michael Brisbin
Charita Cole Brown
Dawn Brown
Miana Bryant
Joyce Burland
Tera Carter
James Chambliss
Diana Chao

Karyl Chastain Beal
Kimberly Comer
Haley Comerford
Mary Ellen Copeland
Robert Cubby
Margaret Curley
Kevin Dedner
Marc DeGregorio
Alexander Donahoe
John Donahoe

Nancy Donahoe
Roselin Dueñas
Carolyn Edwards
Matt Edwards
Nick Emeigh
Lisa Fabian
Joseph Feaster Jr.
Sally Fitlow
Laurie Flynn
Corinne Foxx
Laura Fritz
Carole Furr
Brad Gage
Pam Goldman
Sierra Grandy
Tracy Green
Sarah Greulich
Cathy Guild
Lloyd Hale
Judy Harris
Michael Hauck
Alice Henley
John Henley
Anita Herron
Brenda Hilligoss
Shirley Holloway
Angelina Hudson
Peggy Huppert
Clarence Jordan
George Kaufmann
Patrick Kaufmann
Rosemary Ketchum
George Kohn

Jutta Kohn
Drea Landry
Carlos A. Larrauri
Ray Lay
Philip A. Lederer
Nadine Lewis
Trish Lockard
Kumi Macdonald
Pranita Mainali
Babu George Mathew
Danna Mauch
Nancy-Lee Mauger
Trevor McCauley
Kathryn Cohan
   McNulty
Pooja Mehta
Gary Mihelish
Kurt Mihelish
Lynn Miller
John Moe
Christine Yu Moutier
Chastity Murry
Dante Murry
Elisa Norman
Betsey O'Brien
Jonathan Ordonez
Norman Ornstein
Eleanor Owen
Monique Owens
Denise Paley
Marty Parrish
Kelly Pavelich
Cathleen Payne

Jim Payne
Kenya "The Visionaire"
   Phillips
Jeanne Porter
Ky Quickbane
Jeremiah Rainville
James Ramirez
Karen Ranus
Nikki Rashes
Kristen Roper
Snake Sabo
Kristina Saffran
Josh Santana
Donna Satow
Phil Satow
Susie Seligson
Susan Smiley
Brad Smith
Eric Smith
Mike Smith
Nancy Smith
Richard Smith
Sheryl Smith
Stephen Smith
Christina Sparrock
Kaitlyn Tollefson
Valerie Van Galder
Suzanne Vogel-Scibilia
Caroline Whiddon
Emma Winters
Liam Winters
Bethany Yeiser
Karen Yeiser

Special thanks to Congressman Jamie Raskin and Sarah Bloom Raskin.

RESOURCES

Note: This includes national organizations, books of note, and resources from individuals interviewed in the book presented by chapter.

ONE
Do I Need Help?

Organizations
- The American Foundation for Suicide Prevention (AFSP)
- Anxiety & Depression Association of America
- Bring Change to Mind
- Depression & Bipolar Support Alliance (DBSA)
- Emotions Matter
- Mental Health America
- Mental Health Coalition
- National Association of State Mental Health Program Directors (NASMHPD)
- National Council on Wellbeing / Mental Health First Aid
- National Education Alliance for Borderline Personality Disorder (NEA-BPD)
- National Institute of Mental Health (NIMH)
- One Mind

Books
- *Maybe You Should Talk to Someone* by Lori Gottlieb

Other Resources
- American Association for Marriage and Family Therapy
- American Counseling Association
- American Psychiatric Nurses Association
- College of Psychiatric and Neurologic Pharmacists
- Indian Health Service
- National Association of Social Workers (NASW)
- National Suicide Prevention Lifeline (988)
- Trevor Project Crisis Line 1-866-488-7386

TWO
The Paradox of Diagnosis

Organizations
- American Medical Association
- American Psychiatric Association
- American Psychological Association
- PANDAS Network

Books
- *Brain on Fire: My Month of Madness* by Susannah Callahan

- *The Collected Schizophrenias* by Esmé Weijun Wang
- *The Complete Family Guide to Schizophrenia* by Kim T. Mueser and Susan Gingerich
- *Diagnostic and Statistical Manual of Mental Disorders, DSM-V-TR* by American Psychiatric Association publishing
- *Facing Serious Mental Illness: A Guide for Patients and Their Families* by Oliver Freudenreich et al.
- *The Imp of the Mind: Exploring the Silent Epidemic of Obsessive Bad Thoughts* by Lee Bauer
- *Manic: A Memoir* by Terri Cheney
- *Pathological: The True Story of Six Misdiagnoses* by Sarah Fay
- *The Noonday Demon: An Atlas of Depression* by Andrew Solomon
- *Understanding Mental Illness: A Comprehensive Guide to Mental Health Disorders for Family and Friends* by Carlin Barnes and Marketa Wills
- *An Unquiet Mind: A Memoir of Moods and Madness* by Kay Redfield Jamison

Other Media
- *Depresh Mode with John Moe* (podcast)

THREE
How Do I Find Help? Minding the Many Gaps

Organizations
- 741741 Crisis Text Line
- Creative Crisis Care
- Kennedy Forum
- Parity Track
- SAMHSA 988 Partner Tool Kit
- SAMSHA 988 Suicide And Crisis Lifeline

- State and local NAMI
- State or County Mental Health Authority
- University Of Michigan National Network of Depression Centers

Other Media
- "Acceptance of Insurance by Psychiatrists and the Implications for Access to Mental Health Care" by Tara F. Bishop, Matthew J. Press, Salomeh Keyhani, et al. February 2014, *JAMA Psychiatry*

NAMI Specific
- NAMI Guide "Navigating a Mental Health Crisis"
- NAMI Health Insurance Appeals Guide

FOUR
Pathways to Recovery: First Steps

Organizations
- Advocates for Human Potential (WRAP)
- Copeland Center for Wellness and Recovery
- This is My Brave

Books
- *The Bipolar Disorder Survival Guide* by David Miklowicz
- *The Center Cannot Hold* by Elyn R. Saks
- *Defying the Verdict: My Bipolar Life* by Charita Cole Brown
- *The Hilarious World of Depression* by John Moe
- *ForLikeMinds: Mental Illness Recovery Insights* by Katherine Ponte

- *Spark: The Revolutionary New Science of Exercise and the Brain* by John J. Ratey, MD
- *The Tao of Fully Feeling* by Pete Walker

Other Media
- *Am I Doing this Right? with Corinne Foxx and Natalie McMillan* (podcast)
- *EmotionAL Support with Alessandra Torresani* (podcast)
- *The Me You Cannot See*, produced by Oprah Winfrey and Prince Harry (documentary available on Apple TV)
- NAMI Communicate Instagram page
- "Results of a Randomized Controlled Trial of Mental Illness Self-Management Using Wellness Recovery Action Planning" by Judith A. Cook, Mary Ellen Copeland, et al., March 2011, *Schizophrenia Bulletin*
- State of Mind with Maurice Benard Instagram page

FIVE
Added Complexity: Co-Occurring Substance Use Conditions

Organizations
- Comprehensive Continuous Integrated System of Care Model (CCISC) by Ken Minkoff
- Drug Story Theater
- Dual Diagnosis Anonymous
- National Association for Drug Courts Professionals
- National Institute on Drug Abuse (NIDA)
- Online Communities
  In the Rooms
  Sober Recovery
  Club Soda

r/stop drinking (on Reddit)
Soberistas (for women)
Sober Black Girls Club
Sober Mom Club
- SAMHSA Treatment Locator
- Shatterproof

12-Step Programs
- Alcoholics Anonymous (AA)
- Narcotics Anonymous (NA)

For Families
- Al-Anon
- Alateen
- Nar-Anon

Community-Specific 12-Step Programs
- 12 Steps to Change (Church of Latter-day Saints focus)
- Celebrate Recovery (Christian focus)
- Dual Recovery Anonymous (addiction and mental health conditions)
- JACS (Jewish focus)

Other Approaches to Substance Use Recovery
- HAMS—Harm Reduction, Abstinence, and Moderation Support
- Life Ring Secular Recovery
- The Phoenix
- Secular Organizations for Sobriety
- SMART Recovery (Self-Management and Recovery Training)
- Women for Sobriety

Organizational Books
- *Adult Children of Alcoholics/ Dysfunctional Families* by World Service Organization, Inc.
- *The Big Book* by Alcoholics Anonymous

- *The CRAFT Treatment Manual for Substance Use Problems: Working with Family Members* by Jane Ellen Smith, Robert J. Meyers, and William R. Miller
- *Dual Recovery Book* by anonymous, Hazelden Publishing
- *Empowering Your Sober Self: The LifeRing Approach to Addiction Recovery* by Martin Nicolaus
- *How Al-Anon Works for Families & Friends of Alcoholics* by Al-Anon Family Groups
- *Narcotics Anonymous Basic Text* by Narcotics Anonymous World Services Inc.
- *SMART Recovery Handbook,* 3rd Edition

Books:
Personal Accounts/Memoirs
- *Basketball Junkie: A Memoir* by Chris Herren
- *Beautiful Boy* by David Sheff
- *A Common Struggle: A Personal Journey Through the Past and Future of Mental Illness and Addiction* by Patrick Kennedy
- *Conscious Recovery: A Fresh Perspective on Addiction* by TJ Woodward
- *Dreamland* by Sam Quinones
- *A Drinking Life* by Pete Hamill
- *Drinking: A Love Story* by Caroline Knapp
- *Dry* by Augusten Burroughs
- *In the Realm of Hungry Ghosts: Close Encounters with Addiction* by Gabor Maté
- *Madness: A Bipolar Life* by Marya Hornbacher
- *My Fair Junkie* by Amy Dresner
- *Quit Like a Woman* by Holly Whitaker
- *Sane: Mental Illness, Addiction, and the 12 Steps* by Marya Hornbacher

- *Smashed: Story of a Drunken Girlhood* by Koren Zailckas
- *Tweak* by Nicolas Sheff
- *Understanding Addiction as Self Medication: Finding Hope Behind the Pain* by Edward J. Khantzian and Mark J. Albanese
- *The Weight of Air: A Story of the Lies About Addiction and the Truth About Recovery* by David Poses

SIX
The Impact of Trauma

Organizations
- ACEs Too High
- Centers for Disease Control: Prevention of Adverse Childhood Experiences
- EMDR International Association
- International Society for Neuroregulation & Research
- International Society for Traumatic Stress Studies
- NASMHPD Six Core Strategies to Reduce Seclusion and Restraint Use
- National Center for PTSD
- National Child Traumatic Stress Network

Specifically for Veterans & Their Families
- Coaching Into Care for Friends and Family of a Veteran (888-823-7458)
- Make the Connection
- Veterans Affairs
- Veterans Crisis Line

Books
- *The Body Keeps the Score* by Bessel van der Kolk
- *The Boy Who Was Raised as a Dog* by Bruce Perry

- *Complex PTSD: From Surviving to Thriving* by Pete Walker
- *The Deepest Well: Healing the Long-Term Effects of Childhood Trauma and Adversity* by Nadine Burke Harris
- *Full Catastrophe Living* by Jon Kabat-Zinn
- *Neurofeedback in the Treatment of Developmental Trauma: Calming the Fear-Driven Brain* by Sebern Fisher
- *The Post-Traumatic Growth Guidebook: Practical Mind-Body Tools to Heal Trauma, Foster Resilience and Awaken Your Potential* by Arielle Schwartz
- *The Relaxation Response* by Herb Benson
- *Strengthening Family Resilience* by Froma Walsh
- *Unthinkable: Trauma, Truth, and the Trials of American Democracy* by Jamie Raskin
- *What Doesn't Kill Us: The New Psychology of Posttraumatic Growth* by Stephen Joseph
- *What Happened to You?* by Bruce Perry and Oprah Winfrey
- *Wherever You Go, There You Are* by Jon Kabat-Zinn

Books for Veterans

- *The Battle for Veterans Health Care* by Suzanne Gordon
- *Best Care Anywhere* by Phillip Longman
- *Best Care Everywhere* by David Shulkin et al.
- *Bipolar General: My Forever War with Mental Illness* by Gregg Martin
- *The Wounds of War: How the VA Delivers Health, Healing, and Hope to the Nation's Veterans* by Suzanne Gordon

Other Media

- *Code 9: Officer Needs Assistance*, directed by Deborah Louise Ortiz (documentary, with Robert Cubby)
- Janice Lebel, Nan Stromberg, et al. (2003). "Child and Adolescent Restraint Reduction: A Statewide Initiative to Promote Strength Based Care," *Journal of the American Academy of Child and Adolescent Psychiatry.*
- *The Healing Trauma with Monique Koven* (podcast)
- *Out of the Shadow*, directed by Susan Smiley (documentary)
- SAMSHA Trauma Informed Care in Behavioral Health Services
- V. J. Felitti et al. (1998). "Relationship of Childhood Abuse and Household Dysfunction to Many of the Leading Causes of Death in Adults," the Adverse Childhood Experiences (ACE) Study, *American Journal of Preventive Medicine.*

SEVEN
Helping Your Child, Teen, or Young Adult

Organizations

- AACAP American Academy of Child & Adolescent Psychiatry
- AAP American Academy of Pediatrics
- Active Minds
- Balanced Mind Parent Network
- Center for Youth Wellness
- Center on the Developing Child
- Child Mind Institute
- Clay Center for Young Healthy Minds
- Coordinated Specialty Care / NAVIGATE (1st episode psychosis)
- Families for Depression Awareness
- Fresh Hope for Mental Health

- The JED Foundation, Phil and Donna Satow
- Letters to Strangers, Diana Chao
- The Mental Elephant, Miana Bryant
- NAMI Specific:
  - NAMI "Starting the Conversation: College and Your Mental Health"
  - NAMI Basics
  - NAMI Ending the Silence
  - NAMI Visions for Tomorrow
- Sources of Strength

Books

- *ADHD 2.0 New Science and Essential Strategies for Thriving with Distraction from Childhood through Adulthood* by Ned Hallowell
- *Anxiety Relief for Teens* by Regine Galanti
- *The Behavioral Code: A Practical Guide to Understanding and Teaching the Most Challenging Students* by Jessica Minahan and Nancy Rappaport
- *Borderline Personality Disorder in Adolescents: A Complete Guide to Understanding and Coping When Your Adolescent Has BPD* by Blaise Aguirre
- *The Explosive Child* by Ross Greene
- *More Than a Body* by Lindsay Kite and Lexie Kite
- *Parenting a Bipolar Child: What to Do and Why* by Dr. Gianni Faedda
- *Thinking Differently: An Inspiring Guide for Parents of Children with Learning Disabilities* by David Flink
- *You Are Not Alone for Parents and Caregivers: The NAMI Guide to Navigating Your Child's Mental Health—With Advice from Experts and Wisdom from Real Families* by Christine M. Crawford, MD

Other Media

- *Hiding in Plain Sight* directed by Ken Burns (Film)

EIGHT
Themes of Recovery: Lessons from First-Person Experience

Organizations

- Common Ground by Pat Deegan
- Hearing Voices Network
- National Certified Peer Recovery Support Specialists (NAADAC)
- National Empowerment Center
- The National Mental Health Consumers' Self-Help Clearinghouse

Books

- *Awakenings: Stories of Recovery and Emergence from Schizophrenia* by Bethany Yeiser and Henry A. Nasrallah
- *A Beautiful Mind* by Sylvia Nasar
- *Beyond Borderline: True Stories of Recovery from Borderline Personality Disorder* by John G. Gunderson et al.
- *Building a Life Worth Living* by Marsha Linehan
- *The Comfort Book* by Matt Haig
- *Crazy is My Superpower: How I Triumphed by Breaking Bones, Breaking Hearts, and Breaking the Rules* by AJ Mendez.
- *A First Rate Madness: Uncovering the Links Between Leadership and Mental Illness* by Nassir Ghaemi
- *How to Live with Bipolar Disorder* by Sally Alter
- *Journeys Beyond the Frontier: A Rebellious Guide to Psychosis and Other Extraordinary Experiences* by Mark Ragins

- *Loving What Is: Four Questions That Can Change Your Life* by Byron Katie
- *Meaningful Recovery from Schizophrenia and Serious Mental Illness with Clozapine: Hope & Help* by Dr. Robert S. Laitman, Lewis A. Opler, Ann Mandel Laitman, and Daniel Laitman
- *On Edge: A Journey Through Anxiety* by Andrea Peterson
- *A Peek Inside: Illustrated Journeys in Life with Mental Illness* by Micah Pearson
- *A Practical Guide to Recovery-Oriented Practice: Tools for Transforming Mental Health Care Illustrated Edition* by Larry Davidson et al.
- *Profiles in Mental Health Courage* by Partick Kennedy and Stephen Fried
- *The Quiet Room* by Lori Schiller
- *Reasons to Stay Alive* by Matt Haig
- *Take Charge of Bipolar Disorder: A 4 Step Plan* by Julie Fast and John Preston
- *Turtles All the Way Down* by John Green
- *The Wellness Recovery Action Plan* by Mary Ellen Copeland

Other Media
- *The Anxious Truth: A Panic, Anxiety, and Mental Health Podcast* with Drew Linsalata
- *BP Hope Magazine* (bipolar disorder)
- C. M. Harding et al. "The Vermont Longitudinal Study of Persons with Severe Mental Illness, II: Long-Term Outcome of Subjects Who Retrospectively Met DSM-III Criteria for Schizophrenia." *American Journal of Psychiatry* 6 (June 1987): 727–35.
- *Miyam Bialik's Breakdown* (podcast)
- *The Mental Illness Happy Hour* with Paul Gilmartin (podcast)
- NAMI Blog, includes recovery stories,

tips, and professional perspectives
- *Therapy for Black Girls* with Joy Harden Bradford (podcast)
- *Touched with Fire* directed by Paul Dalio (film)
- *The Trauma Therapist* with Guy McPherson (podcast)

N I N E
The Power of Peers and Community

Organizations
- Clubhouse International
- Depressed Cake Shop
- Emotions Anonymous
- Fountain House
- Me2/Orchestra
- NAMI Specific:
    Connection Recovery Support Group
    Peer-to-Peer
- National Association of Peer Supporters
- SAMHSA's National Model Standards for Peer Support Certification
- Schizophrenia and Psychosis Action Alliance
- Stand Up for Mental Health
- Suicide Anonymous
- Whole Health Action Management (WHAM)

Books
- *Bowling Alone: The Collapse and Revival of American Community* by Robert Putnam
- *Fountain House: Creating Community in Mental Health Practice* by Alan Doyle
- *A Mind That Found Itself* by Clifford Beers

Other Media
- *Orchestrating Change*, produced by Margie Friedman and Barbara Multer-Wellin (documentary)

TEN
Culture and Identity: Barriers and Opportunities

Organizations
- The Association of Black Psychologists
- Black Psychiatrists of America
- Blue Dove (Jewish Mental Health Organization)
- Confess Project
- Hurdle Health
- NAMI Faithnet
- National Eating Disorder Association
- National Latino Behavioral Health Association
- National Medical Association
- Project HEAL
- The Steve Fund
- Trans Lifeline
- The Trevor Project

Books
- *72 Hour Hold* by Bebe Moore Campbell
- *Black Man in a White Coat: A Doctor's Reflections on Race and Medicine* by Damon Tweedy
- *Children of the Land: A Memoir* by Marcelo Hernandez Castillo
- *Hard to Love: Understanding and Overcoming Male Borderline Personality Disorder* by Joseph Nowinski
- *The Joy of the Disinherited: Essays on Trauma, Oppression, and Black Mental Health* by Kevin Dedner

- *Man Down: A Guide for Men on Mental Health* by Charlie Hoare
- *Moving from Shame to Self-Worth, Preaching & Pastoral Care* by Edward P. Wimberly
- *Permission to Come Home: Reclaiming Mental Health as Asian Americans* by Jenny Wang
- *The Protest Psychosis: How Schizophrenia Became a Black Disease* by Jonathan Metzl
- *Psychosocial Research on American Indian and Alaska Native Youth* by Spero Manson
- *The Queer and Transgender Resilience Workbook: Skills for Navigating Sexual Orientation and Gender Expression* by Anneliese Singh
- *The Social Determinants of Mental Health* by Michael T. Compton
- *The Unapologetic Guide to Black Mental Health: Navigate an Unequal System, Learn Tools for Emotional Wellness, and Get the Help you Deserve* by Rheeda Walker, PhD
- *Wrestling with Our Inner Angels: Faith, Mental Illness, and the Journey for Wholeness* by Nancy Kehoe

Other Media
- American Medical Association. "Reckoning with Medicine's History of Racism" by James L. Madara, MD
- American Psychiatric Association. "APA Apologizes for Its Support of Racism in Psychiatry"
- American Psychological Association. "Apology to People of Color for APA's Role in Promoting, Perpetuating, and Failing to Challenge Racism, Racial Discrimination, and Human Hierarchy in U.S."
- National Association of Social Workers. "Undoing Racism through

Social Work: NASW Report to the
Profession on Racial Justice Priorities
and Action"
- NAMI Compartiendo Esperanza
(video series)
- *Real Feels with Brad Gage* (podcast)

ELEVEN
Becoming an Advocate

Organizations
- Carter Center
- CURESZ Foundation
- Hunstman Mental Health Institute
- Kennedy Forum
- NAMI Specific:
  In Our Own Voice
  Provider
  Smarts for Advocacy
- Young Invincibles
- Wellbeing Trust

Books
- *Advocacy Strategies for Health and Mental Health Professions* by Stuart Lustig
- *Fighting for Recovery: An Activists' History of Mental Health Reform* by Phyllis Vine
- *Healing: Our Path from Mental Illness to Mental Health* by Tom Insel
- *Word Play Series 1: Winter: Emotional Spasms* by Kenya Phillips

TWELVE
Family Connection and Communication

Organizations
- National Alliance on Caregiving
- NAMI Related:
  Family & Friends

Family Support Group
Family-to-Family
Homefront

Books
- *Atlas of the Heart: Mapping Meaningful Connection and the Language of Human Experience* by Brené Brown
- *The Forgotten Survivors: A Sister's Journey Through Her Brother's Mental Illness* by Shannon Jaccard
- *Gorilla and the Bird* by Zack McDermott
- *The High-Conflict Couple: A Dialectical Behavior Therapy Guide to Finding Peace, Intimacy, and Validation* by Alan Fruzzetti
- *Loving Someone with Bipolar Disorder* by Julie Fast and John Peterson
- *Motivational Interviewing: Helping People Change* by William Miller and Stephen Rollnick
- *Multifamily Groups in the Treatment of Severe Psychiatric Disorders* by William McFarlane
- *Resilience: Two Sisters and a Story of Mental Illness* by Jessie Close and Pete Earley
- *Still Stepping: A Family Portrait* by Karen Davis
- *Stop Walking on Eggshells* by Paul Mason
- *Taking the War Out of Our Words* by Sharon Ellison
- *Unleashing the Power of Respect: The I-M Approach* by Joseph Shrand

Other Media
- Lisa B. Dixon, Alicia Lucksted, et al. (2011) "Outcomes of a Randomized Study of a Peer-Taught Family-to-Family Education Program for Mental Illness," *Psychiatric Services*

- *Porcupine Love* by Cathleen Payne (blog)
- *We Can Do Hard Things with Glennon Doyle* (podcast)

THIRTEEN
Navigating the Legal System

Organizations
- Academy of Special Needs Planners (ASNP)
- ACLU Prisoners Assistance Directory
- All Rise
- Crisis Intervention Training (CIT) International
- Forensic Peer Support Services
- Forensic-Assertive Community Treatment (F-ACT) Programs
- HIPAA and FERPA: HHS Guide
- HIPAA for Caregivers
- NAMI Specific:
    Divert to What?
    Mental Health Treatment while Incarcerated
    Sharing Your Story with Law Enforcement
- National Guardianship Association
- SAMHSA Resources on Reentry
- SAMHSA Treatment Court Locator
- Special Needs Alliance
- Treatment Advocacy Center (TAC)

Books
- *Crazy: A Father's Search Through America's Mental Health Madness* by Pete Earley
- *Family Guide to Mental Illness and the Law* by Linda Tashbook

Other Media
- *The Definition of Insanity*, produced by Found Object Films (documentary)
- Sequential Intercept Model: SAMHSA

FOURTEEN
The Hardest Family Questions

Organizations
- Henry Amador Center on Anosognosia
- The Matthew Harris Ornstein Memorial Foundation
- National Academy of Elder Law Attorneys (NAELA)
- National Society of Genetic Counselors

Books
- *Birth of a New Brain—Healing from Postpartum Bipolar Disorder* by Dyane Harwood
- *Difficult: Mothering Challenging Adult Children through Conflict and Change* by Judith R. Smith
- *Done with the Crying: Help and Healing for Mothers of Estranged Adult Children* by Sheri McGregor
- *I Am Not Sick, I Don't Need Help* by Xavier Amador
- *You Need Help: A Step-by-Step Plan to Convince a Loved One to Get Counseling* by Mark Komrad and Rosalynn Carter

FIFTEEN
Making Meaning of Loss by Suicide

Organizations
- American Foundation for Suicide Prevention
- Dougy Center for Grieving Children and Families
- Matthew;s Crew
- SAVE.org Suicide Survivor support groups

Books

- *After Suicide Loss: Coping with Your Grief* by Jack Jordan & Bob Baugher
- *By the Time You Read This: The Space between Cheslie's Smile and Mental Illness—Her Story in Her Own Words* by Cheslie Kryst and April Simpkins
- *Devastating Losses: How Parents Cope with the Death of a Child to Suicide or Drugs* by B. Feigelman et al.
- *Do They Have Bad Days in Heaven? Surviving the Suicide Loss of a Sibling* by Michelle Linn-Gust
- *Getting Grief Right: Finding Your Story of Love in the Sorrow of Loss* by Patrick O'Malley and Tim Madigan
- *The Grieving Child* by Helen Fitzgerald
- *Healing the Hurt Spirit: Daily Affirmations for People Who Have Lost a Loved One to Suicide* by Catherine Greenleaf
- *History of a Suicide: My Sister's Unfinished Life* by Jill Bialosky
- *My Son . . . My Son . . . : A Guide to Healing After Death, Loss, or Suicide* by Iris Bolton
- *No Time to Say Goodbye: Surviving the Suicide of a Loved One* by Carla Fine
- *One Friday in April: A Story of Suicide and Survival* by Donald Antrim
- *Saving Ourselves from Suicide—Before and After: How to Ask for Help, Recognize Warning Signs, and Navigate* by Linda Pacha
- *Stepping Back from the Ledge: A Daughter's Search for Truth and Renewal* by Laura Trujillo
- *Suicide Prevention: Stahl's Handbooks* by Christine Yu Moutier, Anthony R. Pisani, et al.
- *Survivors of Suicide* by Rita Robinson and Phyllis Hart
- *The Suicide Index: Putting My Father's Death in Order* by Joan Wickersham
- *Touched by Suicide: Hope and Healing After Loss* by Carla Fine and Michael Myers

Other Media

- Reporting on Suicide: Best Practices for Reporting on Suicide (website)
- Stanford TEMPOS: Tools for Evaluating Media Portrayals of Suicide (website)

SIXTEEN
Family Advocacy

Organizations

- NAMI Smarts for Advocacy

Books

- *Flight from Reason: A Mother's Story of Schizophrenia, Recovery, and Hope* by Karen Yeiser
- *Make a Difference with Mental Health Activism* by Teri Lyon and Trish Lockard
- *Mind Estranged: My Journey from Schizophrenia and Homelessness to Recovery* by Bethany Yeiser
- *Tomorrow Was Yesterday: Explosive First-Person Indictments of the US Mental Health System—Mothers Across the Nation Tell It Like It Is* by Dede Ranahan

Other Media

- *When Medicine Got It Wrong*, directed by Katie Cadigan and Laura Murray (documentary)

SEVENTEEN
Experts Answer the Most Frequently Asked Questions

Organizations
- APA App Adviser
- Bazelon Center for Mental Health Law
- MINT Motivational Interviewing Network of Trainers
- National Disability Rights Network
- National Resource Center for Psychiatric Advanced Directives
- One Mind Cyberguide
- Roadmap to the Ideal Crisis System, Group for the Advancement of Psychiatry
- SMI Adviser—Digital Navigator Training
- SMI Adviser (clozapine and technology)

Books
- *This Is Your Brain on Food* by Uma Naidoo

EIGHTEEN
State-of-the-Art Care and Research for Specific Conditions

Organizations
- AMP Schizophrenia (NIH Foundation)
- The Beck Institute
- Brain and Behavior Research Foundation
- Broad Institute Stanley Center for Psychiatric Research

- Heinz C. Prechter Bipolar Research Program
- MGH Center for Women's Mental Health
- Multidisciplinary Association for Psychedelic Studies (MAPS)
- NOCD: OCD Treatment and Therapy
- OCD International
- PEPPNET (early psychosis; Stanford)
- SAMHSA Early Serious Mental Illness Locator
- Stanley Medical Research Institute

Books
- *Cognitive Behavior Therapy* by Judith S. Beck
- *Cognitive Behavioral Therapy Made Simple: 10 Strategies for Managing Anxiety, Depression, Anger, Panic, and Worry* by Seth J. Gillihan
- *Cognitive Remediation for Successful Employment and Psychiatry Recovery: The Thinking Skills for Work Program* by Susan R. McGurk and Kim T. Mueser
- *DBT Skills Manual* by Marsha Linehan
- *Feeling Good: The New Mood Therapy* by David Burns
- *First, We Make the Beast Beautiful: A New Journey Through Anxiety* by Sarah Wilson
- *Freedom from Obsessive Compulsive Disorder* by Jonathan Grayson
- *Intervening Early in Psychosis a Team Approach* edited by Kate Hardy
- *Surviving Schizophrenia* by E. Fuller Torrey

INDEX

ABOUT THE AUTHOR

DR. KEN DUCKWORTH, MD, is the chief medical officer of the National Alliance on Mental Illness (NAMI) and has worked with NAMI since 2003. Ken is board certified in adult psychiatry and child and adolescent psychiatry, and is an assistant professor of psychiatry at Harvard Medical School. He was previously acting commissioner and medical director at the Massachusetts Department of Mental Health. Ken has worked on an assertive community treatment team, at an early psychosis program, at an elementary school, at a health plan, and with people who are unhoused. His passion for this work comes from his loving dad who had bipolar disorder. Ken lives with his family in Boston.

THE NATIONAL ALLIANCE ON MENTAL ILLNESS (NAMI) is the nation's largest grassroots mental health organization, dedicated to building better lives for the millions of Americans affected by mental illness.

NAMI.ORG | @NAMICOMMUNICATE